ANGINA PECTORIS

Edited by **Federico Piscione**

Angina Pectoris
Edited by Federico Piscione

Published by InTech
Janeza Trdine 9, 51000 Rijeka, Croatia

Publishing Process Manager Romina Krebel

Technical Editor Teodora Smiljanic

Cover Designer InTech Design Team

Additional hard copies can be obtained from orders@intechopen.com

Angina Pectoris, Edited by Federico Piscione
p. cm.
ISBN 978-953-307-359-0

For EU product safety concerns:
IN TECH d.o.o., Prolaz Marije Krucifikse Kozulić 3, 51000 Rijeka, Croatia,
info@intechopen.com or visit our website at intechopen.com.

Meet the editor

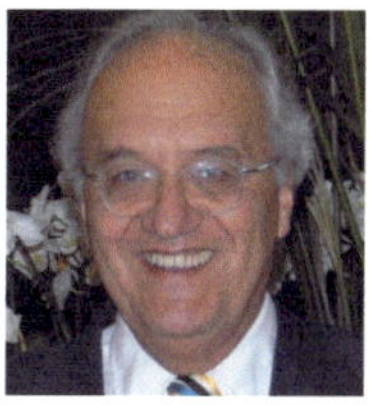

Dr. Federico Piscione, MD, FESC, born in 1948, graduated in 1972 from School of Medicine, University of Naples, Italy. Since 2002, he is Associated Professor at the Department of Medicine, Division of Cardiology, and Head of Cardiac Catheterization Laboratory and Interventional Cardiology, Federico II University in Naples, Italy. Dr. Piscione has written almost 150 articles, 25 chapters in books, and participated in the organization of 18 national and international meetings and congresses. He is a member of Italian Society of Cardiology, Italian Society of Invasive and Interventional Cardiology, New York Academy of Sciences and European Society of Cardiology. Dr. Piscione has received research awards from Italo-American Medical Education Foundation, Clinical Medicine Curriculum, Loyola University, Rome (1976) and National Council of Research, NATO Junior fellowship scheme (1982).

Contents

Preface IX

Chapter 1 **Inflammation and Genetics of Inflammation in Cardiovascular Diseases 1**
Maria Bucova

Chapter 2 **Angina-Like Chest Pain as a Symptom of Digestive Tract Disorders 35**
Jacek Budzyński

Chapter 3 **Conventional and Novel Pharmacotherapy of Angina Pectoris 71**
Solmaz Dehghan

Chapter 4 **Therapy for Angina Pectoris Secondary to Coronary Disease 89**
Antony Leslie Innasimuthu, Sanjay Kumar, Lei Gao, Melaku Demede and Jeffrey S. Borer

Chapter 5 **Beta-Blockers and Coronary Flow Reserve 129**
Maurizio Galderisi

Chapter 6 **The Role of Enhanced External Counterpulsation Therapy in the Management of Coronary Artery Disease 137**
Ozlem Soran

Chapter 7 **Alternative Non-Medical, Non-Surgical Therapies for the Treatment of Angina Pectoris 159**
Maryam Esmaeilzadeh, Bahieh Moradi and Nasim Naderi

Preface

Angina is the most common disorder affecting patients with ischemic heart disease. Indeed, the reported prevalence of angina approximates 10.2 million patients in the USA and it has been estimated that 500,000 new cases of stable angina occur each year. In this book we reviewed the novel mechanisms, such as inflammation factors and genetic determinants, that play a pivotal role in the pathophysiology of angina and that might have potential therapeutic implications in the future (Chapter 1). In addition, because of its prevalence, it is important to distinguish angina due to ischemic heart disease from angina-like chest syndrome, due to digestive tract disorder. At this regard, the pathophisiology, the diagnosis and the treatment of angina-like chest syndrome were carefully reviewed (Chapter 2).

The treatment of angina is based on several conventional agents, nevertheless new drugs with novel mechanism of action, i.e. ranolazine, nicordandil, ivabradine, have been proposed in specific subsets (Chapter 3). However, nitrates, calcium channel blockers and beta adrenergic blockers are the most widely used and studied anti-anginal medications, representing the cornerstone in the treatment of angina secondary to coronary artery disease (Chapter 4 and Chapter 5). Finally, the role of enhanced external counterpulsation and alternative non-medical, non-surgical therapies were also reported, focusing on their potentials, as well as their current limitations.

Therefore, this book provides a thorough review of fundamental principles of diagnosis, pathophysiology and treatment of angina pectoris, representing an invaluable resource not only for cardiologists, but also for general practitioners and medical students.

Professor Federico Piscione
Federico II University
Department of Clinical Medicine, Cardiovascular Sciences and Immunology
Naples - Italy

1

Inflammation and Genetics of Inflammation in Cardiovascular Diseases

Maria Bucova
Institute of Immunology, School of Medicine Comenius University, Bratislava Slovakia

1. Introduction

Inflammation is a complex of defensive mechanisms reacting to the entry of harmful agents to the organism or cells in order to eliminate or at least to dilute the agent, repair damaged cells or tissue and restore homeostasis. From this definition it is clear, that inflammation does not accompany only infectious diseases but also others, causing cell, tissue or organ injury and serves primarily defensively (Table 1). An exaggerated, chronic long lasting or non-adequately regulated inflammatory response could be the cause of adverse reactions and could lead to pathology (Bucova, 2002b).
Inflammation plays an important role also in the etiology of ischemic heart disease (IHD), myocardial infarction (MI), angina pectoris (AP) and hypertension, however, its mechanism in various stages of pathological process is not well understood (Bucova et al., 2008a; Itoh et al., 2007; Kuka et al., 2010; Li, 2005; Pickering et al., 2007, Ross 1999). If the cause of IHD is atherosclerosis or other, it is accompanied by inflammation. Various types of inflammatory cells, cytokines, chemokines and other soluble factors were confirmed to be involved in this process. (Armstrong et al 2006; Aukrust et al., 2001; Brunetti et al., 2006; Bucova et al., 2008a; Ferencik et al., 2007).

1. Infectious - bacteria, fungi, viruses
2. Mechanical – scratching, cutting
3. Physical – burning, radiation
4. Allergic
5. Autoimmune
6. Atherosclerosis and cardiovascular diseases
7. Cancer
8. Nutritional disorders - hypoxia, lack of proteins, vitamins, etc.
9. Other causes

Table 1. Inflammation and its induction agents

2. Immune mechanisms and cardiovascular diseases

Inflammation and **immune system activation** are strongly involved in the pathogenesis of atherosclerosis and cardiovascular diseases. Atherosclerosis is now considered to be a chronic inflammatory disease of the arterial wall where both innate and adaptive immune mechanisms contribute to disease initiation and progression (Table 2).

Non-specific innate immunity	Specific adaptive immunity	Autoimmunity
1. CELLULAR	1. CELLULAR	1. CELLULAR
monocytes, macrophages, neutrophils, eosinophils, NK- cells	T helper cells (Th1, Th2, Th17) T cytotoxic cells (Tc) regulatory T cells (innate and induced)	Tc - lymphocytes
2. HUMORAL	2. HUMORAL	2. HUMORAL
cytokines TNF-α, IL-1, IL-6, chemokines (MCP-1/CCL2, CXCL16, ...) MMP-9, complement, acute phase proteins, histamin, chymase, tryptase, endogenous vasoconstrictors, elastase, ...	cytokines IFN-γ, IL-12, IL-2, IL-4, IL-10, IL-17, IL-33, TGF-β	specific antibodies
3. RECEPTORS (non-specific)	3. Receptors (specific)	
PRR (CD14, TLR, Dectins, TREM-1, RAGE, CR1, CR3, CR4, CRP ...) FcγR, scavenger receptors	T cell receptor (TCR) B cell receptor (BCR)	
4. MECHANISMS	4. MECHANISMS	
inflammation, innate imunity (phagocytosis, complement activation, ...) antigen presentation, potentiation of adaptive immunity	polarization of T cells, activation of specific immunity	antibodies against self, damaged or changed antigens (oxLDL, HSP, ...)

Legend: NK- natural killer, TNF – tumor necrosis factor, IL-1 – interleukin 1, MCP-1 – macrophage chemotactic protein, PRR – pattern recognition receptors, TLR – toll like receptors, TREM-1 (triggering receptor expressed on myelocytes, RAGE – receptor for advanced glycation end product, CR1, CR3, CR4 – complement receptors, FcγR – receptor for Fc fragment of immunoglobulins, IFN-γ - interferon - gama, TGF-β - transforming growth factor beta, oxLDL – oxidized low density lipoprotein, HSP – heat shock protein.

Table 2. Main immune mechanims involved in cardiovascular diseases

To main players of the **innate immune system** belong macrophages, mastocytes and from soluble factors complement components, pro-inflammatory cytokines (tumor necrosis factor (TNF), interleukin-1 (IL-1) and IL-6, chemokines (monocyte chemoattractant protein - MCP-1/CCL2) and acute phase proteins, mainly C-reactive protein (CRP), serum albumin A (SAA) and pentraxins (PTX).

Adaptive immune mechanisms involved in the pathogenesis of cardiovascular diseases are represented predominantly by T helper 1 type (Th1), Th2 and Th17 lymphocytes and immune mechanisms associated with them (Chen et al., 2010; Mostafazadeh et al., 2011) (Table 2). Th1 immunity insures defence against intracellular pathogenic microorganisms, viruses, fungi and tumors, Th2 against extracellular pathogenic microorganisms and helmints and Th17 against extracellular bacterial infection and fungal infection. Exaggerated response of any of mentioned type of immunity contributes to the pathogenesis of various autoimmune inflammatory diseases (Fouser et al., 2008; Mucida et al., 2010; Quian et al., 2010). Cytokines activating these cells and/or produced by these cells and regulating the activity of these cells play a great role in development of atherosclerosis and cardiovascular diseases. The array of cytokines involved in pathogenesis of atherosclerosis is similar to those used by immune effector cells to kill foreign pathogens and damaged or diseased host cells. These are mainly IL-2, interferon-gama (IFN-γ), IL-10, IL-4, IL-17, IL-33 and transforming growth factor-beta (TGF-β) (Chen et al., 2010; Hansson et al., 2005). Regulatory T cells - both innate and induced, controlling the activity of helper T cells are other important components of adaptive immunity (Cheng et al., 2008; George, 2008).

Macrophages belonging to non-specific innate immune mechanisms amplify the adaptive immune response as antigen presenting cells that after having ingested and processed the foreign particle present an immunogenic fragment from it to naive Th0 lymphocytes and start and shift the immune response to the right direction.

Autoimmune response to at least two major autoantigens - oxidized lipoproteins (oxLDL) and heat shock proteins (HSPs) also potentiate inflammation. Namely, HSP60, an endogenous molecule with a chaperone activity, normally located in the mitochondria can be translocated into the cell membrane in response to stress stimuli. It can be released also by stressed or injured cells but also by activated monocytes and macrophages. HSPs in host can likewise be derived from microorganisms during infection, e.g. by *Helicobacter pylori.*

2.1 The innate and adaptive immunity

The innate immune response starts non-specifically as an inflammatory response that develops after pattern recognition receptors (PRR) at the surface of our immune cells (macrophages, dendritic cells, ...) recognize common molecular features originating either from microorganisms - pathogen associated molecular patterns (PAMPs), or from our own body, e.g. from damaged cells - damage associated molecular patterns (DAMPs) (Fig. 1, Table 3). Both PAMPs and DAMPs represent to immune system signals of threatening and bind these molecular patterns by PRR receptors – immune sensors of non-specific innate immunity. To these endogenous DAMPs called also alarmins belong both newly formed (HSPs, heat shock proteins), altered and modified endogenous antigens (oxLDL, oxidized low density lipoprotein cholesterol), or substances released from damaged or necrotic cells. The binding of any PAMPs and DAMPs to concrete PRR results in signal transduction, activation of transcription factors and production of early pro-inflammatory cytokines (TNF-α, IL-1 and IL-6) and chemokines from immune and injured endothelial cells (Chen et al., 2010; Eldfeldt et al., 2002; Ferencik, 2007; Miyake, 2007).

From this point of view the inflammatory response could be triggered directly by infectious but also by some sterile non-infectious stimuli. To the most intensively studied PRR with the involvement in the process of atherosclerosis belong toll like receptors TLR4 and TLR2, CD14 receptor and RAGE (receptor for advanced glycation end products) (Bierhaus et al., 2006; Bucova, 2006; Park et al., 2004).

The expression of adhesive molecules on both endothelial cells and leukocytes increases, chemokines attract monocytes into the vessel wall where they differentiate into

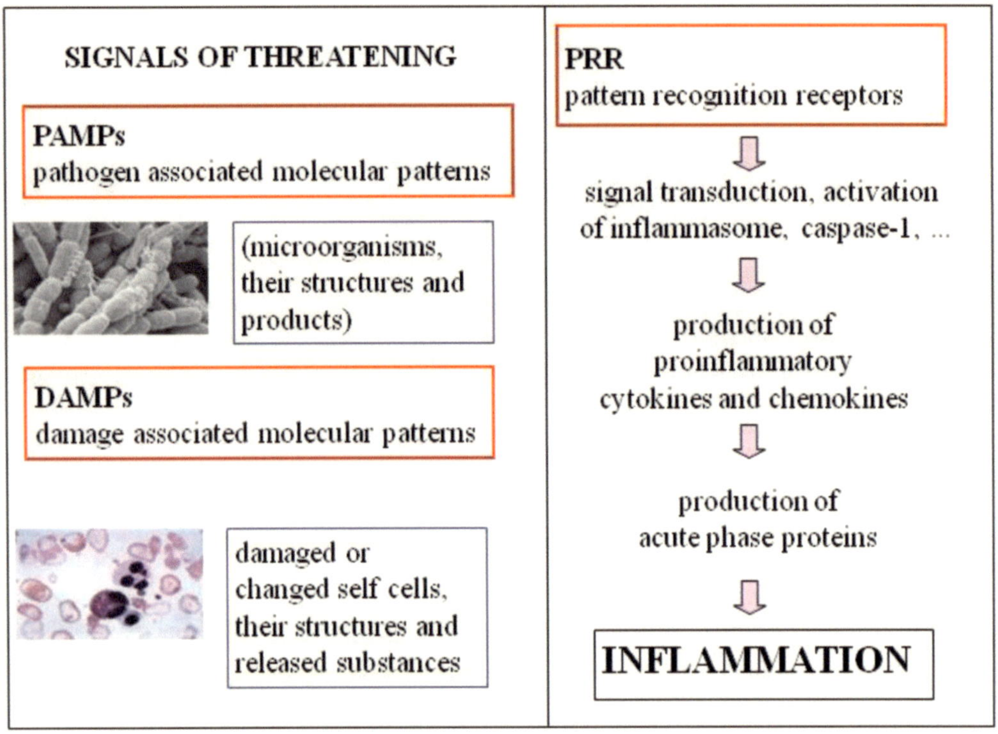

Fig. 1. Infectious and non-infectious inflammation induced by binding exogenous PAMPs and endogenous DAMPs by PRR.

PAMPs (pathogen associated molecular patterns) - microorganisms and their products	DAMPs (damage associated molecular patterns) - damaged or changed self cells and structures, and their products
lipopolysaccharide, peptidoglycan, lipoteichoic acid, lipoarabinomannan, flagelin, zymozan, ssRNA, dsRNA, CpG motifs of DNA, ...	hyaluronic acid, heparan sulfat, extra-domene A of fibronectin, HSP 60, HSP 70, uric acid (crystallic form), HMGB1, IL-33, fibrinogen, hyperglycaemia, hyperkaliemia, ...

Legend: ssRNA - single stranded ribonucleic acid, dsRNA - double stranded ribonucleic acid, DNA - deoxyribonucleic acid, HSP 60 - heat shock protein 60, HMGB1 - high mobility group box 1 protein, IL-33 - interleukin 33

Table 3. Some of the most important PAMPs and DAMPs

macrophages, ingest particles of oxLDL and transform into foam cells. Other substance with strong pro-inflammatory activity that serves also as alarmin or inflammatory mediator of tissue injury is high mobility group box 1 protein (HMGB1). HMGB1 is released both from injured endothelial cells and activated monocytes and macrophages, the next source of this protein are necrotic cells (Chang et al., 2011; Yang et al., 2010).

Released pro-inflammatory cytokines enhance the production of acute phase proteins in the liver and aggravate the inflammation. The pivotal transcription factor involved in the induction of specific pro-inflammatory genes is NF-κB (Barnes & Karin, 1997). Its activation might also represent a mechanism by which CRP amplifies and perpetuates the inflammatory response (Liuzzo et al., 2007) (Fig.1).

Inflammatory process in endothelial cell wall goes along with the activation of adaptive T cell imunity. Macrophages as antigen presenting cells present exogenous or endogenous antigens to naïve helper T cells (Th0), cells of the specific adaptive immunity. After naïve Th0 cells recognize the antigen (oxLDL, HSPs, components of microorganisms, ...), they differentiate into T helper type 1 (Th1) cells that produce interferon-gamma (IFN-γ), the main Th1 type cytokine (Bucova, 2002a; Chen et al, 2010) (Fig. 2, Table 2). IFN-γ further activates macrophages and foam cells, and amounts their production of proinflammatory cytokines and chemokines and the process of atherosclerosis is enhanced. This is the second step or wave of inflammatory response activation. The balance between pro- and anti-inflammatory responses regulates the magnitude of the inflammatory response within the plaque, the plaque instability and thrombus formation.

Th1 cells exhibit a strong pro-atherogenic effect that is balanced by anti-atherogenic effect of regulatory T cells and defined cytokines released from Th2 lymphocytes – interleukin- IL-5 and IL-33. Th2 related IL-4 seems to be pro-atherogenic (Chen et al., 2010; Taleb et al, 2010).

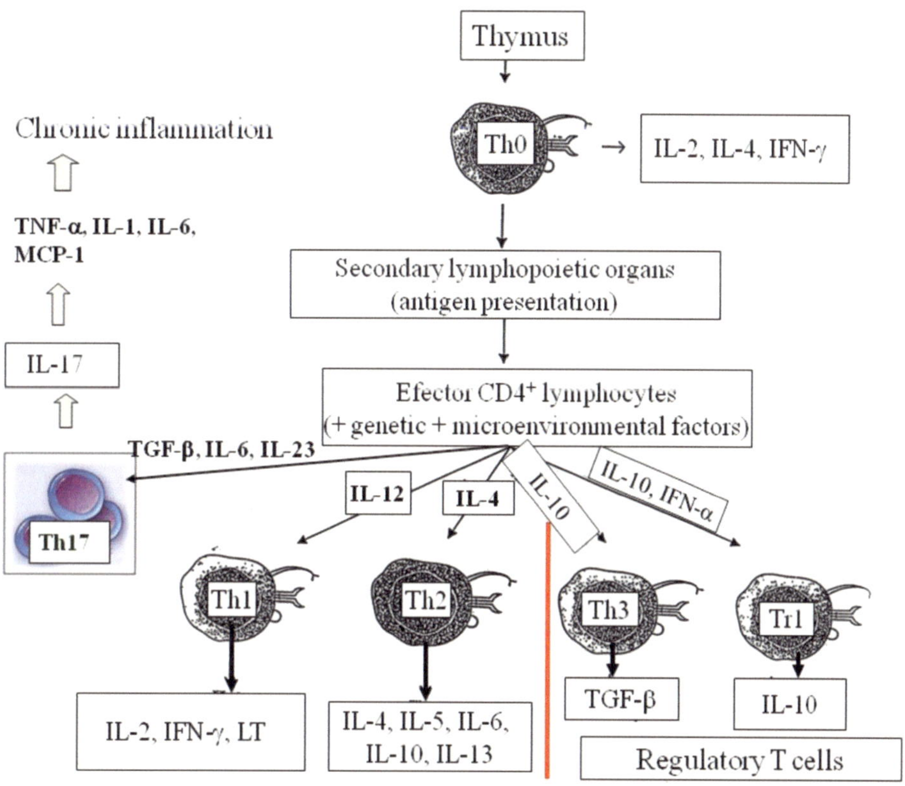

Fig. 2. Th-lymphocytes and cytokines involved in cardiovascular diseases, Polarization of Th-lymphocytes.

Next cells that trigger the inflammatory response in arterial cell wall are Th17 cells, lymphocytes that produce a wast bulk of a strong proinflammatory cytokine IL-17 that leads to elevated production of proinflammatory cytokines TNF-α, IL-1 and IL-6 as well as proinflammatory chemokine MCP-1 (monocyte chemotactic protein) and other neutrophil mobilizing proteins. IL-17 is involved in the pathogenesis of several autoimmune diseases and asthma, its role in atherosclerosis development remains controversial. However, recent studies provide more direct evidence that IL-17 seems to be predominantly pro-atherogenic (Chen et al., 2010).

3. Atherosclerosis and inflammation

Atherosclerosis is an inflammatory disease characterized by vascular injury, lipid accumulation as well as massive infiltration of immune cells in the endothelial wall. Both microbial and self-antigens are responsible for a persistent activation of immune and non-immune cells, thus leading to a condition of chronic smuldering arterial inflammation. At present, atherosclerosis is considered to be an inflammatory disease and atherosclerotic plaque inflammation the cause of intima erosion, rupture and subsequent ischemia (Kraaijeveld et al., 2007; Libby, 2002, Ross, 1999).

Endothelial cell wall inflammation is based on genetic predisposition with mutual interaction between genes and genes, infections and other environmental factors. Repeted inflammatory processes lead to atherosclerosis development, coronary plaque rupture and subsequent ischemia development (Fig. 3).

Endothelial cell wall inflammation - a gradual step-by-step process

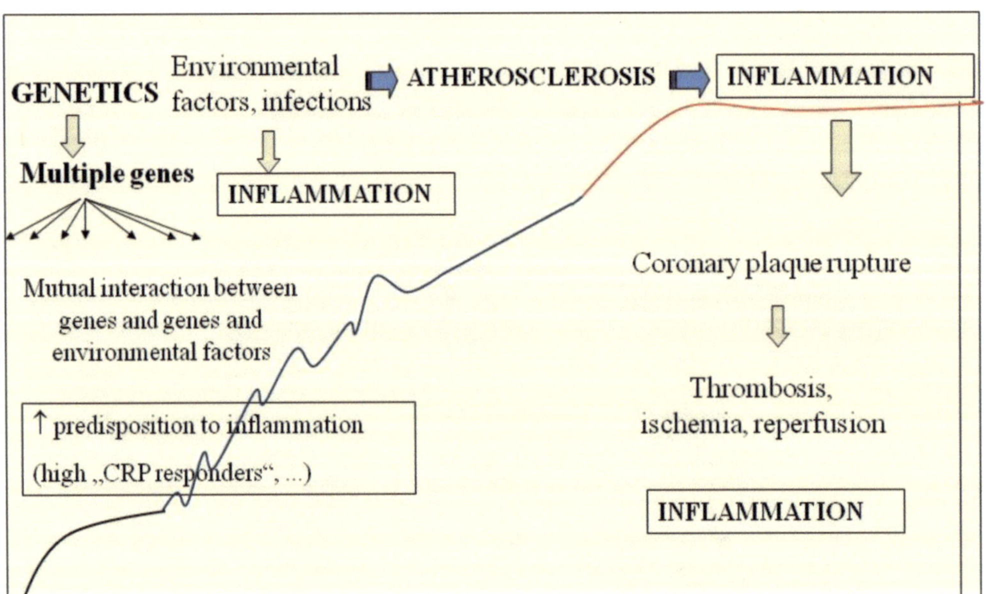

Fig. 3. Inflammation – march to coronary artery disease. A gradual step-by-step process.

The question is, whether the inflammation is the cause or the result of the atherosclerotic plaque rupture. The answer is, both. Intact endothelium is non-sticky and resistant against deposition of any substances into endothelial cell wall (Fig. 4). So, endothelial dysfunction (ED) initiated by both infectious and non-infectious processes (e.g. metabolic syndrome - MetS) is now recognized to play a critical role in the initiation and progression of atherosclerotic vascular disease (Al-Quasi et al., 2008; Bakker et al., 2009; Lamon & Hajjar, 2008). CRP, which levels raise during inflammation contributes to the induction of endothelial cell activation and dysfunction (Deveraj et al., 2010; Grad et al., 2007; Schwartz et al., 2007; Teoh et al., 2008; Venogupal et al., 2003). Patients with MetS have increased plasma levels of oxLDL (Holvoet et al., 2004) and recently it was found that CRP promotes increased oxLDL uptake by vessel wall and cholesterol ester accumulation in Wistar rats (Singh et al., 2008).

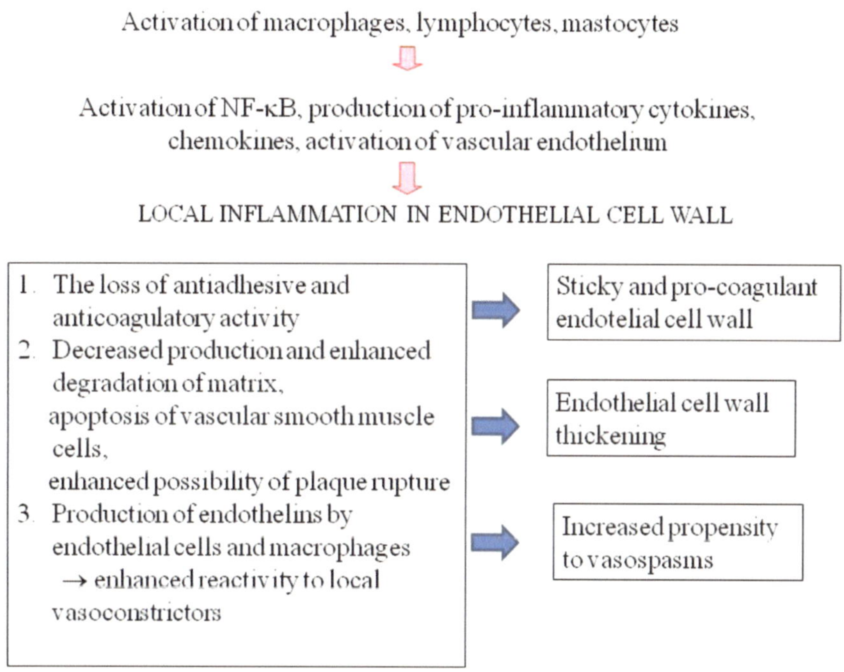

Fig. 4. Local inflammation in endothelial cell wall

Lipid deposition (oxLDL) is accompanied by inflammation - macrophages and T-lymphocytes enter vessel wall and foam cells (macrophages filled with oxLDL particles) develop (Eriksson, 2004). Recruitment of macrophages to the artery wall is one of the first steps in early atherosclerotic lesion formation. Macrophages become activated, produce a large amount of pro-inflammatory cytokines, chemokines and HMGB1 and potentiate inflammation. They release also MMP-9 (matrix metaloproteinase), smooth muscle cells proliferate and intima becomes thickened. Later, fibrosis develops and calcification appears in vessel wall. The more intensive is the inflammation, the higher is the activation of macrophages and atherosclerotic plaque is more unstable, and the thickening of fibrous cap progrediates. In the case of a plaque rupture, tissue factor expressed by activated macrophages facilitate activation of thrombocytes, thrombus formation and subsequent ischemia (Libby, 2002). Critical molecule that is very early released after tisue

ischemia/reperfusion injury is HMGB1 and thereby it functions as early mediator of tissue injury (Chang et al., 2011; Yang et al., 2011).
Chemokines from activated macrophages attract also other immune cells to the site of inflammation – T cells, NK cells and mast cells that aggravate the inflammation. Activated mastocytes support instability of the atherosclerotic plaque by histamine, molecule with pro-inflammatory activity, chymase and tryptase production and support coronary spasm development by the production of endogenous vasoconstrictors. Next mediators are complement components and C-reactive protein (CRP) (Devaraj et al., 2010; Onat et al., 2011).
The ability of macrophages to become activated is extremely important in the atherosclerotic plaque rupture. In subjects with a genetically higher ability of macrophage activation, the rupture and subsequent thrombosis and ischemia may develop in a smaller atherosclerotic plaque, even in a limited coronary atheroma (Kondo et al., 2003). This means that two identical atheromas do not need to be identical and differ in their prognosis. The difference is determined by genetic polymorphisms, e.g. by different ability of macrophages to become activated. In particular, the key role of macrophages in this process has been proven by findings in an animal model - mice deficient for macrophage colony stimulating factor were protected from atherosclerosis.
Inflammation of vascular cell wall is a crucial problem and early proinflammatory cytokines, late proinflammatory cytokine HMGB1, chemokines, and acute phase proteins play a great role in it. Key immune system molecules involved in the process of atherosclerosis and cardiovascular disease development are those involved in the process of inflammation and in the process of antigen presentation, monocytes, macrophages, mastocytes and Th1 immunity activation. Preferentially, these are early proinflammatory cytokines TNF-α, IL-1, IL-6, chemokines MCP-1/CCL2, CXCL16, MIP-1-α, proinflammatory cytokine IL-17, late proinflammatory cytokine HMGB1, INF-γ - main Th1 macrophage activating cytokine, IP-10 (IFN-γ inducing protein) and IL-12, the key Th1 inducing cytokine. On the other hand, IL-10 and TGF-β - mediators with anti-inflammatory, immunoregulatory and immunosuppresive activity control this pathology. It was found that besides Th1 lymphocytes, both T cytotoxic cells and NK cells take part in the process of atherosclerosis (Griva et al., 2010; Wang et al., 2010).
In the last years, other molecules as neopterin and procalcitonin are also studied in relation to inflammation and risk of cardiovascular disease development and prognosis. A great interest is devoted to HMGB1.
While acute inflammation serves to resolve pathogen infection and promotes tissue repair, persistent inflammation results in maladaptive tissue remodelling and damage and often serves as the precursor for arterial remodelling that underlies the increase of age –associated arterial diseases. The inflammation plays also an important role in the development of post-ischemic organ dysfunction in acute coronary syndromes, and in the healing process after myocardial infarction (Dewald et al., 2005). These facts highlight the value of non-specific inflammatory markers in patients with cardiovascular diseases.

4. Nonspecific inflammatory markers and cardiovascular diseases

4.1 C-reactive protein (CRP). Production, regulation of the production and plasma/serum levels of CRP

CRP, a part of an acute phase reaction, previously considered to be a marker of underlying infection or tissue injury, was later found also as a marker of chronic low-grade non-infectious systemic inflammation. Associations between increased levels of CRP and clinical course of the acute MI and other acute coronary syndrome were found (Berk et al., 1990; De Beer et al., 1982; Kardys et al., 2006; Pepys & Hirschfield, 2003).

It was confirmed that CRP is a better risk predictor of the cardiovascular events then LDL levels (Ridker, 2003). Its increased levels are considered a risk factor for atherosclerosis progression and complications even in healthy individuals (Dvorakova & Poledne, 2004). Increased levels of hsCRP were found also in patients with chronic heart failure, diastolic heart failure and dilated cardiomyopathy (Ishikawa et al., 2006; Michowitz et al., 2008; Xue et al., 2006).

At least six major prospective studies support the hypothesis that elevated CRP levels contribute to increased cardiovascular risk (Devaraj et al., 2010; Ridker et al., 2000). These are the Physician's Health Study (PHS) (Ridker et al., 1998), Women's Healthy Study (WHS) (Ridker et al., 2003), Atherosclerosis Risk in Communities (ARIC) study (Ballantyne et al., 2005), and Air Force/Texas Coronary Atherosclerosis Prevention Study (AFCAPS/TexCAPS) (Downs et al., 1998) in the United States and the Monitoring Trends and Determinants on Cardiovascular Diseases/Cooperative Health Research in the Region of Augsburg (MONICA/KORA Augsburg) (Koenig et al., 2008) and the Age Gene/Environment Susceptibility (AGES)-Reykjavik studies in Europe (Eiriksdottir, 2006).

CRP is nowadays added to so called soluble pattern recognition receptors (PRR), sensors of threatening, that recognize some evolutionary conserved substances both from external intruders on the surface of microorganisms and internal structures that originate from our damaged cells, organs or tissues. Some molecules of danger synthesized during threatening of our organism could also be recognized by CRP (Raz, 2007; Sandor & Buc, 2005). After binding to them, the human CRP activates different humoral factors (the complement system), cells (phagocytes) and transducing signals. That evokes the immune response against the intruders and mediates a potent pro-inflammatory pathophysiological effects, too.

Plasma CRP is produced mostly by hepatocytes and is under the regulation of cytokine IL-6. Normal values range round 1,3 mg . L^{-1} in adults (Maruna 2005). Median CRP levels are somehow higher in apparently healthy adults compared to blood donors and are characteristic for a given individual. CRP levels do not demonstrate seasonal neither diurnal variations and are not influenced by food intake (Pepys & Hirschfield, 2003; Szalai et al., 2002). CRP levels have a tendency to increase with age, reflecting an increased incidence of subclinical pathologic processes (Cerovska et al., 2006; Koenig et al., 1999). After a stimulus, plasma CRP levels increase above 5 mg. L^{-1} in 6 hours, and reach the maximum within 48 hours. After that, the level of CRP returns to very low „reference values" in plasma with the same speed.

Gene coding for CRP is localized on the chromosome 1 (1q2.1–2.5) and the main inductor of gene transcription is IL-6. IL-1 and complement act synergically (Buc & Bucova, 2007; Cerovska et al., 2006; Krejsek & Kopecky, 2004). The expression of CRP is regulated mainly at transcription level. Post-transcription mechanisms play also an important regulatory role, e.g. during inflammation CRP stay in the endoplasmatic reticulum is shortened from 18 hours to 75 minutes, enabling a faster CRP production (Krejsek & Kopecky, 2004). The half-life of CRP in plasma is approximately 19 hours and is constant during various conditions in healthy and sick people. Therefore, the only factor determining the level of CRP is its production speed (Aukrust et al., 2007), which directly reflects the intensity of pathological process.

4.2 High sensitive CRP (hsCRP)

In the mid of 1990s, a new method ELISA - imunoassay was established to evaluate the level of high sensitive CRP (hsCRP), which has much higher sensitivity than classic methods used previously. It has been proved that higher levels of hsCRP, previously considered to be within normal range, have a strong predictive value in the development of coronary events in the future. First studies concerned patients with stable, unstable and severe unstable angina. These studies showed the predictive value of hsCRP levels regarding future coronary events (Liuzzo et al., 1994; Thompson et al., 1995) and brought a lot of interest into the predictive values of hsCRP. Studies demonstrating the relationship between higher level of hsCRP and future atherothrombotic events, such as coronary events, stroke, peripheral artery disease, were initiated (Arena et al., 2006; Kraus et al., 2007; Ridker et al., 2000). A cardiovascular risk scale according to hsCRP levels was developed (Pearson et al., 2003) (Table 4).

Cardiovascular risk	hsCRP level
Low	$< 1 \ mg . l^{-1}$
Medium	$1 - 2 \ mg . l^{-1}$
High	$2 - 3 \ mg . l^{-1}$
Infection	$3 - 10 \ mg . l^{-1}$

Table 4. HsCRP scale of cardiovascular risk according to the American Heart Association (Pearson et al., 2003)

4.3 CRP – A contributing factor for increased cardiovascular risk in metabolic syndrome

Metabolic syndrome (MetS) was characterised by a cluster of abnormalities, with insulin resistance and adiposity as central features (Reaven et al., 2005; Eckel et al., 2005; Haffner & Cassells, 2003). Five diagnostic criteria for MetS have been identified by the National Cholesterol Education Program Adult Treatment Panel III (NCEP-ATP III), and the presence of any of these three features – central obesity, dyslipidemia (high triglycerides, low high-density lipoprotein [HDL] cholesterol), hypertension, and impaired fasting glucose – is considered sufficient to diagnose the syndrome (Expert Panel, 2001). About 24% of US adults have MetS, and the prevalence increases with age (44% at age 60 years) (Ford, 2005). 44% of US population over 50 years meeting the NCEP-ATP III criteria has MetS (Alexander et al., 2003).

Metabolic syndrome (MetS) characterised by chronic low-grade inflammation is associated with increased propensity for cardiovascular disease and diabetes development. MetS and cardiovascular disease individuals with MetS have an increased burden of cardiovascular disease (CVD) complications (Devaraj et al., 2010; Lakka et al.; 2002). Men with MetS, even in the absence of baseline coronary artery disease (CAD) or diabetes, had a significantly increased mortality from CAD. It was found that in individuals with MetS, the risk for coronary heart disease (CHD) and stroke was increased threefold ($P<0.001$) and the risk for cardiovascular mortality was increased sixfold ($P<0.001$) (Lakka et al., 2002; Alexander et al., 2003; Devaraj et al., 2004). Individuals with MetS without diabetes had higher CHD prevalence (13.9%), and those with both MetS and diabetes had the highest prevalence of CHD (19.2%) compared with those with neither (Alexander et al., 2003).

Plasma levels of CRP are elevated in individuals with MetS. They were shown to be strongly associated with insulin resistence calculated from the homeostatic model assessment, blood pressure, low HDL, and triglycerides, and also to levels of the proinflammatory cytokines TNF-α and IL-6. Body mass index and insulin resistance were the strongest determinants of the inflammatory state. There is a linear relationship between the number of metabolic features and increasing levels of hsCRP. HsCRP was positively correlated with body mass index, waist circumference, blood pressure, triglycerides, cholesterol, low-density lipoprotein (LDL) cholesterol, plasma glucose, and fasting insulin, and it was inversely correlated with HDL cholesterol and the insulin sensitivity index. The strongest associations were observed between CRP levels, central adiposity, and insulin resistance.

Ridker et al. (2000, 2003) evaluated inter-relationships between CRP, MetS, and incident cardiovascular events among apparently healthy women who were followed for an 8-year period for myocardial infarction, stroke, coronary revascularization, or cardiovascular death. 24% of the cohort had MetS at study entry. They found that women with hsCRP levels of less than 3 mg/L without MetS had the best cardiovascular survival, whereas those with hsCRP levels greater than 3 mg/L with MetS had the worst cardiovascular survival. Other studies also support the hypothesis that an increased hsCRP level in the setting of MetS confers an increased risk of future cardiovascular events.

Thus, it has been proposed that hsCRP should be added as a clinical criterion for MetS and for creation of an hsCRP-modified CHD risk score (Ridker et al., 2000). In addition to the prognostic information that hsCRP evaluation might add to the current definition of MetS, there are several other practical benefits of hsCRP measurement (Devaraj et al., 2010). First, hsCRP is strongly associated with components of MetS that are difficult to measure in routine clinical practice, such as impaired fibrinolysis and insulin resistence (Yudkin et al., 2004, Festa et al., 2000). Also, the widespread availability of commercial assays for hsCRP has made its measurement simple and inexpensive. In addition, as hsCRP does not display diurnal variation and demonstrates long-term stability comparable with cholesterol, it can be reliably evaluated with a single nonfasting measurement. The addition of hsCRP measurement to diagnosis of the MetS may significantly improve the early detection of risk for future diabetes and cardiovascular events in individuals (Ridker et al., 2004).

4.4 CRP, cytokines, chemokines and other nonspecific inflammatory markers

The level of CRP closely correlates with other non-specific inflammatory markers, which show similar although less significant predictive association with future coronary event (Danesh et al., 1998, 1999). Many studies have shown that increased levels of fibrinogen, CRP and IL-6 are associated with the risk of coronary heart disease, clinical course, prognosis and severity of atherosclerosis (Jenny et at., 2007; Sukhija et al., 2007). Similar association was found with the level of IL-8, where the risk of coronary heart diseases was higher in men compared to women and was independent from both traditional risk factors and CRP (Boekholdt et al., 2004). Authors could not exclude the possibility that IL-8 reflected a pre-clinical atherosclerosis. Concentrations of complement components, mainly the C3 to C4 ratio and the level of BNP (brain natrium uretic peptide) could also predict the mortality and severity of cardiovascular disease (Blanghy et al., 2007; Iltumur et al., 2005; Palikhe et al., 2007).

Zouridakis et al. (2004) showed 4 markers predicting rapid progression of coronary heart disease - CRP, sICAM (soluble intercellular adhesive molecules), neopterin and MMP-9 Their levels are higher in „progressors" than in „non-progressors". According to their results the patients with CRP concentration in the medium quartile had 3-fold risk of coronary heart disease progression compared to the patients in the lowest quartile, and patients with sICAM levels higher than 271,4 $ng.ml^{-1}$ (average) had 4-fold increased risk compared to the patients in the lowest quartile. Individuals with neopterin level higher than 7,5 nmol . L^{-1} (medium quartile) have 5-fold increased risk of coronary heart disease development and progression compared to individuals with neopterin levels in the lowest quartile. Patients with MMP-9 concentration higher than 47,9 $\mu g.l^{-1}$ (median) have 3-fold increased risk of coronary heart disease progression compared to the patients in the lowest quartile. As the last two markers are indicators of the activity of macrophages that are key cells playing a causative role in the process of atherosclerosis, the evaluation of their activity seems to be useful in patients at risk. A systemic therapy might prevent development or progression of coronary heart disease.

4.5 CRP and proinflammatory cytokines – The cause and the result of the inflammatory process

It is questionable to what extend are pro-inflammatory cytokines and CRP purely acute phase markers and to what extend are they active inflammatory participants. Increased levels of IL-6 were found in patients with unstable angina, where inflammatory reaction may promote conversion of a stable atherosclerotic plaque to an unstable one (Biasucci et al., 1996). It was also found that plasma CRP level can predict future cardiovascular events or mortality due to coronary heart disease even in healthy individuals (Dvorakova & Poledne, 2004; Kardys et al., 2006; Koenig et al., 2006). CRP predicts cardiovascular risk even in Japanese, who generally have lover levels (Saito et al., 2007). These findings show the possibility that both the progression of atheroma and the plaque rupture might be predicted by a follow-up of CRP levels. The role of TNF-alfa and IL-6 in the atherogenesis and thrombosis was also shown. Pro-inflammatory cytokines TNF-alfa, IL-6, IL-1 and also CRP are in large amounts produced except of liver also by adipocytes (Mohamed et al.,1997; Yudkin et al.,1999). Production of IL-6 in obese patients and approximately 30% of IL-6 in healthy individuals comes from adipocytes. These cytokines inhibit insulin signalization and cause insulin resistance, and also enhance the development of endothelial dysfunction – they increase the expression of adhesive molecules, pro-thrombotic factors, acute phase proteins, which can increase a cardiovascular risk via a feed back mechanism (Conen et al., 2006; Kremen et al., 2006). It was found that, both CRP and pro-inflammatory cytokine levels correlate with blood pressure, dyslipidemia, HDL (high density lipoprotein cholesterol) and level of triglycerides, smoking, diabetes, insulin resistance, markers of endothelial dysfunction and obesity (Bermudez et al., 2002; Cerovska et al., 2006; Chambers et al., 2001; Dvorakova & Poledne, 2004; Ford, 1999; Frohlich et al., 2000). The correlation with BMI (body mass index) was also found, which could partially reflect the fact that the majority of basal CRP and IL-6 is produced in adipocytes (Danesh et al., 1999). Weight decrease was associated with plasma CRP decrease even in healthy individuals (Mohamed-Ali et al., 1997).

In the pathogenesis of coronary heart disease and atherosclerosis, chemokines play an important role, too. The most important are: MCP-1 (monocyte chemotactic protein), MIP-1α (macrophage inflammatory protein), IP-10 (IFN-gama inducible protein, with M_r =10 000), RANTES (regulated on activation normal T-cell expressed and secreted) and eotaxin (Rothenbacher et al., 2006). MCP-1, called also CCL2 (MCP-1/CCL2) is chemotactic to monocytes, T-lymphocytes and NK cells and participates in the development and restoration of diseases characterized with infiltration of monocytes (Gu et al., 1998; 1999). It modulates fibroblasts and endothelial cells function and has an important role in the pathogenesis of myocardial infarction, thrombotic occlusion, myocardial ischemia, and also in the reperfusion and healing process after myocardial infarction (Dewald et al., 2005). Tarzami et al. showed that MCP-1/CCL2 had a dual role in myocardial ischemia - beside chemotactic activity protected myocardial cells against hypoxia induced cell death (Tarzami et al., 2002; 2005).

4.6 Non-specific inflammatory markers in cardiovascular diseases – what do they reflect?

Another question is, what exactly these non-specific markers reflect. Four possibilities can be found and three of them directly or indirectly highlight the role of atherosclerosis: 1. Atherosclerosis, plaque development, its instability, rupture and resulting atherothrombosis are inflammatory events. The first assumption could be that increased levels of inflammatory markers reflects inflammation of the vessel wall. This is possible, but some contradictory results concerning the level of CRP and atherosclerotic plaque size exist. This discrepancy could be explained by genetic polymorphism causing a different ability of macrophages to be activated as it was mentioned above, which explains a possible rupture even in a small atherosclerotic plaque (Kondo et al., 2003). Chronic systemic non-vascular infection is also pro-atherogenic and acute systemic inflammatory episodes are markedly associated with atherosclerotic processes (Rotenbacher et al., 2006). CRP could reflect inflammation in some other part of organism, although the correlation of Chlamydia pneumonie and Helicobacter pylori antibodies with the development of coronary heart disease is not very clear (Danesh et al., 2000). Generally, the above mentioned associations of CRP and IL-6 levels with BMI and IHD risk factors increase the possibility that inflammatory markers associated with the risk of atherothrombosis could reflect a certain metabolic state, which is also pro-atherogenic and is a predisposition to atherothrombotic events, that means it is also pro-inflammatory. In fact, CRP level predicts development of type 2 diabetes independently from traditional risk factors (Freeman et al., 2002). In insulin-resistant obese individuals, increased CRP levels decrease in parallel with the improvement of insulin resistance related to weight loss (Mc Laughlin et al., 2002). The fourth possibility is the fact that individuals differ in their sensitivity to various stimuli leading to acute phase proteins production. Therefore, those who are „higher CRP responders", either due to genetic mechanism or other acquired mechanism (for example, BMI) are simple more sensible to atherosclerosis progression and complications.

4.7 CRP - a cause of cardiovascular disease

CRP has been traditionally thought to be a bystander marker of vascular inflammation, without playing a direct role in CVD. Now, increasing evidence suggests that CRP may directly contribute to the proinflammatory state, and play thus a direct role in vascular injury.

Aggregated CRP binds to and opsonizes LDL and VLDL (very low density lipoprotein), subsequently activates complement and mediates uptake of these particles by macrophages that transforme in foam cells (Pickering et al., 2007; Thomson et al., 1995).

Several reports demonstrated the presence of CRP within atheromatous plaque where it preceeds and mediates monocyte recruitment (Jian-Jun & Chun-Hong, 2004). CRP was found to be widely distributed in early human atherosclerotic lesions of human coronary arteries with two predominant manifestations. First, the majority of foam cells below the endothelium showed positive staining for CRP. This staining was clearly cell associated, mainly along the cell surface. Second, CRP was deposited diffusely rather than focally in the deep fibroelastic layer and the fibromuscular layer of the intima adjacent to the media (Cerovska et al., 2006). CRP activates the classical pathway of complement and has been shown to colocalize with the membrane attack complex (C5b-C9) in early atherosclerotic lesions in the fibromuscular layer of the intima, which contains predominantly smooth muscle cells (Cerovska et al., 2006; Szalai et al., 2002).

CRP can stimulate tissue factor production by macrophages, the main stimulus for initiating coagulation, upregulates the expression of adhesion molecules ICAM-1 and VCAM-1 (vascular adhesion molecule-1) by endothelial cells and mediates proinflammatory factor induction in artery wall as well as circulating monocytes (Aukrust et al., 2007; Liuzzo et al., 1994; Kraus et al., 2007; Pickering et al., 2007). In addition, CRP mediates MCP-1 induction in endothelial cells (Aukrust et al., 2007; Liuzzo et al., 1994).

CRP also stimulates the release of inflammatory cytokines TNF-a, IL-1b, IL-6 and may also directly act as a proinflammatory stimulus to phagocytic cells by binding to the FcRII receptor (Buc & Bucova., 2007). Furthemore, monocytes from healthy subjects were also found to exhibit an enhanced production of IL-6 in response to CRP and this response was significantly inhibited by simvastatin in a dose-dependent manner (Krejsek & Kopecky., 2004). IL-6 production increases very rapidly, 4 h after CRP stimulation and therefore continues to rise at a slower rate, reaching a peak at 24 h.

Devaraj et al. (2009) outlined that CRP contributes to increased cardiovascular risk by inducing endothelial cell dysfunction and activating monocytes.

These data suggest that CRP may indeed be a direct proinflammatory factor involved in the initiation and progression of atherosclerosis.

4.8 HMGB1

HMGB1, formerly known as a nuclear nonhistone protein, that stabilizes nucleosomes, has DNA-binding properties, facilitates gene transcription, and have an essential position in DNA repair (Lange & Vasquez, 2009; Lotze & Tracey, 2005; Wang et al., 2007,). Later studies identified the extracellular form of HMGB1 as a critical mediator of inflammation, mainly sepsis and also as a factor that promotes tissue repair and regeneration (Fink, 2007; De MR et al., 2007; Klune et al., 2008).

HMGB1 is likely to be released into extracellular milieu in two ways - passively from necrotic or injured cells (e.g. after ischemic/reperfusion injury – IRI) and actively by activated monocytes and macrophages (Ulloa & Messmer, 2006). This extracellular HMGB1 acts as alarmin and signaling through RAGE, TLR2 and TLR4 leads to the activation of NF-κB, which induces the production of proinflammatory cytokines and angiogenic factors in both hematopoietic and endothelial cells.

Its key role has been revealed in lethal endotoxemia and sepsis and as it is released later than other pro-inflammatory cytokines (after 16-32 h) it became known as a "late mediator of sepsis" or "late proinflammatory cytokine" (Wang et al., 1999, 2007). Recently identified biological activities of HMGB1 include chemotactic activity, activation of monocytes/macrophages to release proinflammatory cytokines, upregulation of endothelial cell adhesion molecules, stimulation of epithelial cell barrier failure, and mediation of fewer and anorexia (Wang et al., 2004). More recently, HMGB1 was recognized as a proangiogenic factor, and seems to be able to attract also stem cells to the area of injury and inflammation, activate them and promote thus healing and regeneration (De MR et al., 2007; Klune et al., 2008). Interestingly, HMGB1 can act also on local stem cells, activate them, promote their differentiation and facilitate the healing process directly from local sources (Lolmede et al., 2009; Yiang et al., 2010). The discovery of HMGB1 as a critical mediator of inflammation in different inflammatory diseases has stimulated tremendous interest in the field of inflammation research. HMGB1 protein contributes to development of autoimmune diseases, and its role in growth and spread of many types of tumours has also been revealed (Abdulahad et al., 2010; Tang et al., 2010). Thus, HMGB1 represents a potential target in therapy of various disorders related to inflammation (Yang and Tracey, 2010).

HMGB1 is structurally composed of three different domains: two homologous DNA-binding sequences entitled box A and box B and a highly, negatively charged C terminus. The B box domain is responsible for proinflammatory activity of the molecule, whereas the A box region has an antagonistic, anti-inflammatory effect with therapeutic potential. Administration of highly purified, recombinant A box protein or neutralizing antibodies against HMGB1 rescued mice from lethal sepsis (Huang et al., 2010).

Many recent studies demonstrated that HMGB1 played a pivotal role in cardiovascular diseases, such as atherosclerosis, myocardial ischemia/reperfusion injury (IRI), heart failure, and myocardial infarction. Elevated levels of HMGB1 has been detected in patients with coronary artery diseases (CAD), in patients with cerebral and myocardial ischemia, in IRI of the heart and is a novel predictor of adverse clinical outcomes after acute myocardial infarction (Goldstein et al., 2006; Kohno et al., 2009; Yan et al., 2009).

Injury of endothelium is essential for the initiation of atherosclerosis as it leads to the attraction of macrophages. Progression of atherosclerosis goes along with prolonged pro-inflammatory response (Mullaly and Kubes 2004). It was revealed that HMGB1 and RAGE are expressed in endothelial cells, smooth muscle cells, and macrophages of atherosclerotic lesions (Kalinina et al., 2004). Moreover, activated vascular smooth muscle cells are the source of HMGB1 in human advanced atherosclerotic lesions (Innoue et al., 2007). Therefore, up-regulation and secretion of HMGB1 may lead to intensification of inflammatory response in endothelial lesions, promote further atherosclerotic changes and thus may be related to the severity of coronary artery stenosis (Innoue et al., 2007).

4.8.1 HMGB1 in ischemic and reperfusion injury

Many factors have been revealed to be involved in IRI including nitric oxide or plenty of cytokines released under proinflammatory conditions in the afflicted area in many organs i.e. heart, brain, kidney or liver (Matsuki et al., 2006; Hsieh et al., 2007). Recent studies suggest potential implication of HMGB1 in the pathogenesis of IRI (Goldstein et al., 2006). IRI leads to tissue damage and high amounts of HMGB1 protein are released around the central ischemic area (Kim et al., 2006).

4.8.2 HMGB1 in positive feedback mechanism

HMGB1 seems to be involved in positive feedback mechanism, that may help to sustain inflammation and angiogenesis and contribute thus to disease progression. CRP dose dependently induces the production of HMGB1 through the p38 MAPK pathway (Kawahara et al., 2008). In return, HMGB1 triggers the expression of other proinflammatory cytokines and reinforces this way the proinflammatory process (Andersson et al., 2000; Wang et al., 1999). Endothelial cells express HMGB1, as well as its receptors RAGE, TLR2 and TLR4 and signalling through theses receptors leads to activation of NFkappaB, which can subsequently induce the expression of HMGB1 receptors (van Beijnum et al., 2008) These studies suggest that HMGB1 may be a critical proinflammatory cytokine and may play an important role in the pathogenesis of CAD.

Hu et al. (2009) has found markedly increased level of serum HMGB1 that correlated with severity of coronary artery stenosis in patients with stable (SAP) and unstable angina pectoris (USAP), especially in SAP patients. In addition, a strong correlation between angiographic Gensini score and serum level of HMGB1 has been found. However, in subgroup analysis the serum level of HMGB1 was significantly correlated only with angiographic Gensini score in SAP patients, not USAP patients. These results indicated, that the level of serum HMGB1 may predict the degree of coronary artery stenosis in patients with SAP and HMGB1 may be involved in the pathogenesis of USAP (Hu et al., 2009). The serum level of HMGB1 positively correlated with the serum level of hs-CRP, TNF-α and IL-6 in patients with CAD (Hu et al., 2009; Yan et al., 2009). These results are in agreement with previous observations that there is a cross-talk between HMGB1 and other proinflammatory cytokines and CRP.

Passively released from necrotic cells or actively secreted by activated monocytes/macrophages, or other cells, HMGB1 functions as an inflammatory stimulus that upregulates the production of early proinflammatory cytokines TNF-α, IL-1, IL-6, and different inflammatory proteins (MIP- 1α, MIP-1β), and subsequently CRP (Andersson et al., 2000; Sama et al., 2004). Interestingly, HMGB1 alone can directly stimulate the production of CRP which is an independent predictor of coronary artery disease extent in patient with stable and unstable angina pectoris (Arroyo-Espliguero et al., 2009; Niccoli et al., 2008).

4.8.3 HMGB1 and therapy in cardiovascular diseases

HMGB1 is considered as a potential clinical therapy, in association with myocardial infarction. The possibility of evaluating HMGB1 as a regenerative and proliferative agent in the myocardium was first suggested by Palumbo et al. (2004). They demonstrated that HMGB1 induced migration and proliferation of blood vessel mesangioblasts, which are blood vessel stem cells. Later, Limana et al. (2005) discusses the role of HMGB1 in initiating activation and differentiation of endogenous cardiac stem cells in a mouse model of myocardial infarction. The capacity of HMGB1 to promote the development of mouse cardiomyocytes and initiate repair of myocardial infarction is quite remarkable. An exogenous HMGB1 directly injected to peri-infarcted area contributes to increased amount of myocytes inside the area of infarcted cardiomyocytes that goes along with improved outcome confirmed by structural and functional measures (Klune et al., 2008; Limana et al., 2005). These examples support effect of HMGB1 in regenerative processes.

Human cardiac stem cells (CSCs) can be obtained fairly readily from cardiac surgery specimens, and they have been characterized to a very limited extent. As such, it is too early to comment on similarities and differences between mouse and human CSCs, as too little is known about adult human CSCs. Moreover, the use of HMGB1 like any other drugs or molecules that activate resident stem cells in vivo might circumvent the need for „classical" stem cell therapy. Interestingly, the mechanism by which HMGB1 works is not yet clear.

They current working hypothesis is that it functions by interfering with pro-apoptotic pathways (Rosenberg & Oppenheim, 2007).

4.9 Neopterin

Among the immune inflammatory cells, activated macrophages contribute significantly to atherosclerosis plaque progression, fibrous cap disruption and intracoronary trombus formation (Avanzas & Kaski, 2009). Macrophages are a marker of unstable atherosclerotic plaque, may release lytic enzymes that degrade the fibrous cap, produce rupture of the atherosclerotic plaque and therefore play a significant role in the pathophysiology of acute coronary syndrome (Moreno et al, 1994).

IFN-gama - a cytokine produced by activated Th1 cells is centrally involved in atherosclerosis - related inflammation and monocyte/macrophage activation and contributes to this process. In activated macrophages IFN-gama stimulates conversion of tryptophan to kynurenine and production of neopterine (Pedersen et al., 2011). Enhanced tryptophan degradation in patients with coronary heart disease was found to correlate with enhanced neopterin formation.

Neopterin, a pteridine, by-product of the guanosine triphosphate pathway is an activation marker for monocytes/macrophages (Sugioka et al., 2010a, 2010b), marker of inflammation and Th1 immune system activation (Pacileo et al., 2007; Murr et al., 2002). In the past several years, the measurements of neopterin concentrations in body fluids including plasma, serum, urine and cerebrospinal fluid has revealed its potential role in the prediction of long-term prognosis in both patients with viral infections, HIV-1 infection, severe systemic inflammatory diseases, several autoimmune diseases, renal transplant rejection, cancer (Kozłowska-Murawska & Obuchowicz, 2008; Plata-Nazar et al., 2004; Sucher et al., 2010). By neopterin measurements, not only the extent of monocyte/macrophage and Th1 immune system activation but also the extent of oxidative stress could be estimated (Murr et al., 2002).

Elevated plasma/serum levels of neopterin have also been reported in patients with coronary disease compared to controls and in recent years it has become apparent that increased neopterin concentrations are an independent marker for cardiovascular disease (Fuchs et al., 2009). Neopterin serves also as a good biomarker of plaque inflammation, its instability in both coronary and carotid atherosclerotic lesions (Sugioka et al., 2010a), and as a marker for cardiovascular risk (Avanzas & Kaski, 2009). In particular, neopterin predicts future major cardiac and vascular adverse events in patients suffering from coronary artery disease (Avanzas et al., 2005; De Rosa et al., 2011; Pacileo et al., 2007). Serum neopterin is an independent predictor of major adverse coronary events and may also serve as a useful marker for risk stratification in patients with chronic stable angina pectoris.

Coronary angiographic studies have shown a relationship between increased circulating levels of neopterin and the presence of complex coronary lesions in patients with unstable angina pectoris. Moreower, higher prevalence of neopterin-positive macrophages was found in culprit lesions in patients with UAP than in those with stable angina pectoris (SAP), so neopterin could serve as an important biomarker of plaque instability in both coronary and carotid atherosclerotic lesions (Sugioka et al., 2010a, 2010b). However, plasma neopterin levels were significantly higher also in SAP patients with complex carotid plaques than those in noncomplex plaques (Sugioka et al., 2010b). This marker of macrophage activation may be useful for risk stratification even in patients with chronic stable angina (Avanzas et al., 2005).

Left ventricular ejection fraction (LVEF) is the strongest predictor of survival in patients with chronic stable angina (CSA). Baseline neopterin levels - but not CRP - showed a significant inverse correlation with LVEF. Increased serum neopterin concentrations inversely correlate with LVEF values and high neopterin levels are a predictor of LV dysfunction in patients with CSA, irrespective of the extent and severity of coronary artery disease. Neopterin may thus be clinically useful for patient risk stratification (Estévez-Loureiro et al., 2009).

4.10 Procalcitonin

Procalcitonin (PCT) was originally described in 1984 as a 116 amino-acid protein and now is known as a highly selective and specific marker for early diagnosis of sepsis. Procalcitonin (PCT) - prohormon of calcitonin, is under basal condition produced only by C-type cells of thyroid and neuroendocrine cells of the lung. Thus, the basal plasma level of PCT in healthy individuals is very low, under detection limit - below 0.05 ng/ml. Under systemic bacterial infection preferentially of bacterial origin, the levels of PCT raise very quickly because almost all cells of human body start to be the source of PCT and the level of this molecule rapidly increases, it can reach several hundred of ng/ml. That is why is PCT considered as a hormokine, an acute phase marker and an early marker of systemic bacterial infection. The levels of PCT are elevated also under the conditions of non-infectious systemic inflammatory processes, this elevation is not so high. Elevation of PCT is mediated directly by microorganisms or indirectly by pro-inflammatory cytokines (Bucova, 2005).

So far, data on plasma/serum PCT levels in patients with cardiogenic shock and in those with acute coronary syndromes (ACS) are scarce and controversial. While some studies report that PCT levels are increased in ACS patients on admission, other investigations document that plasma PCT concentrations are in the normal range. Ataoğlu et al. (2010) found that higher PCT levels within 48 h post-admission may reflect an inflammatory state that is associated with increased early and 6-month mortality. Picariello et al. (2009) reported that the degree of myocardial ischemia (clinically indicated by the whole spectrum of ACS, from unstable angina to cardiogenic shock following ST-elevation myocardial infarction) and the related inflammatory response are better reflected by C-reactive protein than by PCT, which seems to be more sensitive to a higher degree of inflammatory activation, being positive only in patients with cardiogenic shock. Few studies investigated the dynamics of PCT in cardiac acute patients, and, despite the paucity of data and differences in patients' selection criteria, an increase in PCT values seems to be associated with the development of complications. In acute cardiac patients, the clinical values of procalcitonin rely not on its absolute value, but only on its kinetics over time (Picariello et al., 2009).

5. Genetic background of inflammation in cardiovascular diseases

5.1 Main terms

People differ in the risk of development and death due to various diseases including cardiovascular disease, and differ also in inflammatory reactions (Bucova et al., 2008a; Javor et al., 2007). Inter-individual genetic differences play an important role.

Human diseases are roughly divided into three categories according to genetic factors: 1. „monogenic diseases“ (caused by one gene defect), 2. complex diseases (with multigenic or polygenic predisposition) and 3. diseases without genetic predisposition. The best results were achieved in „monogenic diseases“. Recently, the attention is shifted to complex diseases caused by several genes, including majority of socially burden diseases (Fig. 5).

Single nucleotide polymorphism - SNP:

...AGCAGGATTAGATTACTTTAA... – *allele 1*
...AGCAGGAGTAGATTACTTTAA... – *allele 2*

Repetition polymorphisms:
...GATAGTCTCCTAGTGCGTAC... – *allele 1*
...GATAGTCTCCTCTAGTGCGTAC... – *allele 2*
...GATAGTCTCCTCTCTAGTGCGTAC... – *allele 3*

Fig. 5. The most frequent DNA polymorphisms

Genetic polymorphism means that more than one allele (variant) of gene is present in population. It is referred to when the frequency of the most frequent gene allele in population is lower than 99%, e.g. when the frequency of the rare gene allele is higher than 1%. Single nucleotide polymorphism (SNP) belongs to the most common types of genetic polymorphism, including exchange, insertion or deletion, and repetitive polymorphisms (Fig. 5). The number of SNP polymorphisms in genome is estimated to 10 millions (Hafler et al., 2005). Gene variants, influencing gene expression, are called functional gene polymorphisms. SNP polymorphism may be present in coding, regulatory and in non-coding gene regions (Tsuchiya et al., 2002).

While the polymorphisms in coding regions tend to change the structure of primary protein or result in protein defect, the polymorphisms in regulatory gene areas, influencing gene transcription, may affect gene expression. It is suggested that majority of polymorphisms playing a role in genetic predisposition of complex diseases, are found in regulatory gene areas (Tsuchiya et al., 2002).

Individual genetic susceptibility to complex diseases is present, when an inter-individual difference in disease risk exists, not determined by environmental factors. Regarding diseases, we distinguish susceptibility gene variants (allele), which predispose for disease development (they are more frequently found in patients compared to general population) and protective alleles, which on the contrary, are less common in patients than in healthy subjects.

5.2 Genetics, inflammation and cardiovascular diseases

The inheritance of cardiovascular diseases is polygenic, i.e. several genes can influence their development and clinical course. Except of polymorphisms of genes coding for homocystein, lipid metabolism, factors of coagulation, $\beta 2$ – adrenergic receptors, genes regulating blood pressure and others, inflammatory factors genes play an important role, too (Arnett et al., 2007; Horne et al., 2007; Markovic et al., 2007; Ozanne et al., 2007). These genes are numerous and gene polymorphisms related to different stages of inflammatory response have been found (Andreotti et al., 2002; Bernardo et al., 2006; Espliguero et al., 2005).

5.2.1 Genetics of CRP

The basal level of CRP both in patients and healthy controls are genetically determined. In repetitive measurements in healthy individuals it was found that concentrations of CRP

were relatively stable. It means, that knowledge in CRP genetic component may contribute to the stratification of so far healthy individuals into groups with higher or lower risk for cardiovascular disease development (Crawford et al., 2006; Szalai et al., 2005).
The human CRP gene lies on chromosome 1, within a conserved region that encodes for proteins critical to the immune system and to intercellular communication (Bucova et al., 2008b; D'Aiuto et al., 2005, Suk et al., 2005). Dupuis et al. (2005) found that multiple genes on chromosome 1 may influence inflammatory biomarker levels and may have a potential role in development of cardiovascular disease. They hypothesised that production of biomarkers of vascular inflammation is modulated both genetically and by environmental factors.
Family studies estimates of CRP ranging from 27–40%, and it is hypothesized that genetic variation in the CRP gene may influence plasma CRP levels and subsequent risk of CHD. Several studies have reported individual single nucleotide polymorphisms (SNPs) to be associated with CRP levels and Risk of Incident Coronary Heart Disease in Two Nested Case-Control Studies.
Szalai et al. (2005) sequenced 1156 nucleotides long promoter area of the CRP gene and identified two SNPs - one bi-allelic (-409A/G) and one three-allelic (-390C/T/A), which modulated basal CRP concentration in healthy individuals by influencing transcription factor binding. The results of „Framingham heart study" in 1640 unrelated participants revealed in 9 from 13 studied SNPs a relationship with CRP level (Kathiresan et al., 2006).
Knowing factors, which regulate plasma CRP levels, either basal or induced by infection or other inflammation, is very important also for the cardiovascular risk prediction. It was found that patients with homozygous +1444TT allele of CRP gene had significantly higher plasma CRP levels induced by inflammatory stimulus (D´Aiuto et al., 2005). This effect was independent from IL-6 concentration, IL-6 -174G/C SNP and conventional cardiovascular risk factors.
The production of CRP is except of CRP gene regulated also by other genes coding for IL-6, IL-1 beta and IL-1Ra (Fishman et al., 1998; Kathiresan et al., 2006; Latkovskis et al., 2004; Szalai et al., 2005; Vickers et al., 2002). In 160 patients with angiographically confirmed coronary heart disease, the association of higher plasma CRP level with the presence of IL-1B (+3954)T allele was found as well as a possible relationship between IL-1RN(VNTR)*2 allele and lower CRP concentrations (Latkovskis et al., 2004).
Acute coronary syndrome is associated with the activation of endothelial cells and systemic inflammation. It was found that genetic variations in the IL-1 locus influenced inflammatory processes – the IL-1RN*2 and the –511 alleles, respectively, contributed to changes in the plasma level of soluble markers of endothelial inflammation such as von Willebrand factor (vWF) and E-selectin (Ray et al., 2002). A correlation between higher plasma CRP level and presence of CD14 260TT homozygous allele was also found, which could be associated with the higher ability of macrophages to become activated and produce pro-inflammatory cytokines (Bernardo et al., 2006; Espliguero et al., 2005).
Bucova et al. (2009a) found an association of MCP-1 -2518 A/G single nucleotide polymorphism with the serum level of CRP in Slovak patients with ischemic heart disease, angina pectoris, and hypertension.
Additionally, a genome-wide association study has been performed among 6 345 apparently healthy women in whom 336 108 single nucleotide proteins were evaluated as potential determinants of plasma CRP concentration (Devaraj, 2010). Overall, seven loci that associate with plasma CRP levels were found. It was concluded that common variations in several genes involved in metabolic and inflammatory regulation have significant effects on CRP

levels, consistent with the identification of CRP as a useful biomarker of risk for incident vascular disease and diabetes. Two of these loci (GCKR and HNF1A) are suspected or known to be associated with maturity-onset diabetes of the young, one is a gene-desert region on 12q23.2, and the remaining four loci are in or near the leptin receptor protein gene, the apolipoprotein E gene, the IL-6 receptor protein gene, or the CRP gene itself. The protein products of six of these seven loci are directly involved in MetS, insulin resistance, β-cell function, weight homeostasis, and/or premature atherothrombosis.
Thus, there is a possibility that individuals vary in their sensitivity to intercurrent low-grade acute-phase stimuli to which everybody is exposed, and that those who are higher "CRP responders" through genetic and/or acquired mechanisms, are also more susceptible to progression and complications of atherosclerosis (Dewald et al., 2005).
Understanding the factors that directly or indirectly regulate the CRP release at baseline and during inflammation is very important in context of coronary risk prediction. More scientific groups studied CRP gene polymorphisms and found that basal levels of CRP both in patients and healthy controls are genetically determined and under repeated examination in healthy subjects relatively stable. Thus understanding the genetic background of CRP that regulate basal but also by infection or any type of inflammation induced concentration of CRP might contribute to stratification of healthy subjects to different groups with higher or lower degree of cardiovascular disease development (Cermakova et al., 2005; Pearson at al. 2003; Szalai et al., 2002)

5.2.2 Gene polymorphisms of MCP-1/CCL2 and CCR2 and the risk of cardiovascular disease development

Pro-inflammatory cytokines and chemokines play an important role in the pathogenesis of heart diseases (Rothenbacher et al., 2006). Gene polymorphisms of chemokine MCP-1/CCL2, a molecule that plays an important role in atherosclerosis, and its receptor CCR2 belong to most studied one (Arakelyan et al., 2005; Bucova et al., 2008a; Petrkova et al. 2003). MCP-1/CCL2 is a potent chemoattractant for monocytes, T cells and NK cells. MCP-1 induces the transmigration of $CCR2^{+}$ monocytes from the circulation, promotes their differentiation to lipid-laden macrophages (Gerszten et al., 1999; Tabata et al., 2003) and contributes to the proliferation of arterial smooth muscle cells (Viedt et al., 2002) which, along the macrophages, constitute the key cellular components of atherosclerotic plaques. This chemokine plays a dual role in myocardial ischaemia. In addition to several negative roles in the process of atherosclerosis, thrombotic occlusion of a coronary artery and in the process of reperfusion, this chemokine protects myocytes from hypoxia-induced cell death and has also positive effect in myocardial infarct healing (Dewald et al., 2005; Tarzami et al., 2002, 2005).
Polymorphism of MCP-1 and its receptor CCR2 have been implicated as susceptibility factor for chronic stable angina pectoris, ischemic heart disease and myocardial infarction by several independent investigators (Petrkova et al., 2003; Ortlepp et al., 2003), even in hypertensive ischemic heart disease assymptomatic patients (Penz et al., 2010). An association of CCR2 polymorphisms with the number of closed coronary artery vessels in coronary artery disease was also found (Cha SH et al., 2007). Deletion of MCP-1/CCL2 or CCR2 resulted in a large (50%-80%) reduction in atherosclerotic plaque size (Boring et al.,1998; Gu et al., 1999). However, the data on contribution of the MCP-1 polymorphisms to the pathogenesis of coronary atherosclerosis are not uniform. McDermott et al. found that the presence of MCP-1 -2578G allele in homozygous form was significantly associated with

both myocardial infarction occurrence and higher MCP-1 plasma level. Increased MCP-1 levels were associated with age, smoking, BMI and waist to hip ratio (Mc Dermott et al., 2005). In other study, the plasma MCP-1 level was independently associated with the prognosis of patients with acute coronary syndrome (Deo et al., 2004). Higher levels of MCP-1 were associated with higher age, Caucasian race, early onset of coronary heart disease, smoking, hypertension, hypercholesterolemia and higher hsCRP levels (Deo et al., 2004). Similar association was found in the group of patients with detected calcium in coronary arteries.

It was found that CCR2 -/- mice show smaller area of infarction after ischemic-reperfusion injury, what correlated with decreased oxidative stress of their leucocytes (Hayasaki et al., 2006). So it seems that CCL2/CCR2 axis plays an important role in post-ischemic and post-reperfusion inflammation and could become a new therapeutic goal in selected cardiovascular diseases as well as in stroke in future. It is assumed that CCL2/CCR2 axis inhibition disrupts ischemic-reperfusion injury by decreasing edema, leucocyte infiltration and expression of inflammatory mediators (Dimitrijevic et al., 2007). However, the studies of Tarzami et al. showed that MCP-1/CCL2 played a dual role in myocardial ischemia - beside chemotaxis it also protected myocardial myocytes from hypoxia induced death (Tarzami et al., 2002, 2005). Nevertheless, there is a difference in the role of inflammation in acute and later stages of pathological process (Rosas 2007).

Vascular inflammation plays a central role in atherosclerosis and inflammatory biomarkers, such as CRP, IL-6, MCP and sICAM predict risk of cardiovascular disease (Dupuis et al., 2005). Thus finding genes that influence systemic levels of inflammatory biomarkers may provide insight into genetic determinants of vascular inflammation and cardiovascular disease.

6. Conclusion

Biomarkers of vascular inflammation have genetic, inflammatory and environmental determinants. Identifying genes influencing inflammation, environmental determinants, their interrelationships and early inflammatory biomarkers could help us to improve our understanding of pathophysiology and subsequently carefully consider eventual use of anti-inflammatory agents.

7. References

Abdulahad, D.A. et a al. (2010). HMGB1 in systemic lupus Erythematosus: Its role in cutaneous lesions development. *Autoimmun Rev,* Vol.9, No.10 (August 2010), pp. 661-665

Alexander C.M. et a al. (2003) Third National Health and Nutrition Examination Survey (NHANES III); National Cholesterol Education Program (NCEP). NCEPdefined metabolic syndrome, diabetes, and prevalence of coronary heart disease among NHANES III participants age 50 years and older. *Diabetes,* Vol. 52 pp.1210–1214

Al-Qaisi, M. et al. (2008). Measurement Vol.of endothelial function and its clinical utility for cardiovascular risk. *Vasc Health Risk Manag,* Vol. 4, pp. 647–652

Andersson U. et al. (2000). High mobility group 1 protein (HMG-1) stimulates proinflammatory cytokine synthesis in human monocytes. *J Exp Med,* Vol.192, No4 (August), pp. 565-570

Andreotti, F. et al. (2002). Inflammatory gene polymorphisms and ischaemic heart disease: rewiev of population association studies. *Heart,* Vol.87, No.2, pp. 107–112

Arakelyan, A. et al. (2005). Serum levels of the MCP-1 chemokine in patients with ischemic stroke and myocardial infarction. *Mediators Inflamm,* Vol.3, pp. 175–179

Arena, R. et al. (2006). The relationship between C-reactive protein and other cardiovascular risk factors in men and women. *J Cardiopulm Rehabil,* Vol.26, No.5, pp. 323–327

Arnett DK et al. (2007) Relevance of genetics and genomics for prevention and treatment of cardiovascular disease: a scientific statement from the American Heart Association Council on Epidemiology and Prevention, the Stroke Council, and the Functional Genomics and Translational Biology Interdisciplinary Working Group. *Circulation,* Vol.115, No.22, pp. 2878–2901

Armstrong, E.J. et al. (2006). Inflammatory biomarkers in acute coronary syndromes: part I: introduction and cytokines. *Circulation,* Vol.113, No.6, pp. e72–75

Arroyo-Espliguero, R. P et al. (2009). Predictive value of coronary stenoses and C-reactive protein levels in patients with stable coronary artery disease. *Atherosclerosis,* Vol.204, No.1, (May 2009), pp. 239-243

Ataouglu, H.E. et al. (2010). Procalcitonin: a novel cardiac marker with prognostic value in acute coronary syndrome. *J Int Med Res,* Vol.38, No.1, pp. 52-61

Aukrust, P. et al. (2007). Chemokines in cardiovascular risk prediction. *Thromb Haemost,* Vol.97, No.5, pp. 748–754

Aukrust, P. et al. (2001). Chemokines in myocardial failure - pathogenic importance and potential therapeutic target. *Clin Exp Immunol* , Vol.124, No.3, pp. 343–345

Avanzas, P. et al. (2005). Elevated serum neopterin predicts future adverse cardiac events in patients with chronic angina pectoris. *Eur Heart* J, Vol.26, No5, pp.457-63

Avanzas, P. &, Kaski J.C. (2009). Neopterin for risk assessment in angina pectoris. *Drug News*

Perspect, Vol. 22, No.4, pp. 215-219

Bakker, W. et al. (2009). Endothelial dysfunction and diabetes: roles of hyperglycemia, impaired insulin signaling and obesity. *Cell Tissue Res,* Vol.335, pp.165–189

Ballantyne, C.M., (2005). Lipoprotein associated phospholipase A2, high-sensitivity C-reactive protein, and risk for incident ischemic stroke in middle-aged men and women in the Atherosclerosis Risk in Communities (ARIC) study. *Arch Intern Med,* Vol.165, pp.2479–2484

Barnes, P.J. & Karin, M. (1997). Nuclear factor-kappaB: a pivotal transcription factor in chronic inflammatory diseases. *N Engl J Med,* Vol.336, pp.1066–1071

Berk, B.C. et al. (1990). Elevation of C-reactive protein in "active" coronary artery disease. Am J Cardiol Vol.65, No.3, pp. 168–172

Bermudez, E.A. et al. (2002). Interrelationships among circulating IL-6, C-reactive protein, and traditional cardiovascular risk factors in women. Arterioscler Thromb Vasc Biol, Vol. 22, No.10, pp. 1668–16673

Bernardo, E. et al. (2006). Influence of CD14 C260T promoter polymorphism on C-reactive protein levels in patients with coronary artery disease. *Am J Cardiol,* Vol.98, No.9, pp. 1182–1884

Biasucci, L.M. et al. (1996). Elevated levels of interleukin-6 in unstable angina. *Circulation,* Vol. 94, No.5, pp. 874–877

Bierhaus, A. (2006). RAGE in inflammation: a new therapeutic target? *Curr Opin Investig Drugs*; Vol.7, pp.985-991

Blanghy, H, et al. (2007). Serum BNP, hs-C-reactive protein, procollagen to assess the risk of ventricular tachycardia in ICD recipients after myocardial infarction. *Europace*, Vol.9, No.9, pp. 724–729

Boekholdt, S.M. et al. (2004). IL-8 plasma concentrations and the risk of future coronary artery disease in apparently healthy men and women. The EPIC-Norfolk prospective population study. *Arterioscler Thromb Vasc Biol*, Vol.24, No.3, 1503–1508

Boring, L. et al. (1998). Decreased lesion formation in CCR2 -/- mice reveals a role for chemokines in the initiation of atherosclerosis. *Nature*, Vol. 394, pp. 894–897

Brunetti, N.D. et al. (2006). C-reactive protein in patients with acute coronary syndrome : correlation with diagnosis myocardial damage, ejection fraction and angiografic findings. *Int J Cardiol*, Vol.109, No.2, pp. 248–256

Buc, M. & Bucova, M. (2007). Acute phase proteins – physiology and clinical significance. (in Slovak). *Interna medicina*; Vol.7, No.6, pp. 316–324

Bucova, M. (2005). Procalcitonin, prohormon, hormokine, mediator of inflammation, diagnostic and prognostic marker of systemic inflammation. *Ceskoslovenska fyziologie*, Vol.54, pp. 97-108

Bucova, M. (2002a). Polarization of T-lymphocytes and role of cytokines in the initial process of autoimmunity development. *Rheumatologia*, Vol. 16, No.3, s.117-124

Bucova, M. (2002b). Role of cytokines in the development of local and systemic inflammation and septic shock. *Vnitrni Lekarstvi*, Vol.48, No.8, pp.755-762

Bucova, M. (2006). Sepsa – etiopatogenéza. *Interna med*, Vol.6, No.4, pp. 204-211

Bucova M et al. (2008a). Association of chronic stable angina pectoris with MCP-1 2518 A/G single nucleotide polymorphism in the Slovak population. *Clin Chim Acta*,; 392 (1-2): pp. 71–72

Bucova, M. et al. (2008b). C-reactive protein, cytokines and inflammation in cardiovascular diseases. *Bratisl Lek Listy*, Vol.109, No.8, pp.333-40

Bucova, M. et al. (2009a). Association of MCP-1 -2518 A/G single nucleotide polymorphism with the serum level of CRP in Slovak patients with ischemic heart disease, angina pectoris, and hypertension. *Mediators Inflamm*. 2009:390951.

Cermakova Z et al. (2005). The MCP-1 -2518 (A to G) single nucleotide polymorphism is not associated with myocardial infarction in the Czech population. *Int J Immunogenet*, Vol.32, No.5, pp. 315-318

Cerovska, J. et al. (2006). Prevalence of C-reactive protein levels in adult population in two regions in the Czech Republic and their relation to body. (in Czech) *Vnitrni Lekarstvi*, Vol.52, pp. 1045–1050

Cha, S.H. et al. (2007). Association of CCR2 polymorphisms with the number of closed coronary artery vessels in coronary artery disease. *Clin Chim Acta*; Vol.382, No.1-2, pp. 129–133

Chambers, J.C. et al. (2001). C-reactive protein, insulin resistance, central obesity, and coronary heart disease risk in Indian Asians from the United Kingdom compared with European whites. *Circulation*, Vol.104, No.2, pp. 145–150

Chang, W.J. &Toledo-Pereyra, L.H. (2011)The Role of HMGB1 and HSP72 in Ischemia and Reperfusion Injury. *J Surg Res,Vol*.166, No.2 (April 2011), pp. 219-221

Chen, S. et al. (2010). Emerging role of IL-17 in atherosclerosis. *J Innate immun*, Vol.2, pp. 325-333

Cheng, X. et al. (2008). The Th7/Treg imbalance in patients with acute coronary syndrome. *Clin Immunol*, Vol.127, pp. 89-97

Conen, D. et al. (2006). C-reactive protein and B-type natriuretic peptides in never treated white coat hypertensives. *Hypertens Res*, Vol.29, No.6, pp. 411–415

Crawford DC et al. (2006). Genetic variation is associated with C-reactive protein levels in the Third National Health and Nutrition Examination Survey. *Circulation*, Vol.114, No.23, pp. 2458–2465

D'Aiuto F et al. (2005). C-reactive protein (+1444C>T) polymorphism influences CRP response following a moderate inflammatory stimulus. *Atherosclerosis*, Vol.179, No.2, pp. 413–417

Danesh, J. et al. (2000). Low grade inflammation and coronary heart disease: a prospective study and updated meta-analyses. *BMJ*, Vol.321, No.7255, pp. 199–204

Danesh, J. et al. (1998). Association of fibrinogen, C-reactive protein, albumin, or leukocyte count with coronary heart disease. *JAMA*, Vol.279, No.18, pp. 1477–1482

Danesh, J. et al. (1999). Risk factors for coronary heart disease and acute phase proteins. A population-based study. *Eur Heart J*, 1999, Vol.20, No.13, pp. 954–959

De Beer, F.C. et al. (1982). Measurment of serum C-reactive protein concentration in myocardial ischaemia and infarction. *Br Heart J*, 47 (3): 239–243.

De, M.R. et al. (2007). Multiple effects of high mobility group box protein 1 in skeletal muscle regeneration. *Arterioscler Thromb Vasc Biol*, Vol.27, pp. 2377-2383

Deo, R. et al. (2004). Association among plasma levels of monocyte chemoattractant protein-1, traditional cardiovascular risk factors, and subclinical atherosclerosis. *J Am Coll Cardiol* , Vol. 44, No.9, pp. 1812–1818

De Rosa, S. et al. ((2011). Neopterin; from forgotten biomarker to leading actor in cardiovascular pathophysiology. *Curr Vasc Phamacol*, Vol. 9, No.2, pp. 188-189

Devaraj, S. et al. (2004). Metabolic syndrome: an appraisal of the pro-inflammatory and procoagulant status. *Endocrinol Metab Clin North Am*, Vol.33, pp.431-453

Devaraj, S. et al. (2009). Human C-reactive protein and the metabolic syndrome. *Curr Opin Lipidol*, Vol.20, pp.182-189

Devaraj, S. et al. (2010). Role of C-reactive protein in contributing to increased cardiovascular risk in metabolit syndrome. *Curr Atheroscler Rep*, Vol.12, pp.110-118

Dewald, O. et al. (2005). CCL2/Monocyte chemoatractant protein-1 regulates inflammatory responses critical to healing myocardial infarcts. *Circ Res*, Vol. 96, No.8, pp. 881–889

Dimitrijevic OB et al. (2007). Absence of chemokine receptor CCR2 protects against cerebral ischemia/reperfusion injury in mice. *Stroke*; Vol.38, No.4, pp. 1345–1353

Downs, J.R. et al. (1998). Primary prevention of acute coronary events with lovastatin in men and women with average cholesterol levels: results of AFCAPS/TexCAPS. Air Force/Texas Coronary Atherosclerosis Prevention Study. *JAMA*, Vol.279, pp.1615-1622

Dupuis, J. et al. (2005) Genome scan of systemic biomarkers of vascular inflammation in the Framingham Heart Study : Evidence for susceptibility loci on 1q. *Atherosclerosis*, Vol.182, No.2., pp. 307–314

Dvorakova, A. & Poledne, R. (2004). An ultrasensitive C-reactive protein assay--a new parameter in cardiovascular risk. (in Czech). *Vnitrni Lekarstvi*, Vol.50, No.11, pp. 852–857

Eckel, R.H. et al. (2005), The metabolic syndrome. *Lancet*, Vol.365, No. 9468, pp.1415–1428

Eiriksdottir, G. et al. (2006). Apolipoprotein E genotype and statins affect CRP levels through independent and different mechanisms: AGES-Reykjavik Study. *Atherosclerosis* , Vol.186, pp. 222–224

Eldfeldt, K. et al. (2002). Expression of toll like receptors in human atherosclerotic lesions: a possible pathway for plaque activation. *Circulation*, Vol.105, No.10, pp.1158-1161

Eriksson, E.E. (2004). Mechanisms of leukocyte recruitment to atherosclerotic lesions: future prospects. *Curr Opin Lipidol*; Vol. 15, No.5, pp. 553–558

Espliguero, A.R. et al. (2005). CD14 C(-260)T promoter polymorphism and prevalence of acute coronary syndromes. *Int J Cardiol*, Vol.98, No.2, pp. 307–312

Estévez-Loureiro, R., et al. (2009). Neopterin levels and left ventricular dysfunction in patients with chronic stable angina pectoris. *Atherosclerosis*. Vol.207, No.2, (December 2009), pp. 514-518

Expert Panel on Detection, Evaluation, and Treatment of High Blood Cholesterol in Adults (2001). Executive Summary of the Third Report of the National Cholesterol Education Program (NCEP) Expert Panel on Detection, Evaluation, and Treatment of High Blood Cholesterol in Adults (Adult Treatment Panel III. *JAMA*, Vol.285, pp.2486–2497

Ferencik, M. (2007). Inflammation - a lifelong companion. Attempt at a non-analytical holistic view. *Folia Microbiologica*, Vol.52, No.2, pp. 159–173

Festa, A. et al. (2000). Chronic subclinical inflammation as part of the insulin resistance syndrome: the Insulin Resistance Atherosclerosis Study (IRAS). Circulation, Vol. 102, pp. 42–47

Fink, M.P. (2007). Bench-to-bedside review: High-mobility group box 1 and critical illness.
Crit Care. Vol.11, No.5, pp. 229

Fishman, D. et al. (1998) The effect of novel polymorphisms in the interleukin-6 (IL-6) gene on IL-6 transcription and plasma IL-6 levels, and an association with systemic onset juvenile chronic arthritis. *J Clin Invest*, Vol.102, No.7, pp.1369–1376

Ford, E.S. (1999). Body mass index, diabetes, and C-reactive protein among US adults. Diabetes Care. Vol.22, No.12, pp. 1971–1977

Ford, E.S. (2005). Prevalence of the metabolic syndrome defined by the International Diabetes Federation among adults in the U.S. *Diabetes Care*, Vol. 28, pp. 2745–2749

Fouser, L.A. et al. (2008). Th17 cytokines and their emerging roles in inflammation and autoimmunity. *Immunol Rev*. Vol.226, pp.87-102

Freeman DJ et al. (2002) C-reactive protein is an independent predictor of risk for development of diabetes in the West of Scotland Coronary Prevention Study. *Diabetes*, Vol.51, No.5, pp. 1596–1600

Frohlich M et al. (2000) Association between C-reactive protein and features of the metabolic syndrome: a population based study. *Diabetes care*, Vol.23, No.12, pp. 1835–1839

Fuchs, D. et al. (2009). The role of neopterin atherogenesis and cardiovascular risk assessment. Curr Med Chem Vol. 16, No.35, pp. 4644-53

George, J. (2008). Mechanisms of diseases: the evolving role of regulatory T cells in atherosclerosis. *Nat Clin Pract Cardiovasc Med*, Vol.5, pp.531-540

Gerszten, R.E. et al. (1999). MCP-1 and IL-8 trigger firm adhesion of monocytes to vascular endothelium under flow conditions. *Nature;* Vol.398, pp. 718–723

Goldstein, R.S. et al. (2006). Elevated high-mobility group box 1 levels in patients with cerebral and myocardial ischemia. *Shock.* Vol.25,pp. 571-574

Grad, E. et al. (2007). Transgenic expression of human C-reactive protein suppresses endothelial nitric oxide synthase expression and bioactivity after vascular injury. *Am J Physiol Heart Circ Physiol,* Vol.293, pp. H489–H495

Griva, M. et al. (2010). Potential role of selected biomarkers for predicting the presence and extent of coronary artery disease. *Biomed Pap Med Fac Univ Palacky Olomouc Czech Repub.* Vol.154, No. 3, pp. 219-25

Gu, L. et al. (1998). Absence of monocyte chemoattractant protein-1 reduces atherosclerosis in low density lipoprotein receptor deficient mice. *Mol Cell,* Vol.2, No.2, pp. 275–281

Gu, L. et al. (1999). Monocyte chemoattractant protein-1. *Chem Immunol,* Vol.72, pp. 7–29

Haffner, S. & Cassells, H.B. (2003). Metabolic syndrome - a new risk factor of coronary heart disease? *Diabetes Obes Metab,* Vol.5, pp.359–370

Hafler, D.A. et al. (2005). Applying a new generation of genetic maps to understand human inflammatoty disease. *Nat Rev Immunol,* Vol.5, No.1, pp. 83–91

Hansson, G,K. (2005). Inflammation, atherosclerosis and cardiovascular diseases. *N Engl J Med,* Vol. 352, pp. 1685-1695

Hayasaki T et al. (2006) CC chemokine receptor 2-deficiency attenuates oxidative stress and infarct size caused by myocardial ischemia reperfusion in mice. *Circ J,* Vol.70, No3, pp. 342–351

Holvoet, P. et al. (2004). The metabolic syndrome, circulating oxidized LDL, and risk of myocardial infarction in well-functioning elderly people in the health, aging, and body composition cohort. *Diabetes,* Vol.53, pp.1068–1073

Horne, B.D. et al. (2007). Multiple less common genetic variants explain the association of the cholesteryl ester transfer protein gene with coronary artery disease. *J Am Coll Cardiol,* Vol.49, No. 20, pp. 2053–2060

Hsieh, Y.H. (2007). Resveratrol attenuates ischemia-reperfusion-induced leukocyte - endothelial cell adhesive interactions and prolongs allograft survival across the MHC barrier. *Circ J.* Vol. 71, pp. 423 - 428

Hu, X. et al. (2009). Increased serum HMGB1 is related to the severity of coronary artery stenosis. *Clin Chim Acta,* Vol.406, No.1-2, pp.139-142

Huang, W. et al. (2010). HMGB1, a potent proinflammatory cytokine in sepsis. *Cytokine,* Vol. 51, No.2, pp.119-126.

Iltumur, K. et al. (2005). Complement activation in acute coronary syndromes. *APMIS,* Vol.113, No.3: 167–174

Inoue, K. et al. (2007). HMGB1 expression by activated vascular smooth muscle cells in advanced human atherosclerosis plaques. *Cardiovasc Pathol,* Vol.16, No.3, pp.136-143

Ishikawa C et al. (2006). Prediction of mortality by high-sensitivity C-reactive protein and brain natriuretic peptide in patients with dilated cardiomyopathy. *Circ J,* Vol.70, No.7, pp. 857–863

Itoh, T. et al. (2007).Coronary spasm is associated with chronic low-grade inflammation. *Circ J,* Vol.71, No.7, pp. 1074–1078

Javor, J. et al. (2007). Single nucleotide polymorphisms of cytokine genes in the healthy Slovak population. *Int J Immunogenetics*, Vol.34, No.4, pp. 273–280

Jenny, N.S. et al. (2007). Inflammation biomarkers and near term death in older men. *Am J Epidemiol*, Vol. 165, No. 6, pp. 684–695

Jian-Jun Lia, B & Chun-Hong, F. (2004). C-reactive protein is not only an inflammatory marker but also a direct cause of cardiovascular diseases. *Medical Hypotheses*, Vol. 62, pp. 499–506

Kalinina, N. et al. (2004). Increased expression of the DNA-binding cytokine HMGB1 in human atherosclerotic lesions: role of activated macrophages and cytokines. *Arterioscler Thromb Vasc Biol*, Vol.24, No.12, pp. 2320-2325

Kardys, I. et al. (2006).C-reactive protein and the risk of heart failure. The Rotterdam Study. Br J Nutr, Vol.152, No.3, pp. 514–520

Kathiresan, S. et al. (2006). Contribution of clinical correlates and 13 C-reactive protein gene polymorphisms to interindividual variability in serum C-reactive protein level. *Circulation*, Vol.113, No.11, pp. 1415–1423

Kawahara, K. et al. (2008). C-reactive protein induces high-mobility group box-1 protein release through activation of p38MAPK in macrophage RAW264.7 cells. *Cardiovasc Pathol*, Vol.17, N.3, pp.129-138

Kim, J.B. et al. (2006). HMGB1, a novel cytokine-like mediator linking acute neuronal death and delayed neuroinflammation in the postischemic brain. *J. Neurosci*, Vol.26, pp.6413-6421

Klune, J.R. et al. (2008). HMGB1: Endogenous danger signaling. *Mol Med*, Vol.14, No.7-8, pp.476-484

Koenig, W. et al. (2008). Prospective study of high-sensitivity C-reactive protein as a determinant of mortality: results from the MONICA/KORA Augsburg Cohort Study, 1984–1998. *Clin Chem*, Vol. 54, pp. 335–342

Koenig, W. et al. (1999). C-reactive protein, a sensitive marker of inflammation , predicts future risk of coronary heart disease in initially healthy middle-aged men - results from the MONICA Augsburg, cohort study, 1984 to 1992. *Circulation*, Vol.99, No.2, pp. 237–242

Koenig, W. et al. (2006). Increased concentrations of C-reactive protein and IL-6 but not IL-18 are independently associated with incident coronary events in middle aged men and women. Results from the MONICA/KORA Augsburg case-cohort study, 1984-2002. *Arterioscler Thromb Vasc Biol*, Vol.26, No.12, pp. 2745–2751

Kohno, T. et al. (2009). Role of high-mobility group box 1 protein in post-infarction healing process and left ventricular remodelling. *Cardiovasc Res*, Vol. 81, No. 3, pp.565-573

Kondo T et al. (2003). CD14 promoter polymorphism is associated with acute myocardial infarction resulting from insignificant coronary artery stenosis. *Heart*, Vol. 89, No. 8, pp. 931–932

Kozłowska-Murawska, J. & Obuchowicz. A.K. (2008). Clinical usefulness of neopterin. *Wiad Lek*, Vol.61, No.10-12, pp.:269-72

Kraaijeveld, A.O. et al. (2007). Chemokines and atherosclerotic plaque progression: towards therapeutic targeting? *Curr Pharm Des*, Vol.13, No.10, pp. 1039–1052

Kraus, V.B. et al. (2007). Interpretation of serum C-reactive protein (CRP) levels for cardiovascular disease risk is complicated by race, pulmonary disease, body mass index, gender, and osteoarthritis. *Osteoarthritis Cartilage*, Vol.15, No.8, pp. 966–971

Krejsek, J. & Kopecký, O. (2004). *Clinical immunology* (in Czech). Nucleus, Hradec Králové, 941 pp.

Kremen, J. et al. (2006). Increased subcutanneous and epicardial adipose tissue production of proinflammatory cytokines in cardiac surgery patients: possible role in postoperative insuline resistance. *J Clin Endocrinol Metab,* Vol. 91, No.12, pp. 4620–4627

Kuka. P. et al. (2010). HSP60, oxidative stress parameters and cardiometabolic risk markers in hypertensive and normotensive Slovak females. Bratisl Lek Listy, Vol. 11, No.10, pp.527-34

Lakka, H.M. et al. (2002). The metabolic syndrome and total and cardiovascular disease mortality in middle-aged men. *JAMA*, Vol.288, No.21, pp. 2709–2716

Lamon, B.D. & Hajjar DP (2008). Inflammation at the molecular interface of atherogenesis: an anthropological journey. *Am J Pathol*, Vol.173, pp.1253–1264

Lange, S.S. & Vasquez, K.M. (2009). HMGB1: The Jack-of-all-Trades Protein is a Master DNA Repair Mechanic *Mol Carcinog,* Vol.48, No.7, pp. 571-580

Latkovskis, G. et al. (2004). C-reactive protein levels and common polymorphisms of the interleukin-1 gene cluster and interleukin-6 gene in patients with coronary heart disease. *Eur J Immunogenet,* Vol.31, No.5, pp. 207–213

Li, J.J. (2005). Inflammation: an important mechanism for different clinical entities of coronary artery diseases. *Chin Med J* (Engl), Vol.118, No.21, pp. 817–826

Libby, P. (2002). Inflammation in atherosclerosis. *Nature*, Vol.420, No.6917, pp. 868–874

Limana, F. et al. (2005). Exogenous high-mobility group box 1 protein induces myocardial regeneration after infarction via enhanced cardiac C-kit_ cell proliferation and differentiation. *Circ Res,* Vol. 97, pp. e73–e83.

Liuzzo, G. et al. (1994). The prognostic value of C-reactive protein and serum amyloid A protein in severe unstable angina. *N Engl J Med,* Vol.331, No.7,pp. 417–424

Liuzzo, G. et al. (2007). Persistent activation of nuclear factor kappa-B signaling pathway in patients with unstable angina and elevated levels of C-reactive protein evidence for a direct proinflammatory effect of azide and lipopolysaccharide-free C-reactive protein on human monocytes via nuclear factor kappa-B activation. *J Am Coll Cardiol*, Vol.49, No.2, pp.185-94

Lotze, M.T. &, Tracey, K.J. (2005). High-mobility group box 1 protein (HMGB1): nuclear weapon in the immune arsenal. *Nat Rev Immunol,* Vol.5, pp.331-342

Lolmede, K. et al. (2009). Inflammatory and alternatively activated human macrophages attract vessel-associated stem cells, relying on separate HMGB1- and MMP-9-dependent pathways. *J Leukoc Biol,* Vol.85, No.5, pp.779-787.

Markovic, B.B. et al. (2007). Deletion polymorphism of the angiotensin I-converting enzyme gene in elderly patients with coronary heart disease. *Coll Antropol,* Vol.31, No.1, pp.179–183

Maruna, P. (2005). Acute phase proteins. (in Czech) Maxdorf, Praha, 282 pp.

Matsuki, A. et al. (2006). Early administration of fluvastatin, but not at the onset of ischemia or reperfusion, attenuates myocardial ischemia-reperfusion injury through the nitric oxide pathway rather than its antioxidant property. *Circ J,* Vol.70, pp.1643–1649

Mc Dermott, D.H. et al. (2005). CCL2 polymorphisms are associated with serum monocyte chemoattractant protein-1 levels and myocardial infarction in the Framingham heart study. *Circulation*, Vol.112, No. 8, pp. 1113–1120

Mc Laughlin, T. et al. (2002). Differentiation between obesity and insulin resistance in the association with C-reactive protein. Circulation, Vol.106, No.23, pp. 2908–2912

Michowitz, Y. et al. (2008). Predictive value of high sensitivity CRP in patients with diastolic heart failure. *Int J Cardiol,* Vol.25, No.3, pp. 347–351

Miyake, K. (2007); Innate immune sensing of pathogens and danger signals by cell surface Toll-like receptors. *Semin Immunol,* Vol. 19, pp.3-10.

Mohamed-Ali V et al. (1997). Human subcutaneous adipose tissue releases Il-6 but not TNF-α in vivo. *J Clin Endocrinol Metab*, Vol.82, No.12, 4196–4200

Moreno, P.R. et al. (1994). Macrophage infiltration in acute coronary syndromes.Implications for plaque rupture. *Circulation*, Vol.90, No2, pp. 775-778

Mostafazadeh, A. et al. (2011). Circulating Th1/Th2 cytokines and immunological homunculus in coronary atherosclerosis. *Iran J Allergy Asthma Immunol,* Vol.10, No.1, pp.11-19

Mucida, D. &, Cheroutre, H. (2010). The many face-lifts of CD4 T helper cells. *Adv Immunol,* Vol.107, pp.139-152

Mullaly, S.C. & Kubes, P. (2004). Toll gates and traffic arteries: from endothelial TLR2 to atherosclerosis. *Circ Resp* 95, No.12, pp. 657-659

Murr, C. et al. (2002). Neopterin as a marker for immune system activation. *Curr Drug Metab*, Vol.3, No.2, pp.175-187

Niccoli, G et al. (2008). Independent prognostic value of C-reactive protein and coronary artery disease extent in patients affected by unstable angina. *Atherosclerosis*. Vol.196, No.2, pp. 779-785

Onat, A. et al. (2011). Complement C3 and cleavage products in cardiometabolic risk. *Clin Chim Acta,* Vol.412, No.13-14, pp.1171-1179

Ortlepp JR et al. (2003). Chemokine receptor (CCR2) genotype is associated with myocardial infarction and heart failure in patients under 65 years of age. *J Mol Med*, Vol.81, No.6, pp. 363–367

Ozanne SE et al. (2007). Mechanisms of disease: the developmental origins of disease and the role of the epigenotype. *Nat Clin Pract Endocrinol Metab,* Vol.3, No.7, pp. 539–546

Pacileo, M. et al. (2007). The role of neopterin in cardiovascular disease. *Monaldi Arch Chest Dis*, Vol. 68, No.2, pp. 68-73

Palikhe, A. et al. (2007). Serum complement C3/C4 ratio, a novel marker for recurrent cardiovascular events. *Am J Cardiol*, Vol.99, No.7, pp. 890–895

Palumbo, R. et al. (2004).Extracellular HMGB1, a signal of tissue damage, induces mesoangioblast migration and proliferation. *J. Cell Biol,* Vol.164, No 3, Feb 2, pp. 441–449

Park, J.S. et al. (2004). Involvement of Toll-like receptors 2 and 4 in cellular activation by high mobility group box 1 protein. *J Biol Chem*, Vol.279, pp.7370-7377

Pearson, T. A. et al. (2003). Markers of inflammation and cardiovascular disease: application to clinical and public health practice: A statement for health care professionals from the Centers for Disease Control and Prevention and the American Heart Association. *Circulation,* Vol.107, No.3, pp. 499–511

Pedersen, E.R., et al. (2011). Systemic markers of Interferon-gamma-mediated immune activation and long-term prognosis in patients with stable coronary artery disease. *Arterioscler Thromb Vasc Biol,* Vol. 31, No.3, pp. 698-704

Penz, P. et al. (2010). MCP-1 -2518 A/G gene polymorphism is associated with blood pressure in ischemic heart disease asymptomatic subjects. Bratislava Med J, Vol.111, No.8, pp. 420-425

Pepys, M.B. & Hirschfield, (2003). C-reactive protein: a critical update. *J Clin Invest,* Vol. 111, No.12, pp. 1805–1812

Petrkova, J. et al. (2003). CC chemokine receptor (CCR2) polymorphism in Czech patients with myocardial infarction. *Immunology Letters,* Vol. 88, No.1, pp. 53–55

Picariello, C. et al. (2009). Procalcitonin in patients with acute coronary syndromes and cardiogenic shock submitted to percutaneous coronary intervention. *Intern Emerg Med,* Vol.4. No.5, pp.403-408

Pickering, T.G. et al. (2007). Stress, inflammation, and hypertension. *J Clin Hypertens,* Vol.9, No.7. pp. 567–571

Plata-Nazar, K. et al. (2004). Clinical value of neopterin. Part I. *Med Wieku Rozwoj,* Vol.8, No.2, pp.433-437

Qian, Y. et al. (2010). IL-17 signaling in host defense and inflammatory diseases. *Cell Mol Immunol,* Vol.7, No.5, pp.328-333

Ray, K.K. et al. (2002). Genetic variation at the interleukin -1 locus is a determinant of changes in soluble endothelial factors in patients with acute coronary syndromes. *Clin Sci,* Vol.103, No.3, pp. 303–310

Raz, E. (2007). Organ-specific regulation of innate immunity. *Nature Immunol,* Vol.8, No.1, pp. 3–4

Reaven, G.M. (2005). The insulin resistance syndrome: definition and dietary approaches to treatment. *Annu Rev Nutr,* Vol.25, 391–406

Ridker, P.M. et al. (1998). C-reactive protein adds to the predictive value of total and HDL cholesterol in determining risk of first myocardial infarction. *Circulation,* Vol. 97, pp. 2007- 2011

Ridker, P.M. et al. (2000). C-reactive protein and other markers of inflammation in the prediction of cardiovascular disease in women. *N Engl J Med,* Vol.42, No.12, pp. 836–843

Ridker, P.M. (2003). Clinical application of C-reactive protein for cardiovascular disease detection and prevention. *Circulation,* Vol.107, No.3, pp. 363–369

Ridker, P.M. et al. (2003). C-reactive protein, the metabolic syndrome, and risk of incident cardiovascular events: an 8-year follow-up of 14,719 initially healthy American women. *Circulation,* Vol.107, pp. 391-397

Ridker, P.M. et al. (2004). Should C-reactive protein be added to metabolic syndrome and to assessment of global cardiovascular risk? *Circulation,* Vol. 109, pp. 2818–2825

Rosas, M.M. (2007). Cardiac remodeling and inflammation. *Arch Cardiol Mex,* Vol.77, No.1, pp. 58–66

Rosenberg, H.F. & Oppenheim, J.J. (2007). Interview with Dr. Maurizio C. Capogrossi regarding pivotal advance: High mobility group box 1 protein - a cytokine with a role in cardiac repair. *J Leukoc Biol,* Vol.81, No.1, pp. 38-40

Ross, R, (1999). Atherosclerosis: an inflammatory disease. *N Engl J Med,* Vol.340, No.2, pp. 115–126

Rothenbacher, D. et al. (2006). Differential expression of chemokines, risk of stable coronary heart disease, and correlation with established cardiovascular risk markers. *Arterioscler Thromb Vasc Biol*, Vol. 26, No.1, pp. 194–199

Saito, I. et al. (2007). A low level of C- reactive protein in Japanese adults and its association with cardiovascular risk factors: The Japan NCVC-Collaborative Inflammation Cohort (JNIC) Study. *Atherosclerosis*, Vol.194, pp. 238–244

Sama, A.E. et al. (2004). Bench to bedside: HMGB1-a novel proinflammatory cytokine and potential therapeutic target for septic patients in the emergency department. *Acad Emerg Med*, Vol.11, No.8, pp.867-873

Sandor, F. & Buc, M. (2005). Toll-like receptors. III. Biological significance and impact for human medicine. *Folia Biol (Prague)*. Vol. 51, No.6, pp.198–203

Schwartz, R. et al. (2007). C-reactive protein downregulates endothelial NO synthase and attenuates reendothelialization in vivo in mice. *Circ Res*, Vol.100, pp. 1452–1459

Singh, U. et al. (2008). Human C-reactive protein promotes oxidized low density lipoprotein uptake and matrix metalloproteinase-9 release in Wistar rats. *J Lipid Res*, Vol.49, pp.1015–1023

Sucher, R. et al. (2010). Neopterin, a prognostic marker in human malignancies. *Cancer Lett*, Vol. 287, No.1, pp.13-22

Sugioka, K. et al. (2010a), Neopterin and atherosclerotic plaque istability in coronary and carotid arteries. *J Atheroscler Tromb*, Vol.27, No.11 pp.1115-21

Sugioka, K. et al. (2010b). Elevated levels of neopterin are associated with carotid plaques with complex morphology in patients with stable angina pectoris. *Atherosclerosis*, Vol. 208, No.2, pp. 524-530

Suk, H.J. et al. (2005). Relation of polymorphism within the C-reactive protein gene and plasma CRP levels. *Atherosclerosis*, Vol.178, No.1, pp. 139–145

Sukhija, R. et al. (2007). Inflammatory markers, angiographic severity of coronary artery disease, and patient outcome. *Am J Cardiol*, Vol.99, No.7, pp. 879–884

Szalai, A.J. et al. (2002). Association between baseline levels of C-reactive protein (CRP) and a dinucleotide repeat polymorphism in the intron of the CRP gene. *Genes Immun*ity, Vol. 3, No.1, pp. 14–19

Szalai, A.J. et al. (2005). Single-nucleotide polymorphisms in the C-reactive protein (CRP) gene promoter that affect transcription factor binding, alter transcriptional activity, and associate with differences in baseline serum CRP level. *J Mol Med*, Vol.83, No.6, pp. 440–44

Tabata, T. et al. (2003). Monocyte chemoattractant protein-1 induces scavenger receptor expression and monocyte differentiation into foam cells. *Biochem Biophys Res Commun*, Vol.305, No.2, pp. 380–385

Taleb, S. et al. (2010). Tedgui A, Mallat Z. Adaptive T cell immune responses and atherogenesis. *Current Opin Pharmacol*, Vol.10, pp. 197-202

Tang, D. et al. (2010). HMGB1 release and redox regulates autophagy and apoptosis in cancer cells. *Oncogene*. 2010, Vol.29, No.38, pp.5299-5310

Teoh, H. et al. (2008). Impaired endothelial function in C-reactive protein overexpressing mice. *Atherosclerosis*, Vol.201, pp. 318–325

Tarzami, S.T. et al. (2002). Chemokine expression in myocardial ischaemia: MIP-2 dependent MCP-1 expression protects cardiomyocytes from cell death. *J Mol Cell Cardiol*, Vol. 34, No.2, pp. 209–221

Tarzami, S.T. et al. (2005). MCP-1/CCL2 protects cardiac myocytes from hypoxia induced apoptosis by a $G_{\alpha i}$-independent pathway. *Biochem Biophys Res Commun*, Vol. 335, No.4, pp.1008–1016.

Thompson, S.G. et al. (1995). Hemostatic factors and the risk of myocardial infarction or sudden death in patients with angina pectoris. *N Engl J Med*, Vol.332, No.10, pp. 635–641

Tsuchiya, N. et al. (2002). Variations in immune response genes and their associations with multifactorial immune disorders. *Immunol Rev*, Vol.190, pp. 169–181

Ulloa, L. & Messmer, D. (2006). High-mobility group box 1 (HMGB1) protein: Friend or foe. *Cytokine & Growth Factor Rewiews*. Vol.17, pp. 189-201

van Beijnum, J.R. (2008). Convergence and amplification of toll-like receptor (TLR) and receptor for advanced glycation end products (RAGE) signaling pathways via high mobility group B1 (HMGB1). *Angiogenesis*. Vol.11, pp. 91-99

Venugopal, S.K., et al. (2003). C-reactive protein decreases prostacyclin release from human aortic endothelial cells. *Circulation*, Vol.108, pp.1676–1678

Vickers, M.A. et al. (2002). Genotype at a promoter polymorphism of the interleukin-6 gene is associated with baseline levels of plasma C-reactive protein. *Cardiovasc Res*, Vol. 53, No.4, pp. 681–689

Viedt, C. et al. (2002). Monocyte chemoattractant protein-1 induces proliferation and interleukin-6 production in human smooth muscle cells by differential activation of nuclear factor-κB and activator protein-1. *Arterioscler Thromb Vasc Biol*, Vol.22, No.6, pp. 914–920

Wang, H. et al. (1999). HMG-1 as a late mediator of endotoxin lethality in mice. *Science*, Vol. 285, No. 5125, pp. 248-251

Wang, H. et al. (2004). Extracellular role of HMGB1 in inflammation and sepsis. *J Intern Med*, Vol. 255, No.3, pp. 320-331

Wang, H. et al. (2007). HMGB1 as a potential therapeutic target. *Novartis Found Symp*. Vol. 280, pp.73-85

Wang, H. et al. (2010). Chemokine CXC Ligand 16 serum concentration but not A181V genotype is associated with atherosclerotic stroke. *Clin Chim Acta*, Vol.411, No.19-20, pp.1447-1451

Wang, Q. et al. (2007). The HMGB1 acidic tail regulates HMGB1 DNA binding specificity by a unique mechanism. *Biochem Biophys Res Commun*, Vol.360, No.1, pp.14-19

Xue, C. et al. (2006). Prognostic value of high-sensitivity C-reactive protein in patients with chronic heart failure. *N Z Med J*, Vol.119, No.1245, pp. U2314

Yan, X.X., et al. (2009). Increased serum HMGB1 level is associated with coronary artery disease in nondiabetic and type 2 diabetic patients. *Atherosclerosis*, Vol. 205, No.2, pp. 544-548

Yang, H. & Tracey, K.J. (2010). Targeting HMGB1 in inflammation. *Biochimica et Biophisica Acta*, Vol. 1799, No.1-2. pp. 149-156

Yang, Q.W. et al. (2011). HMBG1 mediates ischemia-reperfusion injury by TRIF-adaptor independent Toll-like receptor 4 signaling. *J Cereb Blood Flow Metab, Vol.* 31, No.2, pp. 593-605

Yudkin, J.S. et al. (2004). The HIFMECH Study Group: Low-grade inflammation may play a role in the etiology of the metabolic syndrome in patients with coronary heart disease: the HIFMECH study. *Metabolism*, Vol.53, pp. 852–857

Yudkin, J.S. et al. (1999). C-reactive protein in healthy subjects: Associations with obesity, insulin resistance, and endothelial dysfunction. A potential role for cytokines originating from adipose tissue? *Arterioscler Thromb Vasc Biol*, Vol.19, No.4, pp. 972–978

Zouridakis, E. et al. (2004). Markers of inflammation and rapid coronary artery disease progression in patients with stable angina pectoris. *Circulation*, Vol.110, No.13, pp.174–153

2

Angina-Like Chest Pain as a Symptom of Digestive Tract Disorders

Jacek Budzyński
[1]University Chair of Gastroenterology, Vascular Diseases and Internal Medicine, Nicolaus Copernicus University in Toruń, Ludwik Rydygier Collegium Medicum in Bydgoszcz
[2]Clinical Ward of Vascular Diseases and Internal Medicine Dr Jan Biziel University Hospital No. 2 in Bydgoszcz
Poland

1. Introduction

Chest pain is a common problem in health care, especially due to its prevalence, the utilization of resources according to the cost of medical procedures, and diagnostic process difficulties. Precordial discomfort occurs in 13-30% of the adult population per year (Cayley, 2005; Dickman & Fass, 2006; Eslick & Talley, 2004; Eslick et al., 2005; Eslick, 2008; Fass, 2008; Fass & Navarro-Rodriguez, 2008; Laird et al., 2004; Ruigómez et al., 2006, 2009), and in 20-40% population during their lifetime (Ruigómez et al., 2006, 2009). About 1.5-5% of the general population seeks a primary care doctor consultation because of chest pain episodes (Cayley, 2005; Erhardt et al, 2002; Eslick, 2008; Fox, 2005; Sheps et al., 2004). Moreover, it is the cause of 634,000 per year cardiologist consultations in the US (Mant et al., 2004), 5% of visits to emergency departments in the UK, and 40% of non-surgical emergency admissions mainly due to acute coronary syndrome suspicion (Ruigómez et al., 2006). Among these patients, only in 15-40% was ischaemic heart disease (IHD) diagnosed on discharge and features of myocardial infarction presented in only 8-10% (Dickman & Fass, 2006; Liuzzo et al., 2005). The analysis by Hollander et al. (2007) has also shown that among patients admitted due to acute coronary syndrome suspicion, myocardial infarction was confirmed in only 4%. Moreover, it has been known for a number of years that about 10-36% of all patients who qualify for coronarography have a normal coronary angiogram (Dickman & Fass, 2006; Dobrzycki et al., 2005; Eslick et al., 2005; Eslick, 2008]. These data corroborate the most recent study by Patel et al. (2010), who conclude that the diagnostic yield of elective coronary angiography (about 20% of all procedures) amounted only to 38% (60% did not influence patients' treatment), in spite of almost 70% of the patients undergoing elective coronary angiography having had positive findings on non-invasive examination (resting electrocardiography, echocardiography, computed tomography, or stress testing). They were also consistent with my recent work, which, among other things, has shown that exercise-provoked chest pain was accompanied by significant ST interval depression in about 60% of subjects with normal coronary angiogram, and 40% of subjects with significant coronary artery narrowing did not present ischaemic-like ECG changes (Budzyński, 2010c).

The above-mentioned data can be summarized as follows:

- non-invasive diagnoses of chest pain and qualification for coronary angiography and percutaneous procedures are still not perfect;
- the most frequent causes of this symptom do not originate in the cardiovascular system; and
- symptom sources other than cardiac should be taken into account more frequently.

On the other hand, these conclusions should not change the prevailing principle that each chest pain episode must be recognized as a potential alarm symptom; the exclusion of life-threatening conditions, including ischaemic heart disease, should remain the basis of chest pain diagnostic procedures. For this reason, it seems a better solution even to overuse coronary angiograms or coronary artery calcification scores (CAC) using multi-slice computer tomography, than miss the detection of severely ill patients. However, it should also always be taken into consideration that invasive cardiological diagnostic procedures give the most benefits to patients with acute chest pain episodes, and in patients with recurrent symptoms, extracardiac sources ought to be more frequently considered (Patel et al., 2010).

It is possible that changes in diagnostic algorithms of chest pain diagnosis and therapy not only decrease the prevalence of this symptom, but might also decrease the costs of health care. Such reductions would be considerable, as the medical procedures connected with chest pain symptoms utilize a noticeable part of health care resources. The annual cost of the medical care of patients with recurrent chest pain in the US ranges from $350 million to $1.8 billion (Leise et al., 2010), and has even reached $3-8 billion (Eslick & Talley, 2004; Eslick et al., 2005; Eslick, 2008; Liuzzo et al., 2005; Mant et al., 2004). In the UK, it consumes approximately 1% of the health care budget (Fox, 2005). However, the real costs of recurrent chest pain are greater because of the social expenditure connected with this symptom (Eslick & Talley, 2004; Eslick et al., 2005; Eslick, 2008; Katerndahl, 2004). Within the one to five-year follow-up period, about 40% of patients with recurrent chest pain are hospitalized at least once due to chest pain, 30% receive a subsequent coronary angiogram (Bugiardini et al., 2005), nearly 30% of patients are unemployed and receive a disability pension, and in 60% of individuals recurrent chest pain limits their physical activity, causing displeasure regarding physicians' competence in 66-81% (Dickman & Fass, 2006).

There may be a number of reasons for unsatisfactory data concerning the prevalence and treatment outcome in patients with recurrent chest pain. To counter this, the many well-known causes of chest pain episodes ought to be analysed, as they have various degrees of clinical importance and may originate from cardiovascular system dysfunction (due to myocardial ischaemia or non-ischaemic reasons), the respiratory system, digestive tract, or begin in the skeleton (Cayley, 2005; Eslick & Talley, 2004; Eslick et al., 2005; Eslick, 2008; Laird et al., 2004). Symptoms deriving from each of these sources may be further aggravated by reactions of depression or panic disorders (Dickman & Fass, 2006; Fass, 2008; Fass & Navarro-Rodriguez, 2008). Moreover, the respective causes of chest pain may coexist and overlap (e.g. the cardiovascular with the gastroenterological or musculoskeletal), and disorders of one system may disturb the function of the others, masking the true cause of symptom evoking. These complicated relationships connected with chest pain make it difficult to diagnose and treat the chest pain source, favour symptom recurrence, and increase resource utilization. Precision in the analysis of symptom characteristics remains the pivotal diagnostic method of chest pain origin because of the aforementioned low diagnostic yield of non-invasive cardiovascular examinations and elective coronarography (Patel et al., 2010). In particular, the localization, radiation and character of chest pain episodes should be evaluated, as well as any aggravating and alleviating factors (Potts & Bass, 1995; Swap & Nagurney, 2005). Angina pectoris is a particular type of chest pain. It is defined as precordial discomfort, sometimes radiating to the jaw or arm, which is provoked by effort, emotional stress, cold or wind, and withdraws after rest or nitroglycerine use. However, too many times it is forgotten that these criteria are applicable to chest pain episodes originating not only from the cardiovascular system, but also from the digestive tract, especially from the oesophagus, stomach and gall bladder. Moreover, angina pectoris may be caused by myocardial ischaemia, resulting not only from coronary artery narrowing, but also from extracardiac disorders, which leads to an imbalance between myocardial oxygen supply and requirement (e.g. anaemia, thyrotoxicosis). Anaemia is frequently secondary to many digestive tract diseases, such as acute and/or chronic bleeding from the alimentary tract (erosions, ulcers, neoplasm), malabsorption, maldigestion, blood sequestration or autoimmunological reactions. In this way, disorders of the digestive tract can also favour angina pectoris exacerbation. Therefore, although certain elements of the chest pain history are associated with increased (radiating to shoulder(s), or arms, or precipitation by exertion) or decreased (pain like stabbing, pleuritic, positional, or reproducible by palpation) likelihoods of a diagnosis of angina pectoris, none of them alone or in combination identify a group of patients, who do not need a further diagnostic testing (Swap & Nagurney, 2005).

To summarize, angina pectoris is an important, prevalent symptom, utilizing enormous quantities of resources, which is considered all too frequently as a typical symptom of coronary artery disease (CAD), but rarely as a symptom of at least two types of digestive tract disease. The first group concerns diseases which evoke angina-like chest pain from the oesophagus, stomach and gall bladder by the stimulation of their chemo-, mechano-, and/or thermoreceptors; the second group manifests clinically as anaemia, which leads to insufficient oxygen supply to the heart. It is important to realize that both these kinds of digestive tract diseases may overlap with CAD, aggravating precordial symptoms or mimicking atherosclerosis progression. These gastroenterological aspects of angina pectoris will be analysed in this chapter in detail.

2. Epidemiology

Coronary artery disease (CAD) is the most frequent cause of morbidity and mortality in developed countries. As a result of such epidemiological data, almost each chest pain episode is considered as originating from the heart. However, recurrent, angina-like chest pain originating from e.g. the oesophagus is also a frequent problem in everyday practice, mainly due to the high prevalence of alimentary tract diseases in the general population. Recurrent chest pain which is non-cardiac in origin is defined as substernal chest pain in the absence of significant epicardial coronary artery stenoses (Eslick & Talley, 2004; Eslick et al., 2005; Eslick, 2008; Dickman & Fass, 2006; Fass, 2008; Hebbard, 2010; Leise et al., 2010). It is reported every year by about 13-30% of adults, without sex preference. It is experienced during a typical lifespan by approximately 20-40% of the population, with a decrease in prevalence with increasing age (Eslick & Talley, 2004; Eslick et al., 2005; Eslick, 2008; Dickman & Fass, 2006; Fass, 2008; Ruigómez et al., 2006, 2009). The majority of patients with recurrent chest pain which is non-cardiac in origin continue to report episodes of long-term symptoms. In the study by Potts and Bass (1995), 75% of the surviving patients with recurrent chest pain and lack of obstructive coronary artery lesions continued to report the occurrence of precordial discomfort 11 years later, and 34% reported weekly chest pain symptoms.

The most prevalent cause of non-cardiac chest pain (NCCP) is gastro-oesophageal reflux disease (GERD), which accounts for up to 60% of cases (Leise et al., 2010). The occurrence of its main symptom, heartburn, at least once per month is reported by about 36-44% of the adult population, 14% once per week, and 7% every day (Lemire, 1997). On the other hand, a chest pain sensation is experienced by about 37% of patients with heartburn occurring once per week, 30% of individuals with more seldom symptom occurrence, and about 8% without the feeling of pyrosis (Fass and Navarro-Rodriguez, 2008).

It is generally estimated that gastroenterological abnormalities have a similar prevalence in patients both with and without significant coronary artery narrowing, which shows a possibility to overlap e.g. GERD and CAD symptoms (Budzyński et al., 2008; Budzyński 2010a, 2010c; Cooke et al., 1998; Dobrzycki et al., 2005; Mehta et al., 1996; Ruigómez et al., 2006, 2009; Schofield et al., 1987, 1989). Only a few authors have suggested a lower coexistence of oesophageal disorders in subjects with CAD (Adamek et al., 1999; Battaglia et al., 2005). On the other hand, the probability of diagnosing the respective functional oesophageal disorders (GERD, motility disorders, visceral hypersensitivity) as a cause of non-cardiac chest pain (NCCP) depends on the location of the patient's consultation. They were the cause of non-cardiac chest pain (NCCP) in 0.6-25% of patients of general practitioners, in 46% of patients admitted to Cardiological Intensive Care Units because of acute chest pain, in 60-70% of patients with angina-like chest pain and a normal coronary angiogram, and in 30-80% of patients with obstructive coronary lesions and chronic precordial discomfort non-responsive to optimal anti-angina therapy (Budzyński et al., 2008; Dobrzycki et al., 2005; Rosztóczy et al., 2007; Świątkowski et al., 2004). Therefore, NCCP caused by gastrointestinal, mainly oesophageal, disorders may coexist with CAD in as many as 30-80% of patients. This is very high but clinically very important, as disease overlapping, which causes a great deal of confusion and clinical doubt, is related to at least three factors: the epidemiological, the pharmacological, and the pathophysiological (Budzyński et al., 2008).

Epidemiological causes of the frequent coexistence of digestive and cardiovascular disorders result from a high prevalence of diseases sourced from both systems and have similar risk factors. Both gastroenterological and cardiovascular diseases are found more frequently in older and obese patients, those suffering from hypertension, diabetes, and obstructive sleep apnoea, as well as in smokers, alcohol drinkers and caffeine over-users (Budzyński et al., 2008; Fass & Dickman, 2006;). The frequent coexistence of gastroenterological and cardiovascular diseases also depends on pharmacological causes due to the adverse effects of drugs recommended in the therapy for both system disorders. It is generally known that calcium channel antagonists (e.g. amlodipine, verapamil and diltiazem), nitrates, blockers of alpha-1 adrenergic receptors, and betamimetics may decrease with lower oesophageal sphincter (LOS) pressure and favour gastro-oesophageal reflux, the most frequent cause of NCCP. It should also be taken into consideration that aspirin-induced gastropathy is a potential cause of NCCP (Hsiao et al., 2009). Its symptoms frequently disappear after empirical therapy with proton pump inhibitors (PPIs), but this has not been confirmed by all authors. Moreover, some medicines used in the treatment of gastroenterological disorders may show pharmacological or pharmacodynamic interactions with drugs recommended for cardiovascular diseases, e.g. omeprazole decreases the bioavailability of digoxin, warfarin and clopidogrel. The last interaction in particular caught the investigator's attention following publication by Juurlink et al. (2009), who reported a greater prevalence of acute coronary syndromes and myocardial infarction in patients taking omeprazole, rabeprazole or lansoprazole for the purpose of preventing gastrointestinal bleeding during dual anti-platelet therapy. Although recent publications have not confirmed the clinical importance of this interaction, their authors and panels of experts have recommended caution in co-prescribing PPIs with clopidogrel (American College of Cardiology Foundation [ACCF], 2010; American Society for Gastrointestinal Endoscopy [ASGE], 2009; Bhatt et al., 2008; de Aquino Lima & Brophy, 2010; Laine & Hennekens, 2010). There is also divergent information concerning the interaction between PPIs and acetylsalicylic acid, showing no effect (Adamopoulos et al., 2009), an increase (Kasprzak et al., 2009), and a decrease (Würtz et al., 2010) in anti-platelet aspirin activity.

Finally, the high prevalence of the coexistence of cardiovascular and gastroenterological chest pain causes may also result from pathophysiological factors, mainly the inflammatory and neural pathways for linked angina (Chauhan et al., 1996; Hoff et al., 2010; Makk et al., 2000; Rosztóczy et al., 2007). They are connected in the mechanism of a vicious circle, in which gastro-oesophageal reflux induces myocardial ischaemia, and products of the anaerobic myocardial metabolism due to ischaemia in turn provoke gastro-oesophageal reflux, dysphagia, or hiccups (Hoff et al., 2010; Krysiak et al., 2008; Stec et al., 2010). These problems are explained in detail in a separate subsection (4b).

3. Prognosis

Patients with recurrent chest pain and normal coronary angiogram (i.e. NCCP) have a relatively good life expectancy prognosis. The 30-day mortality connected with this symptom is estimated at 0.3-1.1% (Eslick & Talley, 2004; Eslick et al., 2005; Eslick, 2008), the risk of major cardiovascular event (death, myocardial infarction) with an odds ratio (OR) amounting to 2.3 (95% CI, 1.3-4.1) (Ruigómez et al., 2006, 2009), and the need for emergency coronary intervention amounting to approximately 4% (Hollander et al., 2007). However, in the recent study by Leise et al. (2010), patients with NCCP which is gastrointestinal in origin displayed less overall survival at all time points compared with their counterparts with NCCP of unknown origin, specifically 70.1% at 10 years and 51.8% at 20 years. This was mainly explained by the overlapping of cardiovascular risk factors in patients with GERD. Whereas, in the paper by Munk et al. (2008), the 10-year relative risk of hospitalization for ischaemic heart disease (a discharge diagnosis of myocardial infarction, angina and/or heart failure) following a normal upper endoscopy among 386 Danish patients with unexplained chest/epigastric pain was 1.6 (95% CI, 1.1-2.2), compared with 3,973 population controls. The adjusted mortality rate ratio was the greatest within the first year after an upper endoscopy and amounted to 2.4 (95% CI, 1.3-4.5). The difference faded with time, and the 10-year adjusted mortality rate ratio amounted to 1.1 (95% CI, 0.9-1.5). The increased mortality among these patients stemmed from alcohol dependence, pneumonia (not as a complication of the endoscopy), and lung cancer, but not IHD.

On the other hand, patients with recurrent chest pain have a poor prognosis in relation to symptoms receding. They also present a high annual rate (50-81%) of chest pain recurrence (Ruigómez et al., 2006, 2009). Unemployment connected with this symptom occurrence concerns 41-50% of patients (Eslick & Talley, 2004; Eslick et al., 2005; Eslick, 2008; Fass, 2008; Fass & Dickman, 2006; Fass & Navarro-Rodriguez, 2008).

The aforementioned data justify undertaking the effort to establish the most precise diagnosis of the source of recurrent chest pain. Such a procedure makes it possible to calm the patient by explaining some of the non-dangerous reasons for chest pain occurrence. Moreover, the diagnosis of the real source of distressing complaints makes possible a specific treatment recommendation. It is effective in different degrees in about 80% of patients, decreasing NCCP episode recurrence and hospitalization necessity, improving patients' health-related quality of life, and reducing the health care costs (Cheung et al., 2009; Dickman & Fass, 2006; Fass, 2008; Fass & Dickman, 2006; Fass & Navarro-Rodriguez, 2008; Laheij et al., 2003; Sheps et al., 2004). The diagnosis of GERD as a source of NCCP and the recommendation of the prolonged use of PPIs has decreased the risk of chest pain recurrence by 46% and the number of patients needing to be treated (NNT) has amounted to 3 (95%CI, 2-4) (Cremonini et al., 2005). Whereas, undiagnosed chest pain has been shown to increase the risk of hospitalization due to CAD and all-cause mortality during 10 years of follow-up (Munk et al., 2008).

4. Pathophysiology

As has been mentioned, angina-like chest pain presents typical features of visceral pain which may be symptomatic of both ischaemic heart diseases and digestive tract disorders. To the first group of diseases belong both patients with coronary artery narrowing, known as patients with CAD, and subjects with a normal or almost normal coronary artery angiogram ("non-visible", "non-obstructive atherosclerotic coronary disease" (Bataglia et al., 2005). Chest pain occurring in patients with a normal coronary angiogram is frequently called NCCP. It may be caused by extracardiac diseases, mainly digestive tract disorders (Labenz, 2010). However, it should also be taken into account that it may also be sourced by missed coronary angiogram lesions, microvascular coronary dysfunction (cardiac syndrome X), coronary spasm, or secondary angina (e.g. aortic valve dysfunction, tachycardia, thyrotoxicosis, anaemia) (Bugiardini et al., 2005).

The relationships between the digestive tract and cardiovascular system are complicated and stem from epidemiological, pharmacological (described above) and pathophysiological factors. Each of them concerns both patients with a normal coronary angiogram and with CAD, and may lead to symptom mimicry and overlapping. There are at least three pathomechanisms evoking angina-like chest pain in the course of digestive tract diseases:

a. chest pain is evoked by stimulation of digestive tract pain receptors and mimics angina;
b. digestive tract diseases via neural and inflammatory pathways disturb myocardial perfusion and evoke chest pain which is cardiac in origin due to myocardial ischaemia, although the true cause of the symptoms is located e.g. in the oesophagus;
c. chest pain, cardiac in origin, is secondary to an imbalance between oxygen supply and myocardial demand due to anaemia, which is frequently secondary to various diseases of the alimentary tract.

4.1 Angina-like chest pain which is digestive tract in origin

The most common example of the first pathophysiological group of chest pain is GERD, responsible for 50-60% of the causes of NCCP (Dickman & Fass, 2006; Eslick & Talley, 2004; Eslick et al., 2005; Eslick, 2008; Fass & Dickman, 2006; Fass & Navarro-Rodriguez, 2008; Hebbard, 2010; Tipnis et al., 2007; Tougas et al., 2001). The main symptoms of GERD are heartburn (pyrosis), regurgitation, or the "reflux chest pain syndrome" distinguished by the definition and classification of GERD developed by the Montreal Consensus Group in 2006 (Vakil et al., 2006). The other diseases which may mimic angina pectoris, frequently known as non-GERD-related NCCP, are as follows: oesophagitis caused by non-reflux-related factors (such as infections or being drug induced); oesophageal motility disorders; hiatal hernia; gastric and duodenal ulcer disease; drug- (aspirin, non-steroidal anti-inflammatory drugs) induced gastropathy; acquired hepato-diaphragmatic migration of the hepatic flexure of the colon (Chilaiditi's syndrome); cholecystitis; and acute pancreatitis (Dickman & Fass, 2006; Drewes et al., 2006; Eslick & Talley, 2004; Eslick et al., 2005; Eslick, 2008; Fass & Dickman, 2006; Fass & Navarro-Rodriguez, 2008; Ruigómez et al., 2006, 2009, , Sorrentino et al., 2005). The Rome Criteria III also distinguish a particular kind of non-cardiac chest pain, called "functional chest pain of presumed esophageal origin", which is defined as midline discomfort which is not of burning quality, lasting at least three months, with an onset at least six months prior to diagnosis, and an absence of GERD and histopathology-based oesophageal motility disorders (Drossman, 2006). My own observations have also shown that exercise-induced oesophageal motility disorders, such as exercise-provoked oesophageal spasm (EPOS) or exercise-provoked gastro-oesophageal acid reflux, may play some role in the pathogenesis of angina-like chest pain in at least 22% of patients with recurrent symptoms (Budzyński, 2010a, 2010b). It is worth underlining that nearly 80% of the patients with functional chest pain simultaneously present symptoms of other functional disorders, primarily irritable bowel syndrome (27%) and abdominal bloating (22%) (Dickman & Fass, 2006; Fass & Navarro-Rodriguez, 2008). Their coexistence with chest pain may help in appropriate diagnoses. The aforementioned mainly oesophageal and gastric abnormalities may be accompanied by endoscopically visible morphological changes in mucosa or not. Some of these differences in the clinical course of GERD have been classified by the Global Consensus Group in Montreal, which, among oesophageal syndromes, enumerates: (a) symptomatic syndromes (without oesophageal erosions) concerning approximately 60% of patients, and (b) syndromes with oesophageal injury (erosive oesophagitis, oesophageal strictures, Barrett's oesophagus, oesophageal adenocarcinoma) (Sarkar et al., 2004; Vakil et al., 2006). In this way, oesophageal erosions are present in 10-70% of patients with NCCP (Fass and Navarro-Rodriguez, 2008); therefore, a lack of endoscopic abnormalities does not exclude both a GERD and an oesophageal origin of NCCP.

The above-mentioned diseases of the oesophagus, stomach, colon, pancreas or gall bladder evoke angina-like chest pain by the activation of local pain receptors, both chemical and mechanical (e.g. ASIC, TRPV, P2X and TREK), by inflammatory mediators, kinins, pepsin, bile acids, changes in oesophageal pH, pressure (oesophageal distension, volume, shear stress), or temperature, and by the induction of a secondary local motility response, expressed by hypermotility, oesophageal long muscle shortening, high amplitude oesophageal peristalsis, oesophageal distension or prolonged oesophageal contractions (Drewes et al., 2006; Sifrim et al., 2007; Tipnis et al., 2007). However, the intensity of the clinical manifestation of these disorders is related to the threshold of receptor stimulation. Its decrease is frequently known as visceral hypersensitivity (Dickman & Fass, 2006; Drewes et al., 2006; Eslick & Talley, 2004; Eslick et al., 2005; Eslick, 2008; Fass & Dickman, 2006; Fass & Navarro-Rodriguez, 2008). It is enumerated as one of the main pathomechanisms of symptoms in the course of cardiac syndrome X, mitral prolapse syndrome, irritable oesophagus, functional dyspepsia, irritable bowel syndrome (IBS), and fibromyalgia (Katerndahl, 2004; Hammet et al., 2003; North et al., 2007). The recently published investigation by Nasr et al. (2010) using a balloon distension test has shown that oesophageal hypersensitivity plays an important role in 75% of patients with functional (non-cardiac and non-reflux) chest pain. The basis of this disorder is a decrease in the pain threshold, both at the central and peripheral perception levels (Dickman & Fass, 2006; Fass & Dickman, 2006; Sheps et al., 2004; Sifrim et al., 2007). The range of the change in this threshold may be modulated by a number of factors influencing the function of the brain-gut axis (Mayer & Tillisch, 2011; Sheps et al., 2004). These factors are as follows:

- personal (female gender, age between 15-34, incorrect response of the autonomic nervous system, psychiatric disorders, stress, sleep disturbances, oesophagitis or gastritis, mucosal mastocyte infiltration, allodynia);
- environmental (stress, *Helicobacter pylori* (Hp) infection, dietary factors, especially a fatty diet) (Remes-Troche, 2010; Sheps et al., 2004; Sifrim et al., 2007; Tougas et al., 2001).

The modulation of the central pain threshold in patients with unexplained chest pain, CAD and occult GERD may also be related to chronic receptor stimulation and/or the coexistence of psychiatric disorder (Drewes et al., 2006; Lenfant, 2010; Remes-Troche, 2010). Sarkar et al. (2004) have reported a decrease in allodynia after therapy with PPIs. Whereas, Makk et al. (2000) have shown a greater oesophageal acid sensitivity (a lower pain threshold) in individuals with a normal coronary angiogram and patients undergoing coronary angioplasty than in those with coronary artery narrowing and undergoing coronary angiography alone. Moreover, in approximately 70% of patients with NCCP, anxiety, depression or somatization have been observed (Dickman & Fass, 2006; Eslick & Talley, 2004; Eslick et al., 2005; Eslick, 2008; Fass & Dickman, 2006; Fass & Navarro- Rodriguez, 2008; Katerndahl, 2004). In these subjects, NCCP amelioration and a decrease in pain hypersensitivity were found after therapy with antidepressants such as imipramine, sertraline or trazodone in controlled and uncontrolled investigations (Dickman & Fass, 2006; Eslick & Talley, 2004; Eslick et al., 2005; Eslick, 2008; Fass & Dickman, 2006; Fass & Navarro-Rodriguez, 2008). Psychiatric disorders, besides decreasing the pain threshold, may also evoke chest pain by hyperventilation and secondary coronary arteries and/or oesophageal spasm (Chauhan et al., 1996). As a result, the following markers of a psychiatric basis for recurrent chest pain were proposed: atypical character of symptoms, female gender, younger age, a high level of anxiety, and a neurotic personality (Ringstrom and Freedman, 2006).

The character of the pain occurring in the course of digestive tract diseases may be similar to that of acute coronary syndrome or recurrent stable angina pectoris. The simple explanation of this fact involves the visceral features of the pain and the anatomical localization of the heart and oesophagus in the chest. The latter factor causes the overlap of the head areas in brain sensory representations of the oesophagus and heart. However, the anatomical relationships between the oesophagus and the heart may produce symptoms in some more immediate way. Namely, the extended left atrium, due to e.g. mitral valve disease or left ventricle cardiac failure, may press the oesophagus, evoking changes in intra-oesophageal pressure, mechanical receptor stimulation or disturbance in the oesophageal passage, known as cardiac dysphagia or odynophagia (angina-like chest pain which is oesophageal in origin). These disorders may also, through pressure receptor stimulation, activate vagal neural reflexes leading to a decrease in myocardial perfusion (angina-like chest pain which is cardiac in origin), described in detail in part b of this section. On the other hand, an enlarged oesophagus, due to e.g. achalasia or oesophageal carcinoma, producing left atrium compression, may also evoke local ischaemia of the atrial muscle and/or activation of mechano-electrical coupling, raising the local dispersion in the functional potential of atrial

muscle cells and producing re-entry loops. These disorders may manifest clinically as chest pain or arrhythmia (Budzyński & Pulkowski, 2009; Duygu et al., 2008; Upile et al., 2006).
To summarize, chest pain originating from the oesophagus may be similar to cardiac-derived angina pectoris. It may be caused by activation receptors in the digestive tract and motor dysfunction of the oesophageal wall. The intensity of the clinical manifestation of these disturbances is modulated by the frequent presence of visceral hypersensitivity. These complicated relationships have explained the confusion and misdiagnosis often accompanying chest pain diagnosis.

4.2 Angina-like chest pain which is cardiac in origin but induced by digestive tract disorders

Apart from the above-mentioned resemblance of chest pain originating from the heart and the oesophagus, as well as the overlapping of symptoms evoked both by cardiovascular and alimentary tract diseases, the clinical doubts concerning the true source of chest pain, whether cardiac or oesophageal, are augmented by the second of the distinguishing pathomechanisms of chest pain caused by diseases of the digestive tract: the activation of neural and inflammatory pathways which in turn may decrease myocardial perfusion.
Neural reflex loops between the heart and oesophagus have been found both in human and animals. Stimulation of oesophageal chemo-, mechano- and thermoreceptors, apart from provoking chest pain of oesophageal origin in about half (49-56%) of patients with a normal coronary angiogram (cardiac syndrome X), coronary artery spasm or obturative lesions in coronarography (patients with CAD), may also activate vagally-mediated, viscero-visceral neural reflexes (e.g. cardio-oesophageal reflex) (Budzyński et al., 2008; Budzyński, 2010c; Charng et al., 1988; Chauhan et al., 1996, Dobrzycki et al., 2005; Drewes et al., 2006; Fass & Dickman, 2006; Makk et al., 2000; Manfrini et al., 2006; Rasmussen et al., 1986; Rosztóczy et al., 2007) or a viscero-somatic neural reflex (Drewes et al., 2006; Jou et al., 2002). The first reflex may evoke ischaemic chest pain, cardiac in origin, resulting from diminished myocardial perfusion and secondary to pre-arteriole contraction (Chauhan et al., 1996; Makk et al., 2000; Rosztóczy et al., 2007); the second, viscero-somatic reflex, causes an increase in the spinotrapezius muscle contractions both after cardiac and oesophageal receptor stimulation via convergent pathways in the sympathetic nerves (Jou et al., 2002). The last reflex is responsible for the somatic component of pain evoked by the stimulation of visceral, cardiac or oesophageal receptors. Moreover, afferent stimulus originating from the oesophagus, stomach or gall bladder may also interfere with stimulus derived from the heart in the spinal cord, which is a further cause of the resemblance of symptoms deriving both from the digestive tract and the cardiovascular system (Sheps et al., 2004).
However, the aforementioned reflexes (neural loops) do not function in all subjects but only in about half (Chauhan et al., 1996; Makk et al., 2000; Mehta et al., 1996; Rosztóczy et al., 2007); this results from the modulation of the impulse transmission along nervous pathways by coexistent mental or psychiatric disorders, the balance between the sympathetic and parasympathetic parts of the autonomic nervous system and the threshold of receptor stimulation, which is decreased in patients with visceral hypersensitivity. These suggestions are supported by papers showing a relatively high prevalence of panic or depressive disorders in approximately half of patients, with both cardiovascular and digestive tract diseases (Lenfant, 2010). Autonomic nervous system imbalance has also been found in up to half of patients with functional chest pain (Nasr et al., 2010; Tougas et al., 2001), *Helicobacter*

pylori infection (Budzyński et al., 2004), functional dyspepsia, irritable bowel syndrome (Mayer & Tillisch, 2011), or chronic heart failure. Modulation of visceral reflex activity by these cofactors may cause the activity of cardio-oesophageal reflexes not to manifest clinically in all subjects. Dobrzycki et al. (2005) have suggested that those most susceptible to the clinically important effect of cardio-oesophageal reflex activity seem to be patients with CAD, because in this patient group even slight coronary reserve impairment may be clinically important. On the other hand, Rosztóczy et al. (2007), using a combination of an oesophageal acid perfusion test and transoesophageal Doppler echocardiographic coronary flow measurement, have shown that 49% of subjects presented coronary spasm in response to oesophageal acidification more frequently than either epicardial coronary artery disease or microvascular coronary disease, probably due to signs of cardio-oesophageal reflex activation. In the gastroenterological work-up, they had higher DeMeester scores, an increased number of reflux episodes, a fraction time below pH 4, and prolonged acid reflux episodes. These data corroborate the paper by Sarkar et al. (2004), who observed the reversible influence of chronic oesophageal mucosa exposure to acid on the visceral pain threshold, one of the mechanisms modulating visceral, vagally-mediated reflex activity. The importance of the role of the parasympathetic nervous system for subjects with NCCP has also been shown by Tougas et al. (2001). In their study, 67% of patients with a normal coronary angiogram presented angina-like chest pain after oesophageal acid infusion. Chest pain in "acid-sensitive patients" was accompanied by a higher baseline heart rate and lower baseline vagal activity (estimated using heart rate variability [HRV] analysis) than "acid-insensitive patients". During acid infusion, vagal cardiac outflow (expressed as a high frequency component of HRV) increased in "acid-sensitive" but not in "acid-insensitive" patients (Tougas et al., 2001).

The endpoint of the aforementioned complicated influence of the nervous system on the interrelationships between the cardiovascular and alimentary systems is myocardial ischaemia, which may manifest clinically in 49-56% of patients as angina pectoris, arrhythmia and syncope (Chauhan et al., 1996; Cubattoli et al., 2009; Cuomo et al., 2006; Makk et al., 2000; Mehta et al., 1996; Rosztóczy et al., 2007). This symptomatic decrease in myocardial perfusion after oesophageal stimulation by acid was produced by epicardial coronary artery spasm (Rosztóczy et al., 2007) or by contraction of the prearterioles (Chauhan et al., 1996). The neural pathway for these effects (so- called linked angina) was proven by the lack of similar perfusion changes in heart transplant recipients (Chauhan et al., 1996). However, the aforementioned reflexive decrease in myocardial perfusion was accompanied by ischaemic electrocardiographic (ECG) changes in only a few works (Budzyński et al., 2008; Dobrzycki et al., 2005; Rosztóczy et al., 2007; Singh et al., 1992; Świątkowski et al., 2004).

However, the above-described mechanism is only the first on the arc of the cardio-oesophageal loop of feedback. The second, opposite arm of this loop may be stimulated by the products of anaerobic myocardial metabolism, mainly bradykinin (Caldwell et al., 1994; Krysiak et al., 2008), invasive cardiac manoeuvres, manipulation, coronary angioplasty (Makk et al., 2000) or cardiac arrhythmia (Stec et al., 2010). Such activation may lead to reflexive oesophageal motility disorders or a decrease in lower oesophageal sphincter (LOS) pressure, which facilitates gastro-oesophageal reflux occurrence, changes in oesophageal pH, potential reflexive activation of a cardio-oesophageal reflex and a reduction in myocardial perfusion (Caldwell et al., 1994). Described as reflexive, bidirectional, neuro-hormonal mechanisms connect the pathogenesis of the digestive tract and cardiovascular diseases in a vicious circle. Moreover, some studies have shown that the described associations between oesophageal and vascular spasm may also result from myogenic mechanisms and may be an overall effect of smooth muscle hypercontractility, depending on the individual concerned (Adamek et al., 1998a, 1998b, 1999; Makk et al., 2000; Manfrini et al., 2006; Rasmussen et al., 1986). The myogenic component of coronary-oesophageal interrelationships has been suggested by the coexistence of oesophageal spasm alongside coronary artery spasm, hypertension, migraine and Raynaud's symptoms.

The occurrence of angina-like chest pain, as well as other cardiac symptoms such as arrhythmia, or syncope may also be secondary to inflammatory factors often deriving from the digestive tract. The role of inflammatory processes in cardiovascular disease pathogenesis has been investigated for many years. At least two mechanisms have been distinguished for the influence of inflammation on cardiac function: local and systemic. The first has been mentioned by Weigl et al. (2003), who have suggested the possibility of local inflammatory process propagation through the oesophageal wall producing local pericarditis or atrial myocarditis. These histological abnormalities can be a substrate of chest pain or arrhythmia (Navarese et al., 2010; Stőlberger & Finsterer, 2003). However, there is more to be said for the role of a systemic inflammatory response in the pathogenesis of chest pain which is cardiac in origin but evoked or intensified by digestive tract diseases. Systemic inflammatory factors known as cytokines (e.g. TNF-alpha, IL-1, IL-6) or adhesion molecules (e.g. VCAM-1, ICAM-1) are involved in the pathogenesis of atherosclerosis, endothelial dysfunction, and cardiac arrhythmia, mainly atrial fibrillation. Their synthesis may be stimulated in the course of many of the diseases of the alimentary tract, such as periodontal diseases, oesophagitis, gastritis, ileitis, inflammatory bowel diseases, liver cirrhosis, pancreatitis, and neoplasm (Shanker & Kakkar, 2009; Stőlberger & Finsterer, 2003). Some reports, including my own data, have also shown the unfavourable effect of *Helicobacter pylori* infection, not only on the course of digestive tract diseases, but also on the course of recurrent angina-like chest pain (Budzyński, 2011), changes in autonomic nervous system balance (Budzyński et al., 2004) and atherosclerosis progression (Franceschi et al., 2009). CagA seropositivity has been significantly and positively associated with the occurrence of acute coronary events, atherosclerosis progression and arrhythmia prevalence (Bunch et al., 2008a, 2008b; Francesci et al., 2009; Miyazaki et al., 2006). The positive relationship between Hp infection and cardiac syndrome X (Celik et al., 2010; Eskandarian et al., 2006; Rasmi & Raeisi, 2009) has also been reported but not confirmed by others (Saleh et al., 2005). Whereas, Sandifer et al. (1996), based on the results of the EUROGAST Study Group, had shown a negative association between the seroprevalence of antibodies to Hp and the death rate from ischaemic heart disease.

Numerous mechanisms for the influence of Hp on atherosclerosis complications have been suggested. They may act directly on atherosclerotic plaques, as suggested by the results of Kowalski et al. (2001), who revealed the presence of Hp DNA in atherosclerotic lesions and an increase in coronary artery diameter after microorganism eradication. It has also been implied that mimicry occurs between the cytotoxin-associated gene-A (CagA) antigen expressed by some Hp strains and the protein presented in atherosclerotic plaques (Franceschi et al., 2009). Hp infection, similarly to periodontal infection (Shanker & Kakkar, 2009) or the hepatitis C virus (Ramdeen et al., 2008), may also act as one amongst a number of factors taking part in the mechanisms of pathogen burden through the following: non-specific inflammatory pathway stimulation (e.g. hs-CRP increase); the induction of endothelial and microvascular dysfunction; an increase in adhesion molecule expression (e.g. VCAM-1, ICAM-1); the over-synthesis of pro-atherogenic cytokines (e.g. IL-1 beta, IL-6, TNF-alpha); changes in autonomic nervous system balance (Budzyński et al., 2004; Budzyński, 2011; Celik et al., 2010; Rasmi & Raeisi, 2009); and the production of metabolic abnormalities, such as hypertriglyceridaemia, increased LDL cholesterol levels, plasma lipid oxidation, hyperfibrinogenaemia, altered blood coagulation and leukocytosis. The role of Hp infection as a cause of myocarditis and ECG changes in patients with persistent chest pain has also been reported (Navarese et al., 2010). Apart from the aforementioned mechanisms, Hp infection may also affect the occurrence of angina-like chest pain which is gastroenterological in origin, being one of the pathogenic factors of gastritis, gastric and duodenal ulcer disease. Hp infection may also play a role in GERD pathogenesis via impaired vagal control of LOS pressure and a decrease in the release of ghrelin, a prokinetic hormone (Thor & Blaut, 2006).

The described systemic inflammatory process mediators, e.g. deriving from the digestive tract, could influence cardiac symptom occurrence, not only by direct action on the vascular wall, but also via neuroimmune- endocrine crosstalk (Collins et al., 2009; Grundy et al., 2006; Marques et al., 2010; Wood, 2007). Inflammation mediators, especially cytokines such as TNF-alpha, interleukin-1 and interleukin-6, may stimulate both the hypothalamus and brain stem. The outcome of the first is the activation of the pituitary-suprarenal axis, which leads to increased cortisol and adrenalin secretion, and of the second is sympathetic activation. The consequence of such neuroendocrine stimulation may be chest pain, myocardial infarction, arrhythmia, sudden death or an increase in intestinal permeability due to digestive tract ischaemia. Its effect may in turn be an increase in cytokine secretion and the activation of immunological cells: lymphocytes, monocytes, macrophages and granulocytes possessing surface receptors for a number of neuroendocrine products. These can then stimulate vessel walls, induce endothelial dysfunction, atherosclerotic plaque instability and in turn produce neuroendocrine imbalance (Marques et al., 2010; Saleh et al., 2005). In this way, the aforementioned relationships involve the cardiological and gastroenterological symptoms in the second neuroimmune-endocrine vicious circle mechanism.

In summary, neural loops, inflammatory processes and neuroimmune-endocrine crosstalk activated by digestive tract disorders may be the second group, in addition to digestive tract abnormalities, of important factors evoking chest pain which is cardiac in origin. It may result from myocarditis and/or a progression or reversible reduction in myocardial perfusion. These processes may play a role in patients both with and without significant coronary artery narrowing.

4.3 Angina-like chest pain which is cardiac in origin but secondary to anaemia caused by diseases of the alimentary tract

The main cause of ischaemic heart disease and its typical symptom of angina pectoris is an imbalance between coronary blood supply and myocardial requirement. This shows that besides a decrease in blood delivery to the myocardium, angina-like chest pain may also be evoked or exacerbated by inadequate oxygen supply due to anaemia. Rapidly or slowly progressing anaemia may be a symptom of many digestive tract diseases, both of the upper and lower parts. It may be an effect of bleeding, malabsorption, maldigestion, blood sequestration or autoimmunological reactions (Zhu et al., 2010). For this reason, diagnostic procedures for the digestive tract, including biochemical and serological examinations, ultrasonography, panendoscopy, colonoscopy, and in special cases capsule endoscopy and single or double balloon enteroscopy, should be recommended for each male, postmenopausal women, and younger females when the quantity of blood loss during menstruation is insufficient to explain the presence of anaemia (Zhu et al., 2010).

However, both cardiologists and gastroenterologists should also take into account that acute bleeding into the digestive tract or slowly progressing iron deficiency anaemia may also be a symptom of the haemorrhagic complications of the anti-thrombotic therapy (e.g. aspirin, clopidogrel, heparin, bivalirudin, etc.) which is fundamental in the treatment of acute coronary syndromes and stable angina pectoris (Dai et al., 2009; Nema et al., 2008). Of these complications, 50% occur in the digestive tract (To et al., 2009). Prior to endoscopic procedures, especially with a high risk of haemorrhagic complications (e.g. polypectomy or mucosal resection), the risk of the discontinuation of dual anti-platelet therapy in particular should be estimated (ASGE, 2009; ACCF, 2010; Bhatt et al., 2008). This is very important, as clopidogrel withdrawal may lead to cardiac stent thrombosis in 15-40% of cases; it is associated with a myocardial infarct rate of 50% and a related death rate of approximately 20% (ASGE, 2009). Therefore, in such clinical situations, consultation between cardiologist and gastroenterologist is needed to avoid patients being treated from a single organ perspective of the relative risks (cardiology vs. gastrointestinal) but with a more global balanced risk assessment instead to optimize patient outcomes.

The above deliberation shows the need for accuracy in evaluating angina pectoris symptom pathomechanisms (primary or secondary) to avoid the iatrogenic, clinically overt or silent haemorrhagic complications of anti-thrombotic drugs. Misdiagnosis or the inadequate taking of a medical history may lead to anaemia occurrence or aggravation, an increase in chest pain severity, unnecessary coronary angiogram performance, or death during haemorrhagic shock. One potential clinical scenario may take the following course: angina pectoris (stable or acute coronary syndrome) + latent digestive tract disease → treatment with aspirin and clopidogrel and/or warfarin or heparin → haemorrhagic complications (clinically overt or silent) → secondary anaemia and/or haemodynamic complications → exacerbation of chest pain severity → coronary angiogram performance, percutaneous coronary intervention and the need for prolonged dual anti-platelet therapy → an increase in the intensity of bleeding from the digestive tract, anaemia aggravation and a further increase in angina pectoris severity. In this way, clinically overt or latent bleeding from the digestive tract and secondary anaemia, besides the aforementioned neural cardio-oesophageal loop and neuroimmune crosstalk, may be the third vicious circle mechanism, in which gastroenterological disorders, exacerbated or complicated by anti-platelet or anti-thrombotic treatment, may increase angina pectoris severity.

5. Diagnosis

According to current opinion, all patients with chest pain should first be evaluated for a cardiac cause of their symptoms (Fass & Dickman, 2006; Potts & Bass, 1995). To make this easier, some authors recommend estimating the probability of cardiac chest pain origin on the basis of tests with nitroglycerine and the number of atherosclerosis risk factors. In spite of some doubts concerning the low specificity of a nitroglycerine test (Fass & Dickman, 2006), chest pain disappearance within five minutes after one dose of 400 mcg of short-acting nitrates, a cardiac or gastroenterological symptom source should be considered, rather than a psychiatric one. Afterwards, if the tests present more than two atherosclerosis risk factors, a cardiological diagnostic pathway should be taken first (an ECG, stress test, stress echocardiography and angiography being the proposed series of steps). However, if patients have fewer than three risk factors, the following sequence of procedures in the diagnosis of angina-like chest pain presumed to be of oesophageal origin is proposed: complete the Carlsson-Dent questionnaire; empirical therapy with proton pump inhibitors (PPIs), known as the "omeprazole test"; endoscopy; 24-hour ambulatory oesophageal pH-metry; 24-hour multichannel intraluminal oesophageal impedance with pH-metry examination, in particular with an analysis of the symptom index (SI) or symptom association probability (SAP); stationary oesophageal manometry; 24-hour oesophageal manometry with SI or SAP evaluation; brain imaging; as well as psychiatric examination (Dickman & Fass, 2006; Eslick & Talley, 2004; Eslick et al., 2005; Eslick, 2008; Fass & Dickman, 2006; Fass & Navarro-Rodriguez, 2008; Hewson et al., 1990; Oranu and Vaezi, 2010; Sheps et al., 2004). The recently proposed diagnostic methods for NCCP presumed to be of oesophageal origin are as follows: a magnifying endoscopy with high resolution imaging (to show oesophageal mucosa microerosions), prolonged oesophageal pH-metry using the wireless Bravo method, high resolution manometry, high frequency intraoesophageal ultrasonography (HFIUS), impedance planimetry, and multi-slice computer tomography. However, their usefulness in the diagnosis of chest pain requires confirmation (Dickman & Fass, 2006; Fass & Dickman; George & Movahed, 2010; Hebbard, 2010).

The Carlsson-Dent questionnaire (CDQ) is a simple but old diagnostic tool for the detection of GERD, the main cause of NCCP without alarm symptoms or the suspicion of the other possible GERD complications (Numans & de Wit, 2003). It has been validated in European patients. In comparison with oesophageal pH-metry and endoscopy, it is estimated as having good sensitivity (89-94%) and a positive predictive value (55-90%) for the detection of GERD.

Empirical therapy with a triple standard dose of PPI (e.g. 40-0-20 mg of omeprazole) gives valuable information about GERD being the reason of NCCP. It is a simple, available, sensitive and cost-effective tool, but the specificity is insufficient to put this test into practice as the single objective diagnostic criterion, mainly due to risks connected with false undiagnosed CAD. Its sensitivity and specificity in the diagnosis of GER-related chest pain in comparison with oesophageal pH-metry reaches 69-95% and 57-86% respectively (Fass & Dickman, 2006; Dickman et al., 2005; Wang et al., 2005). However, this test may be less valuable for patients in whom symptoms appear less frequently than twice a week (Cremonini et al., 2005). On the other hand, taking this limitation into account, testing with PPIs can be used as a diagnostic (lasting 1-2 weeks) and as a diagnostic-therapeutic test (1-4 months of "therapy as investigation"). Chest pain disappearance after the respective period should be interpreted as confirmation of clinical associations between acid regurgitation and symptom occurrence. The economic aspects of NCCP diagnosis also see much of the use of this test in clinical practice. A one-week test with PPI decreased the overall costs of NCCP diagnosis by $573-1,338, mainly due to the reduction in the number of panendoscopies performed (by 81%), 24-hour oesophageal pH-metry (by 79%), and remains the functional diagnostic examination for NCCP (Fass & Navarro-Rodriguez, 2008). Unfortunately, this test was not validated in patients with CAD, in whom GERD symptom prevalence and overlapping seems to be clinically important. Of this group, GERD-related chest pain episodes were found in 30-46% of patients (Budzyński et al., 2008; Dobrzycki et al., 2005). These overlapped with chest pain of cardiac origin, being indistinguishable from angina pectoris resulting from myocardial ischaemia and leading to symptom persistence. In the RITA-3 study, 24% of participants still reported angina in the II-IV class according to the CCS classification over one year after percutaneous coronary intervention (Kim et al., 2005;

Poole-Wilson et al., 2006). In light of this, such empirical testing with PPIs seems to be worth recommending for each patient with refractory angina. Unfortunately, the recent recommendation concerning refractory angina by Kones (2010) does not refer to such a possibility. However, due to possible potential dangerous interactions between clopidogrel and PPIs, this test should be avoided in patients on dual anti-platelet therapy (ACCF, 2010; Bhatt et al., 2008). Our own investigations have also shown the necessity for careful interpretation of testing with PPIs due to an increase found in nitric oxide bioavailability after rabeprazole therapy (Kłopocka et al., 2006) and beta-endorphin plasma levels (Budzyński et al., 2010). These substances produced during therapy with PPIs may mask the true chest pain source, including that of cardiac in origin.

Endoscopy is the most recommendable exploratory procedure in patients with GERD symptoms, fundamentally heartburn and regurgitation, especially when alarm symptoms appear. On the other hand, 50-75% of GERD and 10-70% of NCCP patients have a normal endoscopy examination (non-erosive GERD) (Dickman & Fass, 2006; Fass & Dickman, 2006). The recent report by Dickman et al. (2007a), on the basis of the results of upper endoscopy undergone for NCCP and GERD in a group of respectively 3,688 and 32,981 consecutive patients, has shown a normal upper endoscopy in 44.1% of NCCP patients and 38.8% of those with GERD. Of the NCCP group, 28.6% had a hiatal hernia, 19.4% erosive oesophagitis, 4.4% Barrett's oesophagus, and 3.6% stricture/stenosis. Peptic ulcers were found in 2% of the NCCP patients. Thus, endoscopy does not appear to be dispensable in a large group of patients with NCCP. It is likely that the new generation of endoscopy equipment - magnifying endoscopy - would be helpful in the detection of oesophageal mucosa microerosions, but it is unable to provide certainty of the clinically important association between NCCP and oesophageal lesions found. Therefore, the greatest clinical importance of endoscopy is the possibility of diagnosis, including mucosal biopsy and treatment of the morphologic cause of alarm symptoms and the source of haemorrhaging from the digestive tract. Thus, awareness should be accompanied by the knowledge that normal endoscopy does not exclude a gastroenterological cause of NCCP in patients who also have confirmed CAD.

Twenty-four-hour oesophageal pH-metry has been considered the most sensitive and specific test in the diagnosis of GERD and GER-related chest pain. Although 41-43% of patients with NCCP fulfilled the criteria for pathological GERD (Leise et al., 2010), a significant percentage of patients (about 25%) in whom symptoms corresponded with heartburn had rather normal results for 24-hour pH monitoring examinations (Talaie et al., 2009). This discrepancy resulted from the method limitation, as 24-hour oesophageal pH-metry detects acid reflux, and NCCP may also be provoked by the regurgitation of alkaline or neutral gastric content. Therefore, for NCCP diagnosis, especially in patients who are non-responsive to empirical therapy with PPIs, 24-hour simultaneous oesophageal impedance and pH monitoring seems to be more useful, mainly due to the possibility of non-acid gastro-oesophageal reflux (GER) diagnosis (Sifrim & Blondeau, 2006; Sifrim et al., 2009). An additional but practically the most valuable feature of this tool is the possibility of SI and SAP analysis. These enable the evaluation of the relationships between symptom occurrence and oesophageal function disorders which are not only related to the regurgitation of hydrochlorid acid. Only such a proven relationship gives an acceptable probability that oesophageal disorders are truly the reason for recurrent symptom episodes, and has been the basis of the identification of "GER-related" and "non-GER-related" chest pain (Dickman & Fass, 2006; Fass & Dickman, 2006; Fass & Navarro-Rodriguez, 2008). One of the oldest tests estimating the associations between chest pain occurrence and oesophageal acidification is the Bernstein test. Recently, it has not been practically applied, but formerly it was widely used, not only as a diagnostic tool, but primarily in scientific investigation (Chauhan et al., 1996; Makk et al., 2000; Rosztóczy et al., 2007; Schofield et al., 1987, 1989).

Stationary oesophageal manometry, as well as recently introduced high resolution oesophageal manometry, has minor importance in NCCP diagnosis, mainly due to difficulties with confirming the association between chest pain episodes and motility disorders, and the still unsatisfactory treatment effects (Fass & Dickman, 2006; Hershcovici & Fass, 2010; Nam et al., 2006). However, 24-hour oesophageal function monitoring is potentially more useful, mainly due to the possibility of examining performance during patients' everyday activity, the greater probability of symptom occurrence during examination and the possibility of correlating their presence with oesophageal disorders (using an SI index or SAP). Moreover, there is now the opportunity to evaluate oesophageal pH and motility correlation on the basis of a greater number of analysed parameters in computer software. On the other hand, the usefulness of both oesophageal pH-metry, impedance examination and 24-hour oesophageal manometry is restricted to patients with daily, or at least every two days, symptom prevalence (Singh et al., 1992). Diagnosis of an NCCP source using 24-hour pH-metry or manometry has been obtained in 46% of patients in whom symptoms occurred at least once per day and only in 11% of subjects with chest pain of less frequency (Janssens et al., 1986). In the study by Eslick (2008), following examination of the most numerous population of patients with non-GER-related chest pain to have been assessed in this way, the distribution of oesophageal motility abnormalities was as follows: normal manometry in 70%, nutcracker oesophagus (14.4%), non-specific oesophageal motor disorder (10.8%), diffuse oesophageal spasm (3%), and other (1,8%). In other papers, nutcracker oesophagus was the most prevalent oesophageal dysmotility in patients with chest pain (Fass & Dickman, 2006; Fornari et al., 2008). Some authors have reported a greater prevalence of oesophageal motility disorders in patients admitted due to chest pain having a normal coronary angiogram than in patients with CAD (Adamek et al., 1999; Battaglia et al., 2005). Whereas, it has not only been my own experience, based on patients non-responsive to empirical therapy with PPIs, which has shown a similar frequency of oesophageal dysmotility in patients both with and without significant coronary artery narrowing (Budzyński, 2010b; Cooke et al., 1998).

As has been mentioned, the clinical usefulness of oesophageal motility examination does not seem to be of great value (Dickman & Fass, 2006; Fass & Dickman, 2006; Nam et al., 2006). Trials involving the provocative use of ergonovine, tensilon, bethanechol and pentagastrin, or oesophageal extension with a balloon have not improved diagnostic efficacy either. My own experience has shown the clinical usefulness of exercise-provoked oesophageal dysmotility diagnosis using simultaneous oesophageal manometry and ECG monitoring during a treadmill stress test. Some exercise-provoked oesophageal motility disorder appeared in 22% of patients with recurrent angina-like chest pain non-responsive to empirical therapy with PPIs (Budzyński et al., 2010; Budzyński, 2010a). The occurrence of angina-like chest pain, oesophageal acidification for more than 10 s, and increased simultaneous contractions above 55% during a treadmill stress test had greater than 80% specificity for diagnosing GER-related and non-GER-related chest pain. The practical message coming from these observations was that patients with recurrent chest pain, who did not report e.g. chest pain during a treadmill stress test, have a low (20%) probability of recognizing an oesophageal reason for their symptoms (Budzyński, 2010a).

High frequency intraluminal ultrasound (HFIUS) is an available but rarely used examination, which makes it possible to assess the oesophageal muscle wall thickness in order to evaluate the longitudinal muscle contraction and oesophageal shortening in patients with oesophageal symptoms, including NCCP. Studies conducted using this technique suggest that prolonged oesophageal wall thickening can be connected with chest pain and heartburn episodes (Boesmans et al., 2010; Sifrim & Blondeau, 2006; Sifrim et al., 2009). This examination has also helped to exclude oesophageal ischaemia from the mechanism of chest pain which is gastroenterological in origin (Hoff et al., 2010).

The possibility of having so many gastroenterological examinations for chest pain source diagnoses may lead to problems with making the correct choice. The practical diagnostic algorithm for NCCP presumed to be oesophageal in origin has been proposed by Fass and Navarro-Rodriguez (2008). In all patients with a suspected gastroenterological source of chest pain, after the exclusion of a cardiac origin, they suggest analysing the presence of alarm symptoms (e.g. fever, stomach pain at night, weight loss, anaemia, and signs of bleeding from the digestive tract). If any of these is present, a panendoscopy should first be conducted and treatment should be chosen depending on the diagnosis. In patients without alarm signs, symptom evaluation and testing with PPIs was proposed as the first diagnostic step. In responders to empirical therapy, PPIs should be continued. In patients who fail this test, oesophageal pH-metry "on-therapy", manometry and other gastroenterological investigations, including psychiatric assessment, should be considered.

Careful application of this algorithm in patients with CAD is justified by the proven overlapping of oesophageal chest pain sources in about 30-46% of patients with CAD and cardiac syndrome X (Budzyński et al., 2008; Dobrzycki et al., 2005; Hewson et al., 1990; Oranu & Vaezi, 2010; Singh et al., 1992). Moreover, about 20% of all myocardial ischaemia episodes in patients with CAD correlated with pathological acid gastro-oesophageal reflux episodes, and were recognized as reflexive myocardial silent ischaemia or ischaemic cardiac chest pain due to cardio-oesophageal reflex activation (Dobrzycki et al., 2005). In light of these neurally-mediated cardio- oesophageal interrelationships, a comparison of the coronary reserve in a non-invasive evaluation before and after empirical therapy with PPIs seems to be worth recommending in stable CAD patients, before the next coronarography performance. A decrease in the signs of myocardial ischaemia after one- or two-week-long therapies with PPIs may help to recognize exacerbation of myocardial ischaemia due to oesophageal chemo- receptor activation, which is possible in about half of patients with CAD or cardiac syndrome X (Budzyński et al., 2008; Chauhan et al, 1996; Rosztóczy et al., 2007; Świątkowski et al., 2004). In non-responders to PPI therapy, similarly to patients with NCCP, endoscopy, oesophageal impedance with pH-metry, oesophageal manometry with or without exercise provocation, as well as psychiatric examination, might be helpful (Fass & Navarro- Rodrigues, 2008; Katerndahl, 2004).

6. Treatment

Once the accurate diagnosis of the source of angina-like chest pain has been established, a specific therapy should be recommended. If recurrent chest pain originates only from the heart, due to either ischaemic cardiac or non-ischaemic cardiac disease, typical anti-angina pharmacotherapy and/or myocardial revascularization should be recommended, taking into account the results of the Clinical Outcomes Utilizing Revascularization and Aggressive Drug Evaluation (COURAGE) trial. In patients with refractory angina diagnosed as cardiac in origin, a number of methods have been proposed (Kones, 2010). They are as follows: percutaneous myocardial laser revascularization (PMLR) (McGillion et al., 2010); spinal cord stimulation (SCS) (Lanza et al., 2011); enhanced external counterpulsation (EECP); percutaneous application of low frequency ultrasound, i.e. mechanical shock waves with ECG gating; angiogenesis stimulation by the VEGF gene and CD34+ stem cell therapy; etc.

Individuals with angina-like chest pain with normal coronary angiogram and patients with CAD and overlapping gastroenterological symptoms may achieve symptomatic improvement after therapy oriented to oesophageal disorders (Phan et al., 2009). Such therapy may consist of long-term treatment with PPIs, therapy with calcium antagonists (Budzyński, 2010a; Budzyński et al., 2010), *Helicobacter pylori* eradication (Budzyński, 2011), as well as tricyclic antidepressants (Eslick, 2008; Fass, 2008; Fass & Navarro-Rodriguez, 2008), selective serotonin reuptake inhibitors (citalopram, sertaline) or trazodone (Broekaert et al., 2006). Recent studies have also indicated the favourable effect of theophylline (Rao et al., 2007), botulinum toxin (Achem, 2008; Fass & Navarro-Rodriguez, 2008), acupuncture (Dickman et al., 2007b; Macpherson and Dumville, 2007; Pfab et al., 2011), melatonin due to its positive cardiological and gastroenterological action (Dominiguez-Rodriguez et al., 2009; Konturek et al., 2008; Pereira, 2006), hypnotherapy (Jones et al., 2006; Palsson and Whitehead, 2006), transcutaneous electrical nerve stimulation (TENS) (Borjesson et al., 1998), oesophageal dilatation, oesophagomyotomy and Nissen fundoplication (Achem, 2008; Dickman & Fass, 2006; Phan et al., 2009).

The outcome of long-term therapy with PPIs in patients with NCCP has been widely studied (Bautista et al, 2004; Cremonini et al., 2005, 2010; Dickman et al., 2005; Dickman & Fass, 2006; Liuzzo et al., 2005; Wang et al, 2005). These drugs have shown a favourable effect in 80% of patients with "GER-related" chest pain (Dickman & Fass, 2006). The relative risk reduction for continued chest pain after PPI therapy was 0.54 (95% CI, 0.41-0.71), with an NNT amounting to 3 (Cremonini et al., 2005). The recent meta-analysis by Cremonini et al. (2010) has also shown an advantage with therapy using a PPI over a placebo with an odds ratio of 3.75 (95% CI, 2.78-4.96), as well as a high placebo response amounting to 18.85% (range 2.94%-47.06%). Successful therapy with PPIs is most likely in patients with a GERD diagnosis (Gąsiorowska et al., 2009; Oranu & Vaezi, 2010; Seo et al., 2010). Among these subjects, acid exposure time (AET), symptom association probability (SAP), and the symptom index (SI) obtained from 24-hour oesophageal pH-metry or 24-hour oesophageal impedance with pH analysis are considered the predictors of a favourable therapeutic outcome (Kushnir et al., 2010).

Until now, there have only been a few works evaluating the role of therapy with PPIs in patients with CAD and recurrent chest pain suspected to be non-cardiac in origin and overlapping ischaemic, cardiac-derived chest pain (Budzyński et al., 2008; Dobrzycki et al., 2005; Liuzzo et al., 2005; Mehta et al., 1996; Świątkowski et al., 2004). All of them, including our own work, have evidenced a decrease in chest pain severity and amelioration in health-related quality of life estimated using the SF-36 survey, as well as an improvement in ECG signs of myocardial ischaemia, both during a treadmill stress test (a reduction in subject percentage with a significant decrease in ST interval during the stress test) and during 24-hour ECG Holter monitoring (a decrease in the number of ST-segment depression episodes and total duration of ischaemic episodes-total ischaemic burden) after therapy with PPIs. Liuzzo et al. (2005), studying a veteran patient population with documented CAD, showed through multivariate analysis and proton pump inhibitor therapy that they could independently predict a significant reduction in the prevalence of patients experiencing chest pain (OR = 0.09), emergency department visits (OR = 0.15), and hospitalization (OR = 0.14) for chest pain. On the other hand, our own results have shown that the mentioned favourable PPI effect on the angina pectoris course in patients with CAD should be carefully interpreted because it might not only result from the decrease in cardio-oesophageal reflex activation and therapy with aspirin-induced gastropathy, but also from the increase in nitric oxide bioavailability observed after therapy with rabeprazole in an open-label trial (Kłopocka et al., 2006), as well as the increase in the beta-endorphin plasma level revealed for omeprazole in a randomized, double-blind, placebo-controlled, crossover study (Budzyński et al., 2010).

As has been mentioned, besides a decrease in oesophageal acid exposure time and a reduction in GER-related myocardial ischaemic episodes, PPIs may also improve the course of angina-like chest pain by the alleviation of symptoms related to gastric disease (gastric and duodenal ulcer disease), by preventing and treating aspirin-induced gastropathy, as well as by reducing the risk of haemorrhagic complications from the upper part of the digestive tract and the prevention of secondary anaemia (ACCF, 2010; Bhatt et al., 2008; Hsiao et al., 2009). Tailored PPI prescription should prevail over the generalized in their recommendation for use with patients on dual anti-platelet therapy because of reported and still not definitely excluded potentially life-threatening interactions between PPIs and anti-platelet drugs (clopidogrel, aspirin). Pantoprazole or esomeprazole should be chosen for gastroprotection or time intervals between respective medicines should be recommended (ACCF, 2010; Bhatt et al., 2008). The easiest method for the last option is the recommendation of PPIs in the morning and clopidogrel in the evening.

In patients with recurrent chest pain and GERD diagnosed using oesophageal pH/impedance monitoring and non-responsive to PPIs, many other kinds of therapy have been proposed, including the following: doubling the PPI dose, switching to another PPI, adding histamine type 2-receptor antagonists at night, baclofen recommendation, as well as laparoscopic or open surgery (Dickman & Fass, 2006; Hershcovici & Fass, 2010; Kushnir et al, 2010; Oranu & Vaezi, 2010; Labenz, 2010). The exclusion of eosinophilic oesophagitis in patients with NCCP and aged under 45, atopy or dysphagia might also be helpful (Garcia-Compeăn et al., 2011). Dickman et al. (2007b) found acupuncture added to a single dose of PPI to be more effective than doubling the proton pump inhibitor dose in controlling GERD-related symptoms in patients who had failed with standard dose proton pump inhibitors.

Calcium antagonists, such as verapamil, diltiazem, nifedipine and amlodipine, have mainly been used in therapy for NCCP due to hypertensive oesophageal motility disorders diagnosed using stationary manometry (Dickman & Fass, 2006; Fass & Navarro-Rodriguez, 2006). The reported effects of these drugs in patients with recurrent angina-like chest pain were ambiguous. Some studies have shown a favourable outcome for this group of drugs, some have not confirmed it (Dickman & Fass, 2006; Eslick et al., 2005; Eslick, 2008; Fass & Dickman, 2006). Our own, recently published investigation has shown that patients with recurrent angina-like chest pain non-responsive to treatment with PPIs and an established diagnosis of exercise-provoked oesophageal spasm (EPOS), for whom a calcium antagonist was recommended due to exercise-provoked oesophageal spasm, had a significantly lower risk of hospitalization due to suspected acute coronary syndrome in the 2.7-year follow-up period than the remaining patients (NNT = 3.5) (Budzyński et al., 2010). In my own work it has been documented that Hp eradication had a similar favourable outcome (NNT = 2.7) (Budzyński, 2011). The rationales behind this therapy were the above-cited role of this infection in chest pain pathogenesis both cardiac and gastroenterological in origin.

Psychiatric disorders and anxiety focusing on the heart are common in patients with NCCP (Achem, 2008; Dickmann & Fass, 2006; Fass & Navarro-Rodriguez, 2008; Katerndahl, 2004). They may act as individual factors or via the increase in visceral hypersensitivity. Some studies have shown oesophageal motility abnormalities as markers of depressive or panic disorders. The last were found in 80% of patients with NCCP and oesophageal motor dysfunction and in 30% of subjects with a normal coronary angiogram and oesophageal examinations (Dickman & Fass, 2006). Eslick et al. (2005) have even recommended empirical therapy with tricyclic antidepressants in patients with recurrent chest pain non-responsive to PPIs. The rationale behind such a recommendation is that antidepressants act as pain modulators. In patients with NCCP, behaviour therapy involving trazodone, imipramine, amitriptyline, nortriptyline, citalopram, desipramine and sertraline was used for this purpose (Broekaert et al., 2006; Eslick, 2008; Fass, 2008; Fass & Navarro-Rodriguez, 2008). Their clinical efficacy was confirmed both in uncontrolled and in randomized, placebo-controlled trials. However, the prescribing of these drugs should always be carried out carefully, because of the potential cardiovascular risk of tricyclic antidepressants connected with their adverse effects, such as prolonged QT intervals, hypertension, postural hypotension, and effects on heart rate variability (Hamer et al., 2011). Probably because of this, non-pharmacological methods which could potentially be efficient in subjects with NCCP have been investigated, such as hypnotherapy, behaviour therapy, and acupuncture (Dickman et al., 2007b; Pfab et al., 2011; Yin and Chen, 2010; Zhang et al., 2010). Acupuncture has had a favourable effect on gastric emptying, oesophageal motility, and in patients with GERD, a potential substrate of non-cardiac chest pain. In the study by Macpherson and Dumville (2007), 42% of the patients investigated with a diagnosis of NCCP made in a Rapid Access Chest Pain Unit reported that they would consider acupuncture, 36% reported that they would not, and 22% did not know. Moreover, in the pilot study by Gąsiorowska et al. (2009), a favourable effect of 18 Johrei sessions (a kind of meditation) during six weeks in comparison to waiting-list control patients with functional chest pain was found. The clinical outcome of the mentioned methods is, among other things, explained by a decrease in visceral hypersensitivity, for which one of the mediators may be endogenous opioids, one of the potential pathways of the effect of PPIs (Budzyński et al., 2010). However, it should be checked for each patient as to whether his or her panic or depressive symptoms are the true cause of chest pain recurrence or its cofactor, and not an effect of symptom duration chronicity and the lack of an appropriate diagnosis.

However, particularly in populations with high cardiovascular risk, the appropriate control of cardiovascular risk factors is very important in therapy for patients with angina-like chest pain. The recent study by Leise et al. (2010) has shown that patients with recurrent angina-like chest pain which is gastroenterological but unknown in origin (NCCP-U), in spite of generally being considered as having low cardiac morbidity and mortality, may ultimately show a higher cardiovascular and non-cardiovascular death risk. In this analysis, whose results should still be interpreted with limitations, the NCCP group with a diagnosis of gastrointestinal disorder displayed less overall survival at all time points, specifically 70.1% at 10 years and 51.8% at 20 years, compared with their NCCP-U counterparts. The independent death risk factors in adjusted univariate analysis using Cox's proportional hazards model were as follows: age, the Charlson comorbidity index, previous CABG, and previous valvular disease. No specific cardiac or gastroenterological tests or their absence was associated with mortality. The authors explain their observations by the effect of the coexistence of gastroenterological disorders with latent non-ischaemic cardiovascular disease, coronary artery spasm (Charng et al., 1988; Makk et al., 2000; Manfrini et al., 2006; Rasmussen et al., 1986), microvascular disease (cardiac syndrome X) or at least endothelial dysfunction. An important aspect might also be an overlapping of risk factors for both systems' diseases, such as obesity, obstructive sleep apnoea, hypertension, smoking, and diabetes mellitus.

On the other hand, the study by Leise et al. (2010) has also shown that proper management of patients with recurrent chest pain which is extracardiac in origin is still a great challenge for physicians. During a 20-year follow-up period since an initial visit to an emergency department due to a recurrent chest pain experience, 49% of patients sought subsequent care from the emergency department, 42% had repeated cardiology evaluations, and only 15% were seen by a gastroenterologist. Thirty-eight percent underwent oesophago-gastroduodenoscopy, but very few underwent manometry or a pH probe.

7. Study limitations

The main limitations concerning investigations on the pathogenesis, diagnosis and treatment for patients with recurrent angina-like chest pain, both in patients with and without significant coronary artery narrowing, have been the small number of subject groups, which on average included a little over 100 participants. Only in three studies were the subject groups larger. The other limitations have involved the lack of or a short follow-up period, recommendations of different medication and their doses, non-homogeneous definitions of oesophageal disorders, the establishment of different study endpoints, and only single-centre experience presentations.

8. Future research

Further studies should validate the test of empirical therapy with PPIs in patients with CAD. It would also be significant if the mechanisms for the visceral hypersensitivity leading to a decrease in the chest pain threshold could be identified. The evaluation of some new diagnostic methods, including analysis for cerebral evoked potentials, would also be useful. Moreover, it seems to be important to check once more and re-evaluate the appropriate indications for coronary angiography, both because of its costs and its inseparable exposure to procedure-connected health risks and substantial radiation. All the recommended examinations, both cardiological and gastroenterological, should be connected with precise investigations into cardio-oesophageal and other vagally-mediated reflexes and on the determination of factors predicting their clinical importance. New therapeutic methods for recurrent angina-like non-cardiac chest pain should also be investigated, although critical analysis of relationships between benefits and costs should be performed.

9. Conclusions

- Angina-like chest pain is a common problem in health care because of its prevalence, diagnostic difficulties, resource utilization and potential connection with a reduced health-related quality of life and shorter survival times. This symptom is conditioned by biological, psychological and social factors.
- Angina pectoris may be caused by diseases of the cardiovascular system, digestive tract, and other extracardiac disorders which lead to an imbalance between myocardial blood

supply and oxygen requirement (e.g. anaemia or thyrotoxicosis). In respective patients, potential chest pain causes may overlap and influence each other. Therefore, NCCP may be present in patients both with and without heart diseases. However, the main and first purpose of its diagnostic procedures should be to exclude potentially life-threatening origins.

- Digestive tract diseases may cause angina-like chest pain along at least three pathways. Chest pain may originate from: (1) the oesophagus, stomach or gall bladder, due to stimulation of their chemo-, mechano-, and/or thermoreceptors; (2) the heart due to activation of cardio-oesophageal neural reflexes and secondary diminished myocardial perfusion; as well as (3) the heart due to a decrease in myocardial oxygen supply in the course of anaemia, secondary to acute or chronic alimentary tract bleeding, malabsorption, maldigestion, blood sequestration or autoimmunological reactions. *Helicobacter pylori* infection may play a role in all of these mechanisms.
- The misdiagnosis of cardio-oesophageal interrelationships may lead to the progressive acceleration of the course of the disorders of both systems and the intensity of their symptoms. This occurs in at least three vicious circle mechanisms: neural, inflammatory (neuro-immune crosstalk), and the haemorrhagic complications of anti-thrombotic drugs expressed as anaemia.
- The most frequent causes of NCCP are as follows: GERD, oesophageal motility disorders and panic abnormalities. Their diagnosis needs many times to use more advanced and more specialized diagnostic methods than panendoscopy, such as oesophageal impedance, pH-metry, manometry, or endosonography.
- In the diagnosis of recurrent chest pain of possible oesophageal origin, the most important factor is to confirm the relationship between chest pain episode occurrence and oesophageal disorders. Such a possibility is provided by the test of empirical therapy using PPIs (the "omeprazole test") and, in non-responsive cases, 24-hour oesophageal pH-metry, impedance or manometry with SI or SAP analysis. These help to recognize the source of chest pain in 40-80% of patients.
- The usefulness of exercise-provoked oesophageal disorders, such as exercise-provoked gastro-oesophageal reflux or oesophageal spasm, needs to be evaluated. Any further investigations need also to estimate the interrelationships between the course of cardiovascular and gastroenterological tests as predictors of false positives in their outcomes.
- Therapy for recurrent, angina-like chest pain should be based on the detailed diagnosis of its origin (whether cardiac or extracardiac), an assessment of its possible influence on myocardial perfusion, and the control of cardiovascular risk factors.
- Modern cardiac and gastrointestinal diagnostic methods would probably help to better recognize NCCP pathophysiology, facilitating its diagnosis and treatment. However, they will need to be critically evaluated, not only in relation to potential clinical usefulness, but also in accordance with risk-benefit and benefit-cost ratios.

10. References

Achem, SR. (2008) Noncardiac chest pain-treatment approaches. *Gastroenterology Clinics of North America,* Vol.37, No.4, (December, 2008), pp.859-78, ISSN 0889-8553

Adamek, RJ., Bock, S., & Pfaffenbach, B. (1998a) Oesophageal motility patterns and arterial blood pressure in patients with chest pain and normal coronary angiogram. *European Journal of Gastroenterology and Hepatology*, Vol.10, No.11, (November 1998), pp. 941-5, ISSN 0954-691X

Adamek, RJ., Bock, S., Szymanski, C., Hagemann, D., & Pfaffenbach B. (1998b) Increased occurrence of esophageal hypermotility disorders in patients with arterial hypertension. *Deutsche Medizinische Wochenschrift,* Vol.123, No.12, (March 1998), pp.341-6, ISSN 0012-0472

Adamek, RJ., Roth, B., Zymanski, CH., Hagemann, D., & Pfaffenbach, B. (1999) Esophageal motility patterns in patients with and without coronary heart disease and healthy controls. *Hepatogastroenterology,* Vol.46, No.27, (May-Juni 1999), pp.1759-64, ISSN 0172-6390

Adamopoulos, AB., Sakizlis, GN., Nasothimiou, EG., Anastasopoulou, I., Anastasakou, E., & Kotsi P. (2009) Do proton pump inhibitors attenuate the effect of aspirin on platelet aggregation? A randomized crossover study. *Journal of Cardiovascular Pharmacology,* Vol.54, No.2, (August 2009), pp.163-8, ISSN 0160-2446

American College of Cardiology Foundation (ACCF) Task Force on Expert Consensus Documents, Abraham, N.S., Hlatky, M.A., Antman, EM., Bhatt, DL., Bjorkman, DJ., Clark, CB., Furberg, CD., Johnson, DA., Kahi, CJ., Laine, L., Mahaffey, KW., Quigley, EM., Scheiman, J., Sperling, LS., & Tomaselli, GF. (2010) ACCF/ACG/AHA 2010 Expert Consensus Document on the Concomitant Use of Proton Pump Inhibitors and Thienopyridines. A Focused Update of the ACCF/ACG/AHA 2008 Expert Consensus Document on Reducing the Gastrointestinal Risks of Antiplatelet Therapy and NSAID Use. *Journal of American College of Cardiology,* Vol.56, No.24, (December 2010), pp.2051-2066, ISSN 0735-1097

American Society for Gastrointestinal Endoscopy (ASGE) Standards of Practice Committee, Anderson, MA., Ben-Menachem, T., Gan, SI., Appalaneni, V., Banerjee, S., Cash, BD., Fisher, L., Harrison, ME., Fanelli, RD., Fukami, N., Ikenberry, SO., Jain, R., Khan, K., Krinsky, ML., Lichtenstein, DR., Maple, JT., Shen, B., Strohmeyer, L., Baron, T., & Dominitz, JA. (2009) Management of antithrombotic agents for endoscopic procedures. *Gastrointestinal Endoscopy,* Vol.70, No.6, (December 2009),pp.1060-70, ISSN 0016-5107

Battaglia, E., Bassotti, G., Buonafede, G., Serra, AM., Dughera, L., Orzan, F., Casoni, R., Chistolini, F., Morelli, A., & Emanuelli, G. (2005) Noncardiac chest pain of esophageal origin in patients with and without coronary artery disease. *Hepatogastroenterology,* Vol.52, No.63, (May- Juni 2005), pp.792-795, ISSN 0172-6390

Bautista, J., Fullerton, H., Briseno, M., Cui, H., & Fass, R. (2004) The effect of an empirical trial of high-dose lansoprazole on symptom response of patients with non-cardiac chest pain--a randomized, double-blind, placebo-controlled, crossover trial. *Alimentary Pharmacology and Therapeutics,* Vol.19, No.10, (May 2004), pp.1123-30, ISSN 0269-2813

Bhatt, DL., Scheiman, J., Abraham, NS., Antman, EM., Chan, FK., Furberg, CD., Johnson, DA., Mahaffey, KW., Quigley, EM., Harrington, RA., Bates, ER., Bridges, CR., Eisenberg, MJ., Ferrari, VA., Hlatky, MA., Kaul, S., Lindner, JR., Moliterno, DJ.,

Mukherjee, D., Schofield, RS., Rosenson, RS., Stein, JH., Weitz, HH., Wesley, DJ., & American College of Cardiology Foundation Task Force on Clinical Expert Consensus Documents. (2008) ACCF/ACG/AHA 2008 expert consensus document on reducing the gastrointestinal risks of antiplatelet therapy and NSAID use: a report of the American College of Cardiology Foundation Task Force on Clinical Expert Consensus Documents. *Journal of American College Cardiology,* Vol.52, No.18, (October 2008), pp.1502-17, ISSN 0735-1097

Boesmans, W., Vanden Berghe, P., Farre, R., & Sifrim, D. (2010) Oesophageal shortening: in vivo validation of high-frequency ultrasound measurements of oesophageal muscle wall thickness. *Gut,* Vol.59, No.4, (April 2010), pp.433-40, ISSN 0017-5749

Borjesson, M., Pilhall, M., Eliasson, T., Norssell, H., Mannheimer, C., & Rolny, P. (1998) Esophageal visceral pain sensitivity: effects of TENS and correlation with manometric findings. *Digestive Disease and Sciences,* Vol.43, No.8, (August 1998), pp.1621-8, ISSN 0163-2116

Broekaert, D., Fischler, B., Sifrim, D., Janssens, J., & Tack, J. (2006) Influence of citalopram, a selective serotonin reuptake inhibitor, on oesophageal hypersensitivity: a double-blind, placebo-controlled study. *Alimentary Pharmacology and Therapeutics,* Vol.23, No.3, (February 2006), pp.365-70. ISSN 0269-2813

Budzyński, J., Kłopocka, M., Bujak, R., Świątkowski, M. & Sinkiewicz W. (2004) Autonomic nervous function in Helicobacter pylori infected patients with atypical chest pain studied by analysis of heart rate variability. *European Journal of Gastroenterology and Hepatology,*Vol.16, No.5, (May 2004), pp.451-7, ISSN 0954-691X

Budzyński, J., Kłopocka, M., Pulkowski, G., Suppan, K., Fabisiak, J., Majer, M., & Świątkowski, M. (2008) The effect of double dose of omeprazole on the course of angina pectoris and treadmill stress test in patients with coronary artery disease- a randomised, double-blind, placebo controlled, crossover trial. *International Journal of Cardiology,* Vol.127, No.2, (July 2008), pp.233-239, ISSN 0167-5273

Budzyński, J. & Pulkowski, G. (2009) [Atrial fibrillation, the other arrhythmias and digestive tract.] *Kardiologia Polska* Vol.67, No.11, (November 2009), pp.1268-1273, ISSN 0022-9032

Budzyński, J., Pulkowski, G., Kłopocka, M., Augustyńska, B., Sinkiewicz, A., Suppan, K., Fabisiak, J., Majer, M., & Świątkowski M (2010) The treatment with double dose of omeprazole increases in beta-endorphin plasma level in patients with coronary artery disease. *Archives of Medical Sciences,* Vol.6, No.2, (April 2010), pp.201-207, ISSN 1734-1922

Budzyński, J. (2010a) Exercise-provoked esophageal motility disorder in patients with recurrent chest pain. *World Journal of Gastroenterology,*Vol.16, No.35, (September 2010), pp.4428-35 ISSN 1007-9327

Budzyński J. (2010b) Exertional esophageal pH-metry and manometry in recurrent chest pain. *World Journal of Gastroenterology,*Vol.16, No.34, (September 2010), pp.4305-12, ISSN 1007-9327

Budzyński, J. (2010c) Does esophageal dysfunction affect the course of treadmill stress tests in patients with recurrent angina-like chest pain? *Polskie Archiwum Medycyny*

Wewnętrznej (Polish Archives of Internal Medicine), Vol.120, No.12, (December 2010), pp.484-489, ISSN 0032-3772

Budzyński, J. (2011) The favorable effect of Helicobacter pylori eradicative therapy in patients with recurrent angina-like chest pain and non-responsive to proton pump inhibitors: a preliminary study. *Archives of Medical Science*, Vol.7, No.1, (January 2011), pp.73-80, ISSN 1734-1922

Bugiardini, R., Bairey- Merz, CN. (2005) Angina with 'normal' coronary arteries: a changing philosophy. *JAMA: The Journal of American Medical Association*. Vol.293, No.4, (January 2005), pp.477-84, ISSN 0098-7484

Bunch, TJ., Day, JD., Anderson, JL., Horne, BD., Muhlestein, JB., Crandall, BG., Weiss, JP., Lappe, DL. & Asirvatham, SJ. (2008a) Frequency of Helicobacter pylori seropositivity and C-reactive protein increase in atrial fibrillation in patients undergoing coronary angiography. *American Journal of Cardiology*, Vol.101, No.6, (March 2008), pp.848-51, ISSN 0002-9149

Bunch, TJ, Packer, DL, Jahangir, A., Locke, GR., Talley, NJ., Gersh, BJ., Roy, RR., Hodge, DO. & Asirvatham SJ. (2008b) Long-term risk of atrial fibrillation with symptomatic gastroesophageal reflux disease and esophagitis. *American Journal of Cardiology*, Vol.102, No.9, (August 2008), pp.1207-11, ISSN 0002-9149

Caldwell, MT., Byrne, PJ., Marks, P., Walsh, TN. & Hennessy TP. (1994) Bradykinin, coronary artery disease and gastro-oesophageal reflux. *British Journal of Surgery*, Vol.81, No.10, (October 1994), pp.1462-4, ISSN 0007-1323

Cayley, WE Jr. (2005) Diagnosing the cause of chest pain. American Family Physician, Vol.72, No.10, (November 2005), pp.2012-21, ISSN 0002-838X

Celik, T, Iyisoy, A. & Yuksel, UC. (2010) Possible pathogenetic role of Helicobacter pylori infection in cardiac syndrome X. *International Journal of Cardiology*, Vol.142, No.2, (July 2010), pp.193-4, ISSN 0167-5273

Charng, MJ., Wang, SP., Chang, MS. & Chiang, BN. (1988) Coronary spasm complicating sclerotherapy of esophageal varices. *Chest*. Vol.93, No.1, (January 1988), pp.204-5, ISSN 0012-3692

Chauhan, A., Petch, MC. & Schofield, PM. (1996) Cardio-oesophageal reflex in humans as a mechanism for "linked angina". *European Heart Journal*, Vol.17, No.3, (March 1996), pp.407–413 ISSN 0195-668X

Cheung, TK., Hou, X., Lam, KF., Chen, J., Wong, WM., Cha, H., Xia, HH., Chan, AO., Tong, TS., Leung, GY., Yuen, MF. & Wong, BC. (2009) Quality of life and psychological impact in patients with noncardiac chest pain. *Journal of Clinical Gastroenterology*, Vol.43, No.1, (January 2009), pp.13-8, ISSN 0192-0790

Collins, SM., Denou, E., Verdu, EF. & Bercik P. (2009) The putative role of the intestinal microbiota in the irritable bowel syndrome. *Digestive and Liver Diseases*. Vol.41, No.12, (December 2009), pp.850-3, ISSN 1590-8658

Cooke, RA., Anggiansah, A., Chambers, JB. & Owen WJ. (1998) A prospective study of oesophageal function in patients with normal coronary angiograms and controls with angina. *Gut*, Vol.42, No.3, (March 1998), pp.323-9, ISSN 0017-5749

Cremonini, F., Wise, J., Moayyedi, P. & Talley, NJ. (2005) Diagnostic and therapeutic use of proton pump inhibitors in non-cardiac chest pain: a metaanalysis. *The American Journal of Gastroenterology*, Vol.100, No.6, (Juni 2005), pp.1226-32, ISSN 0002-9270

Cremonini, F., Ziogas, DC., Chang, HY., Kokkotou, E., Kelley, JM., Conboy, L., Kaptchuk, TJ. & Lembo, AJ. (2010) Meta-analysis: the effects of placebo treatment on gastro-oesophageal reflux disease. *Alimentary Pharmacology and Therapeutics*, Vol.32, No.1, (July 2010), pp.29-42, ISSN 0269-2813

Cubattoli, L., Barneschi, C., Mastrocinque, E., Bonucci, P. & Giomarelli, PP. (2009) Cardiac arrest after intragastric balloon insertion in a super-obese patient. *Obesity Surgery*, Vol.19, No.2, (February 2009), pp.253-6, ISSN 0960-8923

Cuomo, R., De Giorgi, F., Adinolfi, L., Sarnelli, G., Loffredo, F., Efficie, E., Verde, C., Savarese, MF., Usai, P. & Budillon, G. (2006) Oesophageal acid exposure and altered neurocardiac function in patients with GERD and idiopathic cardiac dysrhythmias, *Alimentary Pharmacology and Therapeutics*. Vol.24, No.2, (July 2006), pp.361-70, ISSN 0269-2813

Dai, X., Makaryus, AN., Makaryus, JN. & Jauhar, R. (2009) Significant gastrointestinal bleeding in patients at risk of coronary stent thrombosis. *Reviews in cardiovascular medicine*, Vol.10, No.1, (Winter 2009), pp.14-24, ISSN 1530-6550

de Aquino Lima, JP. & Brophy, JM. (2010) The potential interaction between clopidogrel and proton pump inhibitors: A systematic review. *BMC Medicine*, Vol.8, No.1, (December 2010), pp.81, ISSN 1741-7015

Dickman, R., Emmons, S., Cui, H., Sewell, J., Hernández, D., Esquivel, RF. & Fass, R. (2005) The effect of a therapeutic trial of high-dose rabeprazole on symptom response of patients with non-cardiac chest pain: a randomized, double-blind, placebo-controlled, crossover trial. *Alimentary Pharmacology and Therapeutics*, Vol.22, No.6, (September 2005), pp.547-55. ISSN 0269-2813

Dickman, R. & Fass, R. (2006) Noncardiac chest pain. *Clinical gastroenterology and hepatology : the official clinical practice journal of the American Gastroenterological Association*, Vol.4, No.5, (May 2006), pp.558-63, ISSN 1542-3565

Dickman, R., Mattek, N., Holub, J., Peters, D. & Fass R. (2007a) Prevalence of upper gastrointestinal tract findings in patients with noncardiac chest pain versus those with gastroesophageal reflux disease (GERD)-related symptoms: results from a national endoscopic database. *The American Journal of Gastroenterology*, Vol.102, No.6, (June 2007), pp.1173-9, ISSN 0002-9270

Dickman, R., Schiff, E., Holland, A., Wright, C., Sarela, SR., Han, B. & Fass R. (2007b) Clinical trial: acupuncture vs. doubling the proton pump inhibitor dose in refractory heartburn. *Alimentary Pharmacology and Therapeutics*, Vol.26, No.10, (November 2007), pp.1333-44, ISSN 0269-2813

Dobrzycki, S., Baniukiewicz, A., Korecki, J., Skrodzka, D., Prokopczuk, P., Zaremba-Woroniecka, A., Żuk, J. & Łaszewicz, W. (2005) Does gastro-esophageal reflux provoke myocardial ischemia in patients with CAD? *International Journal of Cardiology*, Vol.104, No.1, (September 2005), pp.67-72, ISSN 0167-5273

Dominguez-Rodriguez, A., Abreu-Gonzalez, P. & Reiter, RJ. (2009) Clinical aspects of melatonin in the acute coronary syndrome. *Current Vascular Pharmacology*, Vol.7, No.3, (July 2009), pp.367-73, ISSN 1570-1611

Drewes, AM., Arendt-Nielsen, L., Funch-Jensen, P. & Gregersen, H. (2006) Experimental human pain models in gastro-esophageal reflux disease and unexplained chest pain. *World Journal of Gastroenterology*, Vol.12, No.12, (May 2006), pp.2806-17, ISSN 1007-9327

Drossman, DA. (2006) The Functional Gastrointestinal Disorders & the Rome III Process. *Gastroenterology*, Vol.130, No.5, (April 2006), pp.1377–1390, ISSN 0016-5085

Duygu, H., Ozerkan, F., Saygi, S. & Akyüz, S. (2008) Persistent atrial fibrillation associated with gastroesophageal reflux accompanied by hiatal hernia. *The Anatolian Journal of Cardiology*. Vol.8, No.2, (April 2008), pp.164-5, ISSN 1302-8723

Erhardt, L., Herlitz, J., Bossaert, L., Halinen, M., Keltai, M., Koster, R., Marcassa, C., Quinn, T., van Weert, H. & Task Force on the management of chest pain. (2002) Task force on the management of chest pain. *European Heart Journal*, Vol.23, No.15, (August 2002), pp.1153-76, ISSN 0195-668X

Eskandarian, R., Malek, M., Mousavi, SH. & Babaei, M. (2006) Association of Helicobacter pylori infection with cardiac syndrome X. *Singapore Medical Journal*, Vol.47; No.8, (August 2006), pp.704-6, ISSN 0037-5675

Eslick, GD., Coulshed, DS., & Talley, NJ. (2005) Diagnosis and treatment of noncardiac chest pain. *Nature clinical practice. Gastroenterology and Hepatology*. Vol.2, No.10, (October 2005), pp.463-72, ISSN 1743-4378

Eslick, GD, & Talley NJ. (2004) Non-cardiac chest pain: predictors of health care seeking, the types of health care professional consulted, work absenteeism and interruption of daily activities. *Alimentary Pharmacology and Therapeutics*, Vol.20, No.8, (October 2004), pp.909-15, ISSN 0269-2813

Eslick, GD. (2008) Classification, natural history, epidemiology, and risk factors of noncardiac chest pain. *Disease a Month*, Vol.54, No.9, (September 2008), pp.593-603, ISSN 0011-5029

Fass, R. & Dickman, R. (2006) Non-cardiac chest pain: an update. *Neurogastroenterology and Motility*, Vol.18, No.6, (June 2006), pp.408-17, ISSN 1350-1925

Fass, R. & Navarro-Rodriguez, T. (2008) Noncardiac chest pain. *Journal of Clinical Gastroenterology*, Vol.42, No.5, (May- June 2008), pp.636-46, ISSN 0192-0790

Fass, R. (2008) Evaluation and diagnosis of noncardiac chest pain. *Disease- a- Month*, Vol.54, No.9, (September 2008), pp.627-41, ISSN 0011-5029

Fornari, F., Farré, R., van Malenstein, H., Blondeau, K., Callegari-Jacques, SM. & Barros, SG. (2008) Nutcracker oesophagus: association with chest pain and dysphagia controlling for gastro- oesophageal reflux. *Digestive and Liver Diseases*, Vol.40, No.9, (September 2008), pp.717-22. ISSN 1590-8658

Fox, KF. (2005) Investigation and management of chest pain. *Heart (British Cardiac Society)*, Vol.91, No.1, (January 2005), pp.105-10, ISSN 1355-6037

Franceschi, F., Niccoli, G., Ferrante, G., Gasbarrini, A., Baldi, A., Candelli, M., Feroce, F., Saulnier, N., Conte, M., Roccarina, D., Lanza, GA., Gasbarrini, G., Gentiloni, SN. & Crea F. (2009) CagA antigen of Helicobacter pylori and coronary instability: insight from a clinico-pathological study and a meta-analysis of 4241 cases. *Atherosclerosis*, Vol.202, No.2, (February 2009), pp.535-42, ISSN 0021-9150

García-Compeán, D., González González, JA., Marrufo García, CA., Flores Gutiérrez, JP., Barboza Quintana, O., Galindo Rodríguez, G., Mar Ruiz, MA., de León Valdez, D., Jaquez Quintana, JO. & Maldonado Garza, HJ. (2011) Prevalence of eosinophilic esophagitis in patients with refractory gastroesophageal reflux disease symptoms: A prospective study. *Digestive and Liver Diseases*, Vol.43, No.3., (March 2011), pp.204-8, ISSN 1590-8658

Gąsiorowska, A. & Fass R. (2008) The proton pump inhibitor (PPI) test in GERD: does it still have a role? *Journal of Clinical Gastroenterology*, Vol.42, No.8, (September 2008), pp.867-74, ISSN 0192-0790

Gąsiorowska, A., Navarro-Rodriguez, T., Dickman, R., Wendel, C., Moty, B., Powers, J., Willis, MR., Koenig, K., Ibuki, Y., Thai, H. & Fass R. (2009) Clinical Trial: the Effect of Johrei on Symptoms of Patients with Functional Chest Pain (FCP)-A Pilot Study. *Alimentary Pharmacology and Therapeutics*, Vol.29, No.1, (January 2009), pp.126-34, ISSN 0269-2813

George, A. & Movahed, A. (2010) Recognition of noncardiac findings on cardiac computed tomography examination. *Reviews in Cardiovascular Medicine*, Vol.11, No.2, (Spring 2010), pp.84-91, ISSN 1530-6550

Grundy, D., Al-Chaer, ED., Aziz, Q., Collins, SM., Ke, M., Taché, Y. & Wood JD. (2006) Fundamentals of neurogastroenterology: basic science. *Gastroenterology*. Vol.130, No.5, (April 2006), pp.1391-411, ISSN 0016-5085

Hamer, M., Batty, GD., Seldenrijk, A. & Kivimaki, M. (2011) Antidepressant medication use and future risk of cardiovascular disease: the Scottish Health Survey. *European Heart Journal*, Vol.32, No.4, (February 2011), ISSN 0195-668X

Hammett, RJ., Hansen, RD., Lorang, M., Bak, YT. & Kellow JE. (2003) Esophageal dysmotility and acid sensitivity in patients with mitral valve prolapse and chest pain. *Diseases of the Esophagus*. Vol.16, No.2, (February 2003), pp.73-6, ISSN 1120-8694

Hebbard, G. (2010) Noncardiac chest pain: an unsatisfactory 'diagnosis'? *Journal of Gastroenterology and Hepatology*, Vol.25, No.12, (December 2010), pp.1811-2. ISSN:0815-9319

Hershcovici, T. & Fass R. (2010) An algorithm for diagnosis and treatment of refractory GERD. *Best Practice and Research. Clinical Gastroenterology*, Vol.24, No.6, (December 2010), pp.923-36, ISSN 1521-6918

Hewson, EG., Dalton, CB., Hackshaw BT, Wu, WC. & Richter JE. (1990) The prevalence of abnormal esophageal test results in patients with cardiovascular disease and unexplained chest pain. *Archives of Internal Medicine*, Vol.150, No.5, (May 1990), pp.965-9, ISSN 0003-9926

Hoff, DA., Gregersen, H., Odegaard, S., Liao, D. & Hatlebakk, JG. (2010) Mechanosensation and mucosal blood perfusion in the esophagus of healthy volunteers studied with a multimodal device incorporating laser Doppler flowmetry and endosonography. *Digestive Diseases and Sciences*, Vol.55, No.2, (February 2009), pp.312-20, ISSN 0163-2116

Hollander, JE., Robey, JL., Chase, MR., Brown, AM., Zogby, KE. & Shofer FS. (2007) Relationship between a Clear-cut Alternative Noncardiac Diagnosis and 30-day Outcome in Emergency Department Patients with Chest Pain. *Academic emergency medicine: official journal of the Society for Academic Emergency Medicine*. Vol.14, No.3, (March 2007), pp.210-5, ISSN 1069-6563

Hsiao, FY., Tsai, YW., Huang, WF., Wen, YW., Chen, PF., Chang, PY. & Kuo KN. (2009) A comparison of aspirin and clopidogrel with or without proton pump inhibitors for the secondary prevention of cardiovascular events in patients at high risk for gastrointestinal bleeding. *Clinical Therapeutics*, Vol.31, No.9, (September 2009), pp.2038-47, ISSN 0149-2918

Janssens, J., Vantrappen, G. & Ghillebert G. (1986) 24-hour recording of esophageal pressure and pH in patients with noncardiac chest pain. *Gastroenterology*, Vol.90, No.6, (June 1986), pp.1978-84, ISSN 0016-5085

Jones, H., Cooper, P., Miller, V., Brooks, N. & Whorwell PJ. (2006) Treatment of non-cardiac chest pain: a controlled trial of hypnotherapy. *Gut*, Vol.55, No.10, (October 2006), pp.1403-8, ISSN 0017-5749

Jou, CJ., Farber, JP., Qin, C. & Foreman, RD. (2002) Convergent pathways for cardiac- and esophageal- somatic motor reflexes in rats. *Autonomic neuroscience: basic and clinical.*, Vol.99, No.2, (August 2002), pp.70-7, ISSN 1566-0702

Juurlink, DN., Gomes, T., Ko, DT., Szmitko, PE., Austin, PC., Tu, JV., Henry, DA., Kopp, A. & Mamdani, MM. (2009) A population-based study of the drug interaction between proton pump inhibitors and clopidogrel. *CMAJ: Canadian Medical Association Journal*. Vol.180, No.7, (January 2009), pp.713-8, ISSN 0820-3946

Kasprzak, M., Koziński, M., Bielis, L., Boińska, J., Plażuk, W., Marciniak, A., Budzyński, J., Siller-Matula, J., Rość, D. & Kubica, J. (2009) Pantoprazole may enhance antiplatelet effect of enteric-coated aspirin in patients with acute coronary syndrome. *Cardiology Journal*, Vol.16, No.6, (June 2009), pp.535-544, ISSN 1897-5593

Katerndahl, D. (2004) Panic and Plaques: Panic Disorder and Coronary Artery Disease in Patients with Chest Pain J *The Journal of the American Board of Family Practice* , Vol.17, No.2, (March-April 2004), pp.114–26, ISSN 0893-8652

Kim, J., Henderson, RA., Pocock, SJ., Clayton, T., Sculpher, MJ., Fox, KA. & RITA-3 Trial Investigators. (2005) Health-related quality of life after interventional or conservative strategy in patients with unstable angina or non-ST-segment elevation myocardial infarction: one-year results of the third Randomized Intervention Trial of unstable Angina RITA-3. *Journal of the American College of Cardiology*, Vol.45, No.2, (January 2005), pp.221–8, ISSN 0735-1097

Kłopocka M, Budzyński J, Świątkowski M, Augustyńska B. & Pulkowski, G. (2006) Therapy with rabeprazole increases nitric oxide bioavailability. May it limit usefulness of empirical test with proton pump inhibitor in chest pain diagnosis? *Medical and Biological Sciences*, Vol.20, No.2, (January 2006), pp.57-61. ISSN 1734-591X

Kones, R. (2010) Recent advances in the management of chronic stable angina II. Anti-ischemic therapy, options for refractory angina, risk factor reduction, and revascularization. *Vascular Health and Risk Management*, Vol.6, (September 2010), pp.49-74, ISSN 1176-6344

Konturek, PC., Celiński, K., Słomka, M., Cichoż-Lach, H., Burnat, G., Naegel, A., Bielański, W., Konturek, JW. & Konturek, SJ. (2008) Melatonin and its precursor L-tryptophan prevent acute gastric mucosal damage induced by aspirin in humans. *Journal of Physiology and Pharmacology,* Vol.59, No.Suppl 2, (August 2008), pp.67-75, ISSN 0867-5910

Kowalski, M., Konturek, PC., Pieniążek, P., Karczewska, E., Kluczka, A., Grove, R., Kranig, W., Nasseri, R., Thale, J., Hahn, EG. & Konturek, SJ. (2001) Prevalence of Helicobacter pylori infection in coronary artery disease and effect of its eradication on coronary lumen reduction after percutaneous coronary angioplasty. *Digestive and Liver Diseases,* Vol.33, No.3, (April 2001), pp.222-9, ISSN 1590-8658

Krysiak, W., Szabowski, S., Stepień, M., Krzywkowska, K., Krzywkowski, A. & Marciniak P. (2008) Hiccups as a myocardial ischemia symptom. *Polskie Archiwum Medycyny Wewnetrznej (Polish Archives of Internal Medicine),* Vol.118, No.3, (March 2008), pp.148-51, ISSN 0032-3772

Kushnir, VM., Sayuk, GS. & Gyawali, CP. (2010) Abnormal GERD parameters on ambulatory pH monitoring predict therapeutic success in noncardiac chest pain. *The American Journal of Gastroenterolology,* Vol.105, No.5, (November 2009), pp.1032-8, ISSN 0002-9270

Labenz, J. (2010) Facts and fantasies in extra-oesophageal symptoms in GORD. *Best Practice and Research. Clinical Gastroenterology,* Vol.24, No.6, (December 2010), pp.893-904, ISSN 1521-6918

Laheij, RJ., Van Rossum, LG., Krabbe, PF., Jansen, JB. & Verheugt, FW. (2003) The impact of gastrointestinal symptoms on health status in patients with cardiovascular disease. *Alimentary Pharmacology and Therapeutics,* Vol.17, No.7, (April 2003), pp.881-5, ISSN 0269-2813

Laine, L. & Hennekens, C. (2010) Proton pump inhibitor and clopidogrel interaction: fact or fiction? *The American Journal of Gastroenterology,* Vol.105, No.1, (January 2010), pp.34-41, ISSN 0002-9270

Laird, C, Driscoll, P. & Wardrope, J. (2004) The ABC of community emergency care: chest pain. *Emergency Medicine Journal,* Vol.21, No.2, (March 2004), pp.226-32, ISSN 1472-0205

Lanza, GA, Grimaldi, R., Greco, S., Ghio, S., Sarullo, F., Zuin, G., De Luca, A., Allegri, M., Di Pede, F., Castagno, D., Turco, A., Sapio, M., Pinato, G., Cioni, B., Trevi, G. & Crea F. (2011) Spinal cord stimulation for the treatment of refractory angina pectoris: a multicenter randomized single-blind study (the SCS-ITA trial). *Pain,* Vol.152, No.1, (January 2011), pp.45-52, ISSN 0304-3959

Leise, MD., Locke, GR 3rd., Dierkhising, RA., Zinsmeister, AR., Reeder, GS. & Talley NJ. (2010) Patients dismissed from the hospital with a diagnosis of noncardiac chest pain: cardiac outcomes and health care utilization. *Mayo Clinic Proceedings,* Vol.85, No.4, (April 2010), pp.323-30, ISSN 0025-6196

Lemire, S. (1997) Assessment of clinical severity and investigation of uncomplicated gastroesophageal reflux disease and noncardiac angina-like chest pain. *Canadian Journal Gastroenterology,* Vol.11, Suppl B, (September 1997), pp.37B-40B, ISSN 0835-7900

Lenfant, C. (2010) Chest pain of cardiac and noncardiac origin. *Metabolism: clinical and experimental*. Vol.59, Suppl 1, (October 2010), pp.S41-6, ISSN 0026-0495

Liuzzo, JP., Ambrose, JA. & Diggs, P. (2005) Proton-pump inhibitor use by coronary artery disease patients is associated with fewer chest pain episodes, emergency department visits and hospitalizations. *Alimentary Pharmacology and Therapeutics*,Vol.22, No.2, (July 2005), pp.95-100, ISSN 0269-2813

McGillion, M., Cook, A., Victor, JC., Carroll, S., Weston, J., Teoh, K. & Arthur HM. (2010) Effectiveness of percutaneous laser revascularization therapy for refractory angina. *Vascular Health and Risk Management*, Vol.6, (September 2010), pp.735-47, ISSN 1176-6344

Macpherson, H. & Dumville, JC. (2007) Acupuncture as a potential treatment for non-cardiac chest pain--a survey. *Acupuncture in Medicine: Journal of the British Medical Acupuncture Society*, Vol.25, No.1-2, (June 2007), pp.18-21, ISSN 0964-5284

Makk, LJ., Leesar, M., Joseph, A., Prince, CP. & Wright RA. (2000) Cardioesophageal reflexes: an invasive human study. *Digestive Diseases and Sciences*, Vol.45, No.12, (December 2000), pp.2451-4, ISSN 0163-2116

Manfrini, O., Bazzocchi, G., Luati, A., Borghi, A., Monari, P. & Bugiardini R. (2006) Coronary spasm reflects inputs from adjacent esophageal system. *American Journal of Physiology. Heart and Circulatory Physiology*, Vol.290, No.5, (May 2006), pp.H2085-91, ISSN 0363-6135

Mant, J., McManus, RJ., Oakes, RA., Delaney, BC., Barton, PM., Deeks, JJ., Hammersley, L., Davies, RC., Davies, MK. & Hobbs, FD. (2004) Systematic review and modelling of the investigation of acute and chronic chest pain presenting in primary care. *Health Technology Assessment*, Vol.8, No.2, (February 2004), pp.1-158, ISSN 1366-5278

Marques, AH., Silverman, MN. & Sternberg, EM. (2010) Evaluation of stress systems by applying noninvasive methodologies: measurements of neuroimmune biomarkers in the sweat, heart rate variability and salivary cortisol. *Neuroimmunomodulation*. Vol.17, No.3, (February 2010), pp.205-8, ISSN 1021-7401

Mayer, EA. & Tillisch, K. (2011) The brain-gut axis in abdominal pain syndromes. *Annual Review of Medicine*, Vol.62, (February 2011), pp.381-96, ISSN 0066-4219

Mehta, AJ., de Caestecker, JS., Camm, AJ. & Northfield, TC. (1996) Gastro-oesophageal reflux in patients with coronary artery disease: how common is it and does it matter? *European Journal of Gastroenterology and Hepatology*, Vol.8, No.10, (October 1996), pp.973-8, ISSN 0954-691X

Miyazaki, M., Babazono, A., Kadowaki, K., Kato, M., Takata, T. & Une, H. (2006) Is Helicobacter pylori infection a risk factor for acute coronary syndromes? *The Journal of Infection*, Vol.52, No.2, (February 2006), pp.86-91, ISSN 0163-4453

Munk, EM., Nørgård, B., Dethlefsen, C., Gregersen, H., Drewes, AM., Funch-Jensen, P. & Sørensen, HT. (2008) Unexplained chest/epigastric pain in patients with normal endoscopy as a predictor for ischemic heart disease and mortality: a Danish 10-year cohort study. *BMC Gastroenterology*, Vol.8, (July 2008), pp.28, ISSN 1471-230X

Nam, CW., Kim, KS., Lee, YS., Lee, SH., Han, SW., Hur, SH., Kim, YN., Kim, KB. & Jang, BK. (2006) The incidence of gastro-esophageal disease for the patients with typical chest pain and a normal coronary angiogram. *The Korean Journal of Internal Medicine*, Vol.21, No.2, (June 2006), pp.94-6, ISSN 1226-3303

Nasr, I., Attaluri, A., Hashmi, S., Gregersen, H. & Rao, SS. (2010) Investigation of esophageal sensation and biomechanical properties in functional chest pain. *Neurogastroenterology and Motility: the official journal of the Gastrointestinal Motility Society*, Vol.22, No.5, (May 2010), pp.520-6, e116, ISSN 1350-1925

Navarese, EP., Franceschi, F., Aurelio, A., Natale, L., Rebuzzi, AG. & Gasbarrini, G. (2010) Focal myocarditis mimicking ST-elevation myocardial infarction in a patient with Helicobacter pylori infection: role of magnetic resonance with late gadolinium enhancement. *Recenti progressi in medicina*, Vol.101, No.2, (February 2010), pp.61-3, ISSN

Nema, H., Kato, M., Katsurada, T., Nozaki, Y., Yotsukura, A., Yoshida, I., Sato, K., Kawai, Y., Takagi, Y., Okusa, T., Takiguchi, S., Sakurai, M. & Asaka, M. (2008) Endoscopic survey of low-dose-aspirin-induced gastroduodenal mucosal injuries in patients with ischemic heart disease. *Journal of Gastroenterology and Hepatology*, Vol.23, No.Suppl 2, (December 2008), pp.S234-6, ISSN 0815-9319

North, CS., Hong, BA. & Alpers, DH. (2007) Relationship of functional gastrointestinal disorders and psychiatric disorders: implications for treatment. *World Journal of Gastroenterology*, Vol.13, No.14, (April 2007), pp.2020-7, ISSN 1007-9327

Numans, ME. & de Wit, NJ. (2003) Reflux symptoms in general practice: diagnostic evaluation of the Carlsson-Dent gastro-oesophageal reflux disease questionnaire. *Alimentary Pharmacology and Therapeutics*,Vol.17, No.8, (April 2003), pp.1049-55, ISSN 0269-2813

Oranu, AC. & Vaezi, MF. (2010) Noncardiac chest pain: gastroesophageal reflux disease. The *Medical Clinics of North America*, Vol.94, No.2, (March 2010), pp.233-42, ISSN 0025-7125

Palsson, OS. & Whitehead, WE. (2006) Hypnosis for non-cardiac chest pain. *Gut*. Vol.55, No.10, (October 2006), pp.1381-4, ISSN 0017-5749

Patel, MR., Peterson, ED., Dai, D., Brennan, JM., Redberg, RF., Anderson, HV., Brindis, RG. & Douglas, PS. (2010) Low diagnostic yield of elective coronary angiography. *New England Journal Medicine*, Vol.362, No.10, (March 2010), pp.886-95, ISSN 0028-4793

Pereira, Rde S. (2006) Regression of gastroesophageal reflux disease symptoms using dietary supplementation with melatonin, vitamins and aminoacids: comparison with omeprazole. *Journal of Pineal Research* Vol.41, No.3, (October 2006), pp.195-200, ISSN 0742-3098

Pfab, F., Winhard, M., Nowak-Machen, M., Napadow, V., Irnich, D., Pawlik, M., Bein, T. & Hansen, E. (2011) Acupuncture in critically ill patients improves delayed gastric emptying: a randomized controlled trial. *Anesthesia and Analgesia*, Vol.112, No.1, (January 2011), pp.150-5, ISSN 0003-2999

Phan, A., Shufelt, C. & Merz, CN. (2009) Persistent chest pain and no obstructive coronary artery disease. *JAMA: the Journal of the American Medical Association*, Vol.301, No.14, (April 2009), pp.1468-74, ISSN 0098-7484

Poole-Wilson, PA., Pocock, SJ., Fox, KA., Henderson, RA., Wheatley, DJ., Chamberlain, DA., Shaw, TR., Clayton, TC. & Randomised Intervention Trial of unstable Angina

Investigators. (2006) Interventional versus conservative treatment in acute non-ST elevation coronary syndrome: time course of patient management and disease events over one year in the RITA 3 trial. *Heart,* Vol.92, No.10, (October 2006), pp.1473-9, ISSN 1355-6037

Potts, SG. & Bass, CM. (1995) Psychological morbidity in patients with chest pain and normal or near-normal coronary arteries: a long- term follow-up study. *Psychological Medicine,* Vol.25, No.2, (March 1995), pp.339–347, ISSN 0033-2917

Ramdeen, N, Aronow, WS., Chugh, S. & Asija, A. (2008) Patients undergoing coronary angiography because of chest pain with hepatitis C virus seropositivity have a higher prevalence of obstructive coronary artery disease than a control group. *Archives of Medical Sciences,* Vol.4, No.4, (December 2008), pp.452–454, ISSN 1734-1922

Rao, SS., Mudipalli, RS., Remes-Troche, JM., Utech, CL., Zimmerman, B. (2007) Theophylline improves esophageal chest pain- a randomized, placebo- controlled study. *The American Journal of Gastroenterology,* Vol.102, No.5, (May 2007), pp.930-8, ISSN 0002-9270

Rasmi, Y. & Raeisi, S. (2009) Possible role of Helicobacter pylori infection via microvascular dysfunction in cardiac syndrome X. *Cardiology Journal,* Vol.16, No.6, (June 2009), pp.585-7, ISSN 1897-5593

Rasmussen, K., Funch-Jensen, P., Ravnsbaek, J., & Bagger, J.P. (1986) Oesophageal spasm in patients with coronary artery spasm. *Lancet,* Vol.I, No.8474, (January 1986), pp.174-176, ISSN 0140-6736

Remes-Troche, JM. (2010) The hypersensitive esophagus: pathophysiology, evaluation, and treatment options. *Current Gastroenterology Reports,* Vol.12, No.5, (October 2010), pp.417-26, ISSN 1522-8037

Ringstrom, E. & Freedman, J. (2006) Approach to undifferentiated chest pain in the emergency department: a review of recent medical literature and published practice guidelines. *The Mount Sinai Journal of Medicine, New York,* Vol.73, No.2, (March 2006), pp.499-505, ISSN 0027-2507

Rosztóczy, A., Vass, A., Izbéki, F., Nemes, A., Rudas, L., Csanády, M., Lonovics, J., Forster, T. & Wittmann, T. (2007) The evaluation of gastro-oesophageal reflux and oesophagocardiac reflex in patients with angina-like chest pain following cardiologic investigations. *International Journal of Cardiology,* Vol.118, No.1, (May 2007), pp.62-8, ISSN 0167-5273

Ruigómez, A., Massó-González, EL., Johansson, S., Wallander, MA. & García-Rodríguez, LA. (2009) Chest pain without established ischaemic heart disease in primary care patients: associated comorbidities and mortality. *The British Journal of General Practitioners: the Journal of the Royal College of general Practitioners,* Vol.59, No.560, (March 2009), pp.e78-86, ISSN 0960-1643

Ruigómez, A., Rodríguez, LA., Wallander, MA., Johansson, S. & Jones, R. (2006) Chest pain in general practice: incidence, comorbidity and mortality. *Family Practice,* Vol.23, No.2, (April 2006), pp.167-74, ISSN 0263-2136

Saleh, N., Svane, B., Jensen, J., Hansson, LO., Nordin, M. & Tornvall, P. (2005) Stent implantation, but not pathogen burden, is associated with plasma C-reactive protein and interleukin-6 levels after percutaneous coronary intervention in patients with stable angina pectoris. *American Heart Journal*, Vol.149, No.5, (May 2005), pp.876-82, ISSN 0002-8703

Sandifer, QD., Vuilo, S. & Crompton, G. (1996) Association of Helicobacter pylori infection with coronary heart disease. Association may not be causal. *British Medical Journal*, Vol.312, No.7025, (January 1996), pp.251, ISSN 0959-8138

Sarkar, S., Thompson, DG., Woolf, CJ., Hobson, AR., Millane, T. & Aziz Q. (2004) Patients with chest pain and occult gastroesophageal reflux demonstrate visceral pain hypersensitivity which may be partially responsive to acid suppression. *American Journal of Gastroenterology*, Vol.99, No.10, (October 2004), pp.1998-2006, ISSN 0002-9270

Schofield, PM., Bennett, DH., Whorwell, PJ., Brooks, NH., Bray, CL., Ward, C. & Jones, PE. (1987) Exertional gastro-oesophageal reflux: a mechanism for symptoms in patients with angina pectoris and normal coronary angiograms. *British Medical Journal (Clin Res Ed)*, Vol.294, No.6585, (June 1987), pp.1459-61, ISSN 0267-0623

Schofield, PM., Whorwell, PJ., Brooks, NH., Bennett, DH. & Jones PE. (1989) Oesophageal function in patients with angina pectoris: a comparison of patients with normal coronary angiograms and patients with coronary artery disease. *Digestion*, Vol.42, No.2, (February 1989), pp.70-8, ISSN 0012-2823

Seo, TH., Kim, JH., Lee, JH., Ko, SY., Hong, SN., Sung, IK., Park, HS. & Shim, CS. (2010) Clinical distinct features of noncardiac chest pain in young patients. *Journal of Neurogastroenterology and Motility*, Vol.16, No.2, (April 2010), pp.166-71, ISSN 2093-0879

Shanker, J. & Kakkar, VV. (2009) Role of Periodontal Infection in Cardiovascular Disease: a Current Perspective. *Archives of Medical Sciences, Vol.*5, No.2, (April 2009), pp.125-134, ISSN 1734-1922

Sheps, DS., Creed, F. & Clouse, RE. (2004) Chest pain in patients with cardiac and noncardiac disease. *Psychosomatic Medicine.* Vol.66, No.6, (November- December 2004), pp.861-7, ISSN 0033-3174

Sifrim, D. & Blondeau, K. (2006) Technology insight: The role of impedance testing for esophageal disorders. *Nature Clinical Practice. Gastroenterology and Hepatology*, Vol.3, No.4, (April 2006), pp.210-9, ISSN 1743-4378

Sifrim, D., Blondeau, K. & Mantillla, L. (2009) Utility of non-endoscopic investigations in the practical management of oesophageal disorders. *Best Practice and Research. Clinical Gastroenterology*, Vol.23, No.3, (March 2009), pp.369-86, ISSN 1521-6918

Sifrim, D., Mittal, R., Fass, R., Smout, A., Castell, D, Tack, J. & Gregersen, H. (2007) Review article: acidity and volume of the refluxate in the genesis of gastro-oesophageal reflux disease symptoms. *Alimentary Pharmacology and Therapeutics*, Vol.25, No.9, (May 2007), pp.1003-17, ISSN 0269-2813

Singh, S., Richter, JE., Hewson, EG., Sinclair, JW. & Hackshaw, BT. (1992) The contribution of gastroesophageal reflux to chest pain in patients with coronary artery disease. *Annals of Internal Medicine*, Vol.117, No.10, (November 1992), pp.824-30, ISSN 0003-4819

Sorrentino, D., Bazzocchi, M., Badano, L., Toso, F. & Giagu, P. (2005) Heart-touching Chilaiditi 's syndrome. *World Journal of Gastroenterology, Vol.11, No.29,* (August 2005), pp.4607-4609, ISSN 1007-9327

Stec, S., Tarnowski, W., Kalin, K., Sikora, K. & Kołakowski P. (2010) High-resolution esophageal manometry with ECG monitoring for management of premature ventricular complexes-associated dysphagia. *Dysphagia*, Vol.25, No.1, (March 2010), pp.66-9, ISSN 0179-051X

Stöllberger, C. & Finsterer, J. (2003) Treatment of esophagitis/vagitis-induced paroxysmal atrial fibrillation by proton-pump inhibitors. *Journal of Gastroenterology,* Vol.38, No.11, pp.1109, ISSN 0944-1174

Swap, CJ. & Nagurney, JT. (2005) Value and limitations of chest pain history in the evaluation of patients with suspected acute coronary syndromes. *JAMA: Journal of American Medical Association.* Vol.294, No.20, (November 2005), pp.2623-9, ISSN 0098-7484

Świątkowski, M., Budzyński, J., Kłopocka, M., Pulkowski, G., Suppan, K., Fabisiak, J., Morawski, W. & Majer M. (2004) Suppression of gastric acid production may improve the course of angina pectoris and the results of treadmill stress test in patients with coronary artery disease. *Medical Science Monitor,* Vol.10, No.9, (September 2004), pp.CR524-529, ISSN 1234-1010

Talaie, R., Forootan, M., Donboli, K., Dadashzadeh, N., Sadeghi, A., Poorsaadat, S., Moghimi, B., Alizadeh, AH. & Zali MR. (2009) 24-hour ambulatory pH-metry in patients with refractory heartburn: a prospective study. *Journal of Gastrointestinal and Liver Diseases*, Vol.18, No.1, (March 2009), pp.11-5, ISSN 1841-8724

Thor, PJ. & Błaut, U. (2006) Helicobacter pylori infection in pathogenesis of gastroesophageal reflux disease. *Journal of Physiology and Pharmacology,* Vol.57, Suppl 3, (September 2006), pp.81-90, ISSN 0867-5910

Tipnis, NA., Rhee, PL. & Mittal, RK. (2007) Distension during gastroesophageal reflux: effects of acid inhibition and correlation with symptoms. *American Journal of Physiology Gastrointestinal Liver Physiology,* Vol.293, No.2, (August 2007), pp.G469-74, ISSN 0193-1857

To, AC., Armstrong, G., Zeng, I. & Webster MW. (2009) Noncardiac surgery and bleeding after percutaneous coronary intervention. *Circulation. Cardiovascular Interventions,* Vol.2, No.3, (April 2009), pp.213-21, ISSN 1941-7640

Tougas, G., Spaziani, R., Hollerbach, S., Djuric, V., Pang, C., Upton, AR., Fallen, EL. & Kamath, MV. (2001) Cardiac autonomic function and oesophageal acid sensitivity in patients with non-cardiac chest pain. *Gut* Vol.49, No.5, (November 2001), pp.706–12, ISSN 0017-5749

Upile, T., Jerjes, W., El Maaytah, M., Singh, S., Hopper, C. & Mahil, J. (2006) Reversible atrial fibrillation secondary to a mega-oesophagus. *BMC Ear Nose Throat Disord,* Vol.6, No.15, (December 2006), pp.1-4, ISSN 1472-6815

Vakil, N., van Zanten, SV., Kahrilas, P., Dent, J., Jones, R. & Global Consensus Group. (2006) The Montreal definition and classification of gastroesophageal reflux disease: a global evidence-based consensus. *American Journal of Gastroenterology,* Vol.101, No.8, (August 2006), pp.1900-20, ISSN 0002-9270

Wang, WH., Huang, JQ., Zheng, GF., Wong, WM., Lam, SK., Karlberg, J., Xia, HH., Fass, R. & Wong, BC. (2005) Is proton pump inhibitor testing an effective approach to diagnose gastroesophageal reflux disease in patients with noncardiac chest pain?: a meta-analysis. *Archives of Internal Medicine*, Vol.165, No.11, (June 2005), pp.1222-8, ISSN 0003-9926

Weigl, M., Gschwantler, M., Gatterer, E., Finsterer, J. & Stöllberger, C. (2003) Reflux esophagitis in the pathogenesis of paroxysmal atrial fibrillation: results of a pilot study. Southern Medical Journal, Vol.96, No.11, (November 2003), pp.1128-32, ISSN 0038-4348

Wood, JD. (2007) Neuropathophysiology of functional gastrointestinal disorders. *World Journal of Gastroenterology*, Vol.13, No.9, (March 2007), pp.1313-32, ISSN 1007-9327

Würtz, M., Grove, EL., Kristensen, SD. & Hvas, AM. (2010) The Antiplatelet Effect of Aspirin is Reduced by Proton Pump Inhibitors in Patients With Coronary Artery Disease. *Heart*, Vol.96, No.5, (November 2009), pp.368-71, ISSN 1355-6037

Yin, J. & Chen, JD. (2010) Gastrointestinal motility disorders and acupuncture. *Autonomic Neuroscience: basic and clinical*, Vol.157, No.(1-2), (October 2010), pp.31-7, ISSN 1566-0702

Zhang, CX., Qin, YM. & Guo, BR. (2010) Clinical study on the treatment of gastroesophageal reflux by acupuncture. *Chinese Journal of Integrated Medicine*, Vol.16, No.4, (August 2010), pp.298-303, ISSN 1672-0415

Zhu, A., Kaneshiro, M. & Kaunitz, JD. (2010) Evaluation and treatment of iron deficiency anemia: a gastroenterological perspective. *Digestive Diseases and Science*, Vol.55, No.3, (March 2010), pp.548-59, ISSN 0163-2116.

3

Conventional and Novel Pharmacotherapy of Angina Pectoris

Solmaz Dehghan
School of Pharmacy and Pharmaceutical Sciences,
Mashhad University of Medical Sciences, Mashhad
Iran

1. Introduction

As it has been mentioned in the previous chapters, Angina pectoris, commonly known as angina, is severe chest pain and discomfort due to myocardial ischemia. A lack of blood, hence a lack of oxygen supply for heart muscle, will cause this pain which can be because of narrowed and blocked coronary arteries. In other words, angina can be assumed to play the role of a protective mechanism to signal myocardial ischemia.

There are different kinds of angina. Stable, unstable, Prinzmetal's or variant angina and latterly discovered type called microvascular angina which is caused by small blood vessels, not artery damage.

Although the amount of mortalities and morbidities of heart diseases and additionally the diagnostic techniques in this field underwent drastic improvements, still there are many patients complaining about angina pectoris mostly as a restricting pain. Due to the report of American Heart Association statistics committee and stroke statistics subcommittee in 2010, the prevalence of angina pectoris has become 9.8 million, translating to almost 30 thousand per million. This amount in Europe has been estimated to be around 20 - 40 thousand per million (Fox, Garcia et al. 2006; Fernandez, Tandar et al. 2010; Lioyd-Jones, Adams et al. 2010). In another study performed in US, it has been mentioned that 1 in 4 patients is experiencing angina pectoris following myocardial infarction. With regard to the annual occurrence of MI in US which is 1.5 million cases, there are significant amount of people in each year suffering from angina. Therefore, curing angina pectoris is of high importance (Plomondon, Magid et al. 2007).

Although one of the main goals in angina treatment is relief of symptoms, amelioration of the position, especially pain, will unexpectedly cause the ischemia to proceed and so, the consequence will be cardiac injury. Considering this problem, due to American and European drug regulators the anti-anginal medicines also needs to possess anti-ischemia effects, as well. Other purposes of angina pectoris treatment are slowing progression of the disease and reduction of future events, especially heart attacks and, of course, death by treating the underlying heart condition. Treatments for angina include lifestyle changes, medicines, medical procedures, cardiac rehabilitation, and other therapies and will depend on the severity of the symptoms, severity of the underlying disease, and extent of damage to the heart muscle, if any (Parker and Parker 2002; Fernandez, Tandar et al. 2010).

In recent decades, pharmaceutical scientists focus has been on design of systems which can manage to release the medication with a steady or a controlled speed. These delivery systems are called "novel".
The application of novel drug delivery systems in angina therapy show their importance through controlling release of a medication with short therapeutic index or decreasing the drug dosage intervals which can increase patients' compliance in following up the therapy or even it can control the release of drug according to the chronobiology (Dehghan, Aboofazeli et al. 2010; Mandal, Biswas et al. 2010).
In this chapter, medications and pharmacotherapy of angina pectoris will be mainly discussed. At the end of chapter one will be informed of conventional and novel medications for treatment of angina.

2. Anti-angina currently used medicines

In angina therapy drugs are playing an important role. A variety of medicines with different dosage forms and amounts are prescribed in each type of angina. Since the main cause of angina is lack of oxygen supply in the coronary arteries, the anti-anginal agents usually play their roles through increasing oxygen delivery or decreasing oxygen requirement of the tissue or both. Obviously, ascending the amount of oxygen delivery is possible with vasodilation and reduced oxygen demand can be caused by cardioinhibitors which reduce heart rate and contractility. There are still other mechanisms that may occur in treating angina pectoris. For instance, anti-thrombotic drugs which avoid formation of thrombus, like anticoagulants, are involved in angina therapy. Figure 1 shows a schematic classification of conventional anti-anginal medications.
Regularly, in angina pharmacotherapy, medications are prescribed for three different purposes. 1) To reduce the number of angina attacks by daily use of certain drugs over a

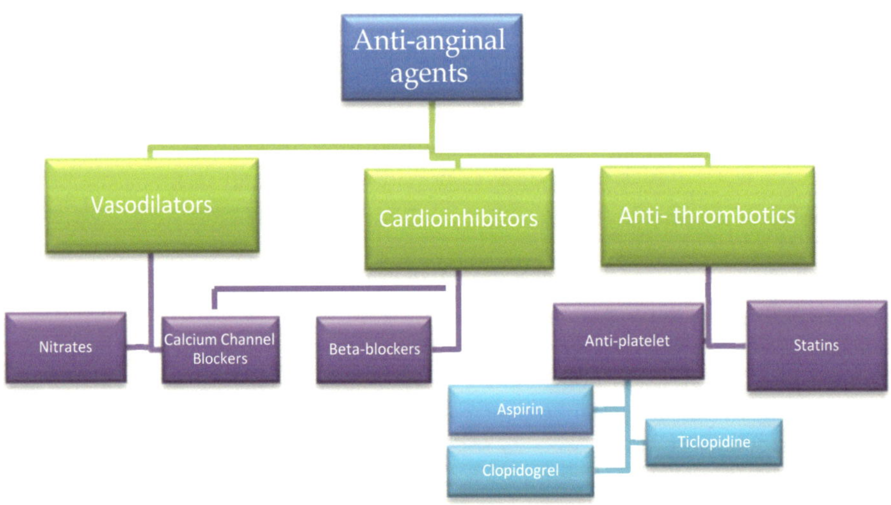

Fig. 1. Conventional medicines used in treatment of angina pectoris

long period. 2) To prevent attacks before some exercises or robust activities. 3) To relief the pain and pressure of an attack when it begins.
Generally, there are five main types of medicines, which help to relief, control symptoms and increase blood flow and oxygen supply to the heart muscle:

- Nitrates
- Beta-blockers
- Calcium channel blockers
- Anti-platelets
- Statin drugs

Moreover, due to the patient's condition, other medications can be prescribed by the specialist, as well. And also these drugs can be prescribed in combination which in most cases it works more efficiently than monotherapy.

2.1 Nitrates and nitrites

Here the term "nitrates" is taken to include both nitrates and nitrites avoiding repetition. But it is presumed that the nitrates can only reduce to nitrites for exerting their action.
Nitrates are one of the oldest medications for angina. They are potent vasodilators that open up the arteries, improving blood flow to the body (including heart) which raises the oxygen supply of myocardium. There are two kinds of nitrates: short acting nitrate preparation and long acting nitrate preparation. Short acting ones usually are used to ease angina pains and/or to prevent developing an anginal attack before an exercise that is likely to cause one. Whilst the long acting productions are prescribed in a regular daily basis for the patients with frequent anginal pains and it is not useful for rapid pain relief.
The most important drug of this group is Nitroglycerin (glyceryl trinitrate) which was the first medication used in 1879 by William Murrell for the treatment of angina pectoris and, its immediate release forms, still remains the therapeutic mainstay for patients suffering from classic and variant angina. Nitroglycerin is often administered sublingually for rapid relief of angina sudden attack (Murrell 1879). The main drugs of this group include: nitroglycerin or glyceyl trinitrate (GTN), isosorbide dinitrate, isosorbide mononitrate, pentaerythritol tetranitrate (PETN) and amyl nitrite.

2.1.1 Mechanism of action

Nitrates in the smooth muscle of both venous and arterial beds, are denitrated into nitric oxide (NO) which is a potent vasodilator. This vasodilatation relieves anginal pain through different mechanisms. Veins dilation will reduce cardiac workload and consequently, oxygen demand. Coronary dilation will increase blood flow to ischemic areas. And finally dilation of arterioles will lower the afterload and so cardiac workload.
The released NO from nitrates activates guanylate cyclase and increases the amount of cyclic guanine monophosphate (cGMP). cGMP which is a second messenger, activates protein kinase. Myosin light chains dephosphorylate by protein kinase. As a result, the smooth muscle becomes relaxed. Additionally, decreased intracellular calcium levels by cGMP are another mechanism of smooth muscle relaxation (Katzung, Masters et al. 2009).

2.1.2 Pharmacokinetics

The nitrates undergo first-pass effect in liver excluding isosorbide mononitrate. Thus, despite their high absorption from the GI, nitrates absorption into the systemic circulation is

incomplete; i.e., oral preparations have slow onset of action (except sublingual tablets) which is not pleasant when quick relief is required. So, there are available dosage forms with short onset time.
Nitrates distribute extensively throughout the body and their bonding to plasma protein has been estimated to be around 60%.
Nitrates undergo metabolism in liver by the enzyme glutathione organic nitrate reductase. For example the yielded active metabolites for nitroglycerin are glyceryl dinitrates and mononitrates.
The metabolites of nitrates are excreted in urine, except isosorbide moninitrate, that less than 1% of it is eliminated in urine. Elimination half-lives of nitrates differ depending on the kind of nitrate and administration route. Table 1 indicates elimination half-lives of some preparation of nitrates.

2.1.3 Adverse reactions

Acute side effects: Throbbing headache and dizziness are the most common side effect of nitrates (these are probably consequences of blood vessles vasodilation). Orthostatic hypotension is another common side effect of using nitrates. There is a rare situation named "nitrite syncope". In which the nitrate-induced hypotension is severe and thus, the lowered blood pressure will cause slowing of heart rate, nausea, shivering and syncope. The adverse effects of gastrointestinal tract include nausea and vomiting.
Nitrate tolerance: Continuous uptake of nitrates (any kind) in high dose may cause tolerance. In tolerance, the nitrate's effect will become weak or disappear completely. Although, the mechanism of tolerance has been poorly understood but diminished amount of nitric oxide and systemic compensation can be partly responsible for this phenomenon. The well-known so called "Monday disease" is a touchable example of nitrate tolerance that has happened in industries, especially where explosives are manufactured(Rutherford 1995; Munzel, Daiber et al. 2005).

2.1.4 Dosage forms

According to different indications of nitrates, considering two main groups of long- and short- acting nitrates, there are a wide range of preparation forms to fulfill the patients' demands (table 1).
Short acting and long acting anti-anginal agents are being prescribed due to their onset and duration of action. For rapid cardiac response, nitroglycerin formulations with short onset (sublingual tablets or pump sprays) are administered. At the commencement of an attach, exactly when the patient starts to feel the chest pain or before starting an activity, one 0.3 or 0.4 mg pill or one metered dose of spray can be taken and patient can repeat it every 5 minutes, if necessary, up to maximum three doses. These dosage ranges for isosorbide dinitrate is fairly different. In this case, sublingual 2.5 to 10 mg tablets should be taken. The repetition dose is every 2-3 hours during acute phase and 4-6 hours for prophylaxis.
Long acting nitroglycerin sustained-release tablets are prescribed 2.5-13 mg every 6-12 hours. Alternatively, the topical form or the patches can be used instead. Isosorbide dinitrate extended-release formulations are administered 40-80 mg twice daily.
In any case, it is necessary to have 10-12 hours nitrate-free interval per day due to prevention of nitrate tolerance (Cutler, Eff et al. 1995; Katzung, Masters et al. 2009).

Kind of nitrate	Dosage form	Amount of active agent	Elimination half-life
Nitroglycerin	Tablets (sublingual)	0.15, 0.3, 0.4 and 0.6 mg	1/2-1 hr
	Tablets (buccal and controlled-release)	1, 2 and 3 mg	3-5 hr buccal
	Capsules (sustained-release)	2.5, 6.5, 9 and 13 mg	5 hr
	Aerosol (lingual)	0.4 mg/metered spray	1/2-1 hr
	I.V.	0.5, 0.8 and 5 mg/ml	3-5 min
	I.V. premixed solutions in dextrose	100, 200 and 400 mcg/ml	
	Topical	2% ointment	2-12 hr
	Transdermal (patches)	0.1, 0.2, 0.4, 0.6 and 0.8 mg/hour systems	24 hr
Isosorbide dinitrate	Tablets	5, 10, 20, 30 and 40 mg	5-6 hr
	Tablets (sublingual)	2.5, 5 and 10 mg	1/2-2 hr
	Tablets (extended-release)	40 mg	5-6 hr
	Tablets (chewable)	5 and 10 mg	1/2-2 hr
	Capsules (extended-release)	40 mg	5-6 hr
Isosorbide mononitrate	Tablets	10 and 20 mg	Unknown
	Tablets (extended-release)	30, 60 and 120 mg	
Amyl nitrite	Solution (inhalation)	50 mg	5 min

Table 1. Commercialized dosage forms of nitrates (Christensen, Comerford et al. 2003).

2.2 Beta blockers

Beta blockers have been used for over 35 years to treat both angina and high blood pressure (hypertension). These medications through beta blockade slow the heart rate, decrease blood pressure, and lessen the force of contraction of the heart muscle, however, the third generation of beta blockers show to have vasodilatory effects through different pathways which will be discussed more in section 2.2.1. When taken regularly, beta-blockers are proven to prevent heart attacks and mortality and reduce the frequency of angina attacks (reinfarction). Because of their effects on the respiratory system, beta-blockers are unsuitable for angina sufferers who have asthma or bronchitis. Carvedilol, propranolol and atenolol are some of most important beta blockers.

2.2.1 Mechanism of action

There are three types of beta receptors in the body that control several different functions. Beta-1 receptors are located mostly in heart muscle and also in eye and kidneys, whilst the prominent part of beta-2 receptors are in upper respiratory system (bronchial vascular smooth muscle); however, there are a few beta-2 receptors in heart muscle. And finally beta-3 receptors are distributed in adipose tissue. The beta receptors are targets of cathecolamines, especially noradernaline (norepinephrine) and adernaline (epinephrine). In fact, beta blockers induce their effect by preventing the normal ligand (cathecolamines) from binding to beta receptors. Due to their distribution sites in body, beta-1 and beta-2 blockers are of interest in angina therapy. Preventing adrenaline's performance on heart by beta blockers causes lower heart rate, contractility and blood pressure and in one words reduced heart's workload. Thus, the myocardial oxygen demand will decrease and this final effect is assumed to be the most important effect of beta blockers in angina treatment. The final function of beta blockers owing to their ability to be selective or nonselective, cause them to have different indications. The nonselective beta antagonists, blockade both beta-1 and beta-2 receptors, whereas, the selective ones only block beta-1 receptors (cardioselective beta blockers). These two groups of agents that are used in angina pharmacotherapy are listed in table 2, seperately.

Nonselective Beta blockers useful in angina treatment	Selective Beta blockers useful in angina treatment
Carvedilol	Acebutolol
Labetalol	Atenolol
Nadolol	Betaxolol
Penbutolol	Bisoprolol
Pindolol	Metoprolol
Propranolol	
Timolol	

Table 2. Selective and nonselective anti-anginal beta blockers

As it was mentioned before, the third generation of beta-adrenoceptor antagonists comprises drugs with extra ability of vasodilatation. Most of them play their role by blocking alpha-1 receptor (labetalol, carvedilol and bucindolol). Nebivolol is the exception of third generation; because, the vasodilatation mechanism of this beta-1 highly selective blocker is by stimulating nitric oxide release (Weiss 2006; Karter 2007).

2.2.2 Pharmacokinetics

Most of beta blockers are quickly absorbed after oral administration (generally from small intestine). Moreover, their systemic absorption after topical application has been confirmed to be without significant delay. However, there are pharmacokinetical differences in the

drugs of this category which is mostly because of their hydrophilic or lipophilic affinities. For example the absorption of hydrophilic beta blockers such as nadolol and atenolol from GI is incomplete. Furthermore, this characteristics influence beta blockers indications, as well. Since, the lipophilic beta antagonists can pass blood brain barrier and enter CNS (propranolol), they are used in prophylactic treatment of migraine or vascular headache.
Beta adrenoceptor antagonists' distribution in body is also influenced by this quality. The lipophilic beta blockers are more detected in biologic fluids.
Due to solubility of beta blockers in water or lipid, their metabolism and elimination can be through liver or kidneys; i.e. drugs with low lipophilicity are excreted from kidneys, whilst more lipophilic substances are metabolized in liver.

2.2.3 Adverse reaction

Beta blockers are widely prescribed throughout the world in several remedies and they do not seem to have many severe side effects. Nevertheless, their most important unpleasant effects are due to inhibitory effect of nonselectives on beta-2 receptors. Since beta-2 receptors are mainly in bronchi, beta-2 antagonists hinder opposing the alpha 1 receptor-mediated vasoconstructor tone. Thus the patients with any dysfunction in their airways will experience serious problems. To overcome this disadvantage, new class of beta blockers with beta-1 selectivity and partial beta-2 agonist ability, has emerged. Beta-1 antagonists are preferable to the prior beta blockers, however, since bronchospasm was reported in certain individuals followed by selective beta blockers uptake, they are not considered completely "safe".
Other adverse effects experienced by the patients are dizziness and lightheadedness accompanied by blurred vision. Some people may feel cold in their hands and feet as a result of decreased blood pressure, especially to the extremities. Moreover, beta blocker consumption may cause some allergic reactions like rashes and itching.

2.2.4 Dosage forms

Available formulations of beta blockers have been summarized in table 3.
Among these drugs, betaxolol, bisoprolol, nadolol and penbutolol are prescribed for angina prophylaxis, while others are used in treatment of angina attacks.

Generic name of beta receptor antagonist	Dosage form	Amount of active agent	Dosage range
Acebutolol	Capsules	200 & 400 mg	200 mg twice daily up to 800 mg and even higher, if necessary
Atenolol	Tablets	25, 50 & 100 mg	50 mg once daily and can be adjusted after one week. Maximum daily dose is 200 mg

Generic name of beta receptor antagonist	Dosage form	Amount of active agent	Dosage range
Betaxolol	Tablets (film-coated)	10 & 20 mg	10-20 mg once a day. Can be increased to 50 mg/day after one or two weeks of inadequate response
Bisoprolol	Tablets	5 & 10 mg	5 mg per day, can be increased every three days, up to 20 mg
Carvedilol	Tablets		Started with 6.25mg twice a day and can be continued up to 50mg per day
Labetalol (Quyyumi, Wright et al. 1985)	Tablets (film-coated)	100, 200 & 300 mg	
Metoprolol	Tablets	50 & 100 mg	100 to 400 mg in divided doses
	Tablets (extended-release)	25, 50, 100 & 200 mg	100 to 400 mg daily
Nadolol	Tablets	20, 40, 80, 120 & 160 mg	40 mg per day. Can be increased up to even 240 in certain time intervals
Penbutolol	Tablets	20 mg	20-40 mg once a day
Pindolol	Tablets	5 & 10 mg	15 to 40 mg divided doses per day
Propranolol	Capsules (extended-release)	60, 80, 120 & 160 mg	Tablets or solution can be administered 40-320 mg in three or four doses daily and the long-acting forms are given once a day, however, it can increase
	Tablets	10, 20, 40, 60 & 80 mg	
	Solution	4, 8 & 80 mg/ml	
Timolol	Tablets	5, 10 & 20 mg	10-30 mg twice daily(Arronow, 1980)

Table 3. Beta blockers dosage forms which are used as anti-anginal agents (Christensen, Comerford et al. 2003)

2.3 Calcium channel blockers (CCBs)

Calcium channel blockers, also called slow calcium channel antagonists or slow channel blockers, inhibit calcium ion movement through slow channels in cardiac and smooth muscles. CCBs are mostly used for treatment of classic and variant angina. Also, they are particularly beneficial if angina is caused by arterial spasms (Prinzmetal's variant angina) rather than blockage.

Drugs of this category are classified into two classes, dihydropyridines (DHPs) and non-dihydropyridines (non-DHPs). The non-DHPs are again comprises of three further compounds: phenylalkylamines, benzothiazepines and tertralols (Ryman and Gurk-Turner 1999). The most selective calcium channel blockers belong to dihydropyridines.

2.3.1 Mechanisms of action

CCBs blockade the calcium ion influx into vascular smooth muscle cells and cardiac myocytes across the voltage gated slow channels. Thus the intracellular calcium levels will diminish. Since, the most important ion for muscle contractility is assumed to be calcium, as a result of decreased calcium levels, vasodilatation of both coronary and peripheral arteries and lower cardiac conduction will be observed. Vasodilatations will cause low blood pressure and consequently, less heart afterload and oxygen demand.

2.3.2 Pharmacokinetics

CCBs are usually well absorbed following oral administration, although they can have different bioavailability due to their metabolism.

They are widely distributed in body fluids with a high protein-binding affinity. It is proved that protein binding percentage of dihydropyridines is higher than non-dihydropyridines.

Most of Calcium channel blockers are metabolized and cleared hepatically and less than 5% is secreted unchanged in urine. And some of them undergo extensive first-pass metabolism which will influence drug's plasma level and half life. Thus, it should be taken into account in dose adjustment.

Elimination half-lives of old CCBs are rather short (3-8 hours), whereas the newer ones (esp. new DHPs) have been designed to last longer in body (Opie 1989; Piepho 1991).

2.3.3 Adverse reactions

Generally, the side effects of CCBs are not really common but still the incidence of some adverse reactions has been reported in a number of patients. Peripheral vasodilatation accounts for the major side effects of DHPs like flushing, headache, rashes, excessive hypotension, peripheral edema (esp. Pedal edema) and palpitation (reflecting reflex tachycardia) (Sirker, Missouris et al. 2001). The later effect is the reason that most of DHPs are not preferred in treatment of angina pectoris.

Non-DHPs side effects are mostly because of the muscle relaxation effect; for instance, they can cause severe bradycardia, or can influence electrical conduction system of heart. This relaxation in smooth muscles of intestine and colon may cause constipation. Constipation is followed by verapamil administration.

2.3.4 Dosage forms

Two main classes of slow channel blockers, have different mode of actions and thus, diverse indications. Although all calcium channel blockers seem to be effective in treatment of stable

angina, causing reflex tachycardia, the dihydropyridines usually are not administered for this purpose. The only FDA approved DHPs as the treatments for angina are nifedipine, amlodipine, nicardipine and biperidil of which nifedipine and amlodipine are used in both vasospastic and chronic stable angina, while biperidil and nicardipine's application is limited to just chronic stable angina (Ryman and Gurk-Turner 1999; Helms, Quan et al. 2006). Table 4 displays dosage forms of some CCBs which are used in angina therapy.
Mibefradil, of tertralol subgroup, was used as an anti-anginal agent but was withdrawn from the market because of serious interactions with other drugs.

Dihydropyrodines			
Generic name of beta receptor antagonist	Dosage form	Amount of active agent	Dosage range
Amlodipine	Tablets	2.5, 5 & 10 mg	5-10 mg daily
Nicardipine	Capsules	20 & 30 mg	20-40 mg three times a day
Nifedipine	Capsules	10 & 20 mg	10-20 mg three times a day, can increase due to patients position
	Tablets (extended-release)	30, 60 & 90 mg	30 to 60 mg once daily
Bepridil	Tablets (film-coated)	200 & 300 mg	200 up to maximum 400 mg daily
Non-dihydropyridines			
Generic name of beta receptor antagonist	Dosage form	Amount of active agent	Dosage range
Diltiazem	Tablets	30, 60, 90 & 120 mg	Start with 30 mg three times a day and can be increase up to 360 mg divided doses per day
	Capsules (extended-release) (Containing multiple 60-mg units of diltiazem)	120, 180 & 240 mg	120-480 mg once daily(Cutler, 1995)
	Capsules (sustained-release)	60, 90, 120, 180, 240, 300, 360 & 420 mg	
Verapamil	Tablets	40, 80 & 120 mg	
	Tablets (sustained-release and extended-release)	120, 180 &240 mg	

	Capsules (sustained-release)	100, 120, 180, 200,240, 300 & 360 mg
	Capsules (extended-release)	120, 180 & 240 mg

Table 4. Calcium channel blockers administered in angina therapy (dosage forms and dosing ranges) (Christensen, Comerford et al. 2003)

2.4 Anti-platelets

These anti-thrombotic drugs prevent platelet clumping and so thrombus formation in blood circulation. There are several subgroups of antiplatelets such as: cyclooxygenase inhibitors, adenosine diphosphate (ADP) receptor inhibitors (contains thienopyridines), glycoprotein IIB/IIIA inhibitors and adenosine reuptake inhibitors. Anti-plateletes, dislike anti-coagulants, have the most anti-clot effect in arterial circulation. Since aspirin and clopidogrel are this group's mainly prescribed drugs in angina, in this section they will be discussed in details. Ticlopidine is another thienopyridine that has been shown to have effects on treatment of unstable angina. But according to the results of some studies, ticlopidine have more adverse effects than clopidogrel (Hankey, Sudlow et al. 2000).

Aspirin has clot-preventing properties within the coronary arteries or other blood vessels. Daily aspirin therapy is advised to patients, unless they have problems tolerating it. In this case, clopidogrel can be used instead. However, one recent study showed that in patients suffering stable angina, treatment with aspirin and clopidogrel indicates greater platelet formation blockade rather than monotherapy with aspirin alone (Saha, Berglund et al. 2008).

2.4.1 Mechanism of action

Since aspirin has many indications, it can act through different biologic pathways. Aspirin anti-platelet and with less importance anti-inflammatory effects are believed to be the main mechanisms in treating angina pectoris.

Anti-platelet and anti-inflammatory: While administered in low doses, aspirin inhibits prostaglandin synthetase action and therefore avoid clotting followed by preventing thromboxane A_2, the platelet-aggregating substance, formation. Aspirin owes this ability of prostaglandins and thromboxanes suppression to irreversible inactivation of the cyclooxygenase (COX) enzyme. As the chemical structure of aspirin can be observed in fig.2, its free acetyl group is attached to a serine residue in the active site of COX enzyme through a covalent bond. This is the reason of difference between aspirin and the similar anti-inflammatory NSAIDs group which are reversible inhibitors.

Although if the dose of aspirin rises, it will interferes with prostacyclin production and so this will negate the anticlotting properties.

The exact mechanism of aspirin's anti-inflammatory action is not completely understood but it is mostly believed that the ability to inhibit prostaglandin synthesis can influence synthesis or action of other mediators of inflammation by restraining them.

Clopidogrel is a selective adenosine diphosphate (ADP) antagonist. It irreversibly blocks the ADP receptor on the platelet cell membrane and consequently the glycoprotein IIb/IIIa cannot be activated and so platelet aggregation will be avoided (Savi, Nurden et al. 1998).

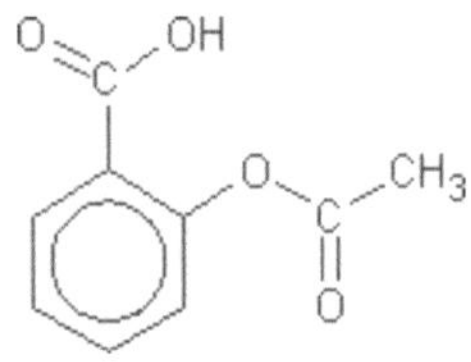

Fig. 2. Chemical structure of aspirin

2.4.2 Pharmacokinetics

Since aspirin is a weak organic acid with a pK_a equal to 3.5, in oral dosage form it is expected to absorb in stomach and proximal small intestine in nonionized form; because in these areas the acidic environment dominates.

Suddenly after absorption it is metabolized into acetic acid and salicylate. This rapid metabolism is resulting in high concentrations of salicylates in most body liquids and fluids. Therapeutic salicylate blood level for anti-inflammatory effect is 150 to 300 mcg/ml. Salicylates have rather high protein binding ranged from 75 to 90% depending on blood level.

Salicylate is excreted by the kidneys with first-order kinetics and its elimination half-life has estimated to be between 2 and 4.5 hours depending on the aspirin administered dose (in toxic doses this range reaches 15 to 30 hours) (Hartwig-Otto 1983).

Clopidogrel is a prodrug and after rapid oral absorption, it is converted to the active agent in liver. The half life of this active agent is 8 hours.

Clopidogrel is eliminated almost equally from urine and feces.

2.4.3 Adverse reactions

One of the main adverse effects of aspirin is gastric upset. Especially when taken in high doses the risk of gastrointestinal bleeding increases. Aspirin uptake can be also accompanied by nausea and heartburn.

The patient taking aspirin is advised to be monitored frequently; the main reason is because it may cause leucopenia, thrombocytopenia and prolonged bleeding time.

Other rare but severe side effects include Rey's syndrome, anaphylaxis and angioedema.

Some of clopidogrel's side effects are neutropenia, hemorrhage and skin rash.

2.4.4 Dosage forms

There are several dosage forms of these medications available in the market. As aspirin is considered to be multifunctional, the only forms that can be used in treatment of angina are in table 5.

2.5 Statins

Statins or HMG CoA reductase inhibitors, lower cholesterol and have been shown to stabilize the fatty plaque on the inner lining of the coronary artery, even when the blood cholesterol is normal or minimally increased. Due to recent research statins can atorvastatin, fluvastatin, lovastatin, pravastatin, and simvastatin (Dehghan, Aboofazeli et al. 2010; Dvir and Battler 2010).

2.5.1 Mechanisms of action

Since hyperlipidemia has been proved to be one of the main reasons for coronary heart diseases, lowering lipid levels in bloods can decrease the incidence of cardiovascular

disease. The most effective impact of statins on the patients suffering from anginal attacks is believed to be through lowering the LDL cholesterol level in plasma (Khan 2006).
HMG CoA reductase is an enzyme responsible for mevalonate production. In lipid forming pathway, mevalonate is finally transformed to cholesterol. Statins which have some structural similarities with this HMG CoA, can competitively attach to the enzyme and block it. Therefore, the speed of cholesterol biosynthesis will decline. Statins play their role in angina therapy through other mechanisms, as well.
Researchers have defined some other modes of actions for statins, rather than lipid lowering, in managing heart related diseases like anti-inflammatory, plaque stability and prevention of clotting. These beneficial effects are independent from lipid lowering characteristics (Furberg 1999).

Name	Drug Form	Amount of Active Agent	Dosage Ranges
Aspirin	**Tablets**	81 and 325 mg	Prevention doses: 81 to 325mg daily or every other day; Treatment doses: 160 to 325mg once daily
	Tablets (enteric-coated)	81, 100, 162, 165 and 325 mg	
	Tablets (chewable)	81 and 100 mg	
	Tablets (effervescent)	100 mg	
	Suppositories	120, 125, 200 and 300 mg	
Clopidogrel	**Tablets**	75 mg	75 mg once a day

Table 5. Available dosage forms of aspirin and clopidogrel for angina treatment

2.5.2 Pharmacokinetics

The pharmacokinetic characteristics of statins vary widely due to their different structures which determine their water or lipid solubility. Quite lipophilic statins are atorvastatin, simvastatin, lovastatin, fluvastatin, cerivastatin and pitavastatin; whereas pravastatin and rosuvastatin are relatively hydrophilic. Obviously, the lipophilic compounds have rapid absorption and distribute easily in biologic fluids.
Almost all of lipophilic statins are metabolized hepatically by cytochrome P450 enzymes and due to their efficient first-pass effect their bioavailability varies from 5% to 60%. Whilst, the hydrophilic statins have longer half lives and excreted both through liver and kidneys.
HMG CoA reductase inhibitors have half lives ranged from less than 5 hours in simvastatin up to 22 hours in pravastatin and 20 - 30 hour in some metabolites of atorvastatin (Garcia, Reinoso et al. 2003; Schachter 2004).

2.5.3 Adverse reactions

Although statins considered being among the safest drugs, the most important but infrequent side effect of statins is because of their metabolism pathway (cytochrome P450) which can cause myopathy and hepatotoxicity and of course serious interactions with other substances. Myopathy appears as pain and weakness in muscles and rarely rhabdomyolysis. One of statins called cerivasatin was withdrawn from the market due to fatal rhabdomyolysis reports, in 2001.

Other side effects address the liver. Statins can increase amount of hepatic enzymes. This increase, if severe, will cause liver damage. Therefore, the medication can be changed to another statin.

2.5.4 Dosage forms

Atorvastatin, fluvastatin, pravastatin, rosuvastatin and simvastatin are frequently prescribed as treatments of angina pectoris. More information about the different formulations and dosage of these drugs can be found in table 6.

Generic name of beta receptor antagonist	Dosage form	Amount of active agent	Dosage range
Atorvastatin	Tablets (film-coated)	10, 20, 40 & 80 mg	Starting with 10-40 mg once a day, can be increased up to 80 mg daily for maintenance dose
Fluvastatin	Capsules	20 & 40 mg	20 to 80 mg divided doses
	Tablets (extended-release)	80 mg	80 mg once a day
Pravastatin	Tablets	10, 20, 40 & 80 mg	Usually 40 or 80 mg/day, however, it can be 10 or 20 mg in renal or hepatic dysfunction
Rosuvastatin	Tablets	5, 10, 20 & 40 mg	5 to 40 mg once daily (max starting dose is 20 mg)
Simvastatin	Tablets	5, 10, 20, 40 & 80 mg	Starting from 5 or 10 mg and continue with up to 80 mg

Table 6. Statins used in angina therapy.

3. New drugs with novel mechanisms of action

3.1 Ranolazine

Ranolazine is a piperazine derivative which has been proved as an anti-anginal and anti-ischemic agent. Although its mode of action is totally different from other anti-anginal medications and is not clearly understood, some studies show that ranolazine main mechanism in angina is through blockade of late Na current in sarcolemma (late I_{Na}).

In patients with heart failure and chronic angina, in addition to normal Na flow into cells there is a late Na ion current which increases intracellular Na levels. Elevated levels of Na in the cell influence Ca flow and finally contractility of myocardium, leading to incomplete

relaxation and heart muscle dysfunction. Ranolazine by inhibition of late Na current helps the ischemic condition to recover (Maier 2009).
Ralolazine has a variable absorption after oral administration. It is highly metabolized in liver and intestine. Ranolazine excreted into both feces and urine.
This drug is available as extended-release tablets and usually is prescribed 500 to 1000 mg once daily (FDA 2006; Dvir and Battler 2010).

3.2 Nicorandil

Nicorandil is a nicotinamide ester that is classified as an ATP- sensitive potassium channel opener and it has also some nitrate-like activating effects. This medication is a vasodilator able to dilate both arterial and venous systems resulting in reduced pre- and afterload.
Nicorandil's nitrate component is responsible for venous vasodilatation and the arteries and arterioles vasodilatation is developed by opening K^+ channels.
This potassium channel agonist is highly absorbed from GI. It is not seriously undergo first-pass effect thus it is expected to have high bioavailability (75-100%). Its major route of elimination is kidneys.
Gastrointestinal ulceration and discomfort, headache, flushing and weakness have been reported to be main adverse reactions to nicorandil (Frydman 1992; Hiremath, Valluru et al. 2010).

3.3 Ivabradine

Ivabradine is the first specific and selective inhibitor of the I_f channel in the sinus node become commercialized (I_f is a name for mixed Na+-K+ inward flow). This drug has bradycardic effects and lowers the heart rate that may prevent myocardial ischemia and angina pectoris; however its pharmacologic benefits have not been proved to be useful in the whole patients suffering from stable angina. It may be used in patients who have beta-blockers intolerance.
Ivabradine is being absorbed completely and has a bioavailability around 40% due to first-pass effect. Its elimination is mainly through hepatic metabolism.
Since the f channels are located in the retina as well, the major side effects accompanying ivabradine consumption are visual symptoms like headache, dizziness and luminous/visual phenomenon. Thus, ivabradine may influence driving task (Macher and Levy 2009; Dvir and Battler 2010; Farrer 2010; Fernandez, Tandar et al. 2010).

3.4 Trimetazidine

Trimetazidine is a metabolic agent which is considered as the first cytoprotective anti-ischemic compound. This drug inhibits fatty acid metabolism by partially blocking 3-ketoacyl CoA thiolase. And by this means, enhances the glucose consumption of myocardium, exactly opposed to what happened in ischemia. Therefore, increased glucose oxidation will result in decreased oxygen demand.
Trimetazidine is widely used outside North America as an effective agent for treatment of stable angina; however it is not proved to be used in US (Di Napoli and Taccardi 2009; Fernandez, Tandar et al. 2010).

3.5 Fasudil

Fasudil is a potent rho-kinase inhibitor, Ca^+ antagonist and vasodilator. Inhibiting rho-kinase will influence the contractility of vascular smooth muscle.

One of indications of fusadil is in adjunct therapy of vasospasdic and stable angina (Vicari, Chaitman et al. 2005).
More anti-anginal drugs are under development and further studies and longer follow ups are required to establish their place in treatment of patients with coronary artery disease.

4. Current researches

Traditional therapies for angina pectoris have focused largely on heart rate reduction and coronary vasodilation. On the other hand, considering the pharmaceutical aspect, the conventional dosage forms are not sufficient for all medications and in some cases there are progressive demands on novel drug formulations to reduce the dose intervals, to obtain drug levels constant in patients' blood and release the medication following biological rhythm. Additionally, route of administration plays an important role in efficacy and even toxicity of the drug.

4.1 Timed-release drug delivery system

Drug delivery systems (DDS) that can precisely control the release rates have had an enormous impact on the health care system. Of this category controlled-release or sustained-release drug delivery systems are one of the most beneficial and advantageous drug delivery technologies that are used in particular medications to control their release. In the last two decades there has been a remarkable improvement in the field of novel drug delivery systems. Carrier technology offers an intelligent approach for drug delivery by coupling the drug to a carrier particle such as microspheres, nanoparticles, liposomes, etc, which modulates the release and absorption characteristics of the drug (Vasir, Tambwekar et al. 2003; Dehghan, Aboofazeli et al. 2010).
The candidates for being embedded in these systems should meet some qualifications, of which, short half life, narrow therapeutic index and high first-pass effect can be mentioned.
As it was shown previously in this chapter, there are several timed-controlled formulations available for use in angina therapy.

4.2 Pulsatile drug delivery system

It has been proved that in cardiovascular disease there are some morning increases in capillary resistance, vascular reactivity and platelet agreeability which decrease latter in the day. Therefore, there is a higher possibility (or risk) of myocardial infarction and sudden cardiac death before noon rather than evening. Furthermore, the obtained data from several studies show that the time of medication administration can influence its pharmacodynamic and pharmacokinetic.
Considering these facts, scientists have developed a novel drug delivery system named pulsatile drug delivery based on chronobiology in which drug is released from supporting carriers in response to different stimuli. The carriers can react to pH, temperature, magnetic or electric field, ultrasound, light and mechanic forces. Carriers are usually polymers which own certain characteristics such as safety, biocompatibility ability to respond to external stimuli.
There are some FDA approved chronotherapeutic products. Verapamil and propranolol are two samples of this category which is specifically designed to lower morning increased blood pressure. In the near future, there will be medications possessing this technology for treatment of angina (portaluppi, 2007 & Mandal, 2010).

5. Conclusion

Decades of research in these fields results in promising achievements. Still there are several studies aiming to develop new agents with novel mechanisms of action, to develop agents overcoming the problems and limitations of traditional and conventional medications and or their dosage forms more, to carry clinical trials focusing on combination therapy for reduction of adverse effects and finally to select the new agents which have mortality benefit when added to standard therapy.

6. References

Christensen, L., K. Comerford, et al., Eds. (2003). AHFS Drug Handbook, Lippincot Williams & Wilkins.

Cutler, N. R., J. Eff, et al. (1995). "Dose-ranging study of a new, once-daily diltiazem fofrmulation for patients with stable angina." J Clin Pharmacol 35(2): 189-195.

Dehghan, S., R. Aboofazeli, et al. (2010). "Formulation optimization of nifedipine containing microspheres using factorial design." African J Pharm and Pharamcol 4(6): 346-354.

Di Napoli, P. and A. A. Taccardi (2009). "Trimetazidine: the future of cardiac function?" Future Cardiol 5(5): 421-424.

Dvir, D. and A. Battler (2010). "Conventional and novel drug therapeutics to relief myocardial ischemia." Cardiovasc Drugs Ther 24: 319-323.

Farrer, F. (2010). "New or novel drugs 2009." SA Pharm J: 29-33.

FDA. (2006). "Ranexa (ranolazine) extended-release tablets." from http://www.accessdata.fda.gov/drugsatfda_docs/label/2008/021526s004lbl.pdf.

Fernandez, S. F., A. Tandar, et al. (2010). "Emerging medical treatment for angina pectoris." Expert Opin. 15(1): 283-298.

Fox, K., M. A. Garcia, et al. (2006). "Task force on the management of stable angina pectoris of the European Society of Cardiology. ESC committee for practice guidelines (CPG). Guidelines on the management of stable angina pectoris: executive summarry: the Task Force on the Management of Stable Angina Pectoris of the European Society of Cardiology." Eur Heart J 27: 1341-1381.

Frydman, A. (1992). "Pharmacokinetic profile of nicorandil in humans: an overview." J Cardiovasc Pharmacol 20 Suppl 3: S34-44.

Furberg, C. D. (1999). "Natural statins and stroke risk." Circulation 99: 185-188.

Garcia, M. J., R. F. Reinoso, et al. (2003). "Clinical pharmacokinetics of statins." Methods Find Exp Clin Pharmacol 25(6): 457-481.

Hankey, G. J., C. L. M. Sudlow, et al. (2000). "Thienopyridines or aspirin to prevent stroke and other serious vascular events in patients at high risk of vascular disease?: A systematic review of the evidence from randomized trials." Stroke 31: 1779-1784.

Hartwig-Otto, H. (1983). "Pharmacokinetic considerations of common analgesics and antipyretics." Am J Med 75(5A): 30-37.

Helms, R. A., D. J. Quan, et al. (2006). Textbook of therapeutics. Philadelphia, Lippincott Williams & Wilkins.

Hiremath, J. G., R. Valluru, et al. (2010). "Pharmaceutical aspects of nicorandil." Int J Pharm and Pharm Sci 2(4): 24-29.

Karter, Y. (2007). "Nebivolol: more than a highly selective Beta blocker." Recent Pat Cardiovasc Drug Discov 2(2): 152-155.

Katzung, B., S. Masters, et al. (2009). Basic and clinical pharmacology, McGraw-Hill Medical.

Khan, M. G. (2006). Encyclopedia of heart diseases, Elsevier Academic Press.

Lioyd-Jones, D., R. Adams, et al. (2010) "2010 update: a report from the American Heart Association statistics committee and stroke statistics subcommittee. Circulation." American Heart Association statistics committee and stroke statistics 119, 480-486.

Macher, J. P. and S. Levy (2009). "Effect of ivabradine, a novel antiaginal agent, on driving performance: A randomize, double-blind, placebo-controlled trial in healthy volunteers." Clin Drug Investig 29(5): 339-348.

Maier, L. S. (2009). "A novel mechanism for the treatment of angina, arrhythmias, and diastolic dysfunction: Inhibition of late I_{Na} using ranolazine." J Cardiovasc Pharmacol 54: 279-286.

Mandal, A. S., N. Biswas, et al. (2010). "Drug delivery system based on chronobiology- A review." Journal of Controlled Release 147: 314-325.

Munzel, T., A. Daiber, et al. (2005). "Explaining the phenomenon of nitrate tolerance." Circ Res 97(7): 618-628.

Murrell, W. (1879). "Nitroglycerine as a remedy for angina pectoris" Lancet 1: 80.

Opie, L. H. (1989). "Calcium channel antagonists, Part VI: clinical pharmacokinetics of first and second-generation agents." Cardiovasc Drugs Ther 3: 482-497.

Parker, J. N. and P. M. Parker (2002). The 2002 official patient's soure book on angina. San Diego, ICON Group International.

Piepho, R. W. (1991). "Heterogeneity of calcium channel blockers." Hosp Pharm 26: 856-864.

Plomondon, M. E., D. J. Magid, et al. (2007). "Association between angina and treatment satistaction after myocardial infarction." J Gen Intern Med 23(11): 1-6.

Quyyumi, A. A., C. Wright, et al. (1985). "Effects of combined alpha and beta adrenoceptor blockade in patients with angina pectoris. A double blind study comparing labetalol with placebo." Br Heart J 53(1): 47-52.

Rutherford, J. D. (1995). "Nitrates tolerance in angina therapy. How to avoid it." Drugs 49(2): 196-199.

Ryman, K. and C. Gurk-Turner (1999). "Calcium channel blocker review." BUMC Proceedings 12(1): 34-36.

Saha, S., M. Berglund, et al. (2008). "Clopidogrel inhibits platelet aggregation in patients on aspirin with stable chronic angina pectoris." Int J Cardiol 123(2): 195-196.

Savi, P., P. Nurden, et al. (1998). "Clopidogrel: a review of its mechanism of action." Platelets 9(3-4): 251-255.

Schachter, M. (2004). "Chemical, pharmacokinetic and pharmacodynamic properties of statins: an update." Fundam Clin Pharmacol 19: 117-125.

Sirker, A., C. G. Missouris, et al. (2001). "Dihydropyridine calcium channel blockers and peripheral side effects." J Hum Hypertens 15: 745-746.

Vasir, J. K., K. Tambwekar, et al. (2003). "Bioadhesive microspheres as a controlled drug delivery system." Int J Pharm 255: 13-32.

Vicari, R. M., B. Chaitman, et al. (2005). "Efficacy and safety of fasudil in patients with stable angina. A double-blind, placeo-controlled, phase 2 trial." J Am Coll Cardiol 46(10): 1803-1811.

Weiss, R. (2006). "Nebivolol: a novel beta-blocker with nitric oxide-induced vasodilatation." Vasc Health Risk Manag 2(3): 303-308.

4

Therapy for Angina Pectoris Secondary to Coronary Disease

Antony Leslie Innasimuthu, Sanjay Kumar, Lei Gao, Melaku Demede and Jeffrey S. Borer
State University of New York Downstate Medical Center and College of Medicine, Brooklyn and New York, N.Y. United States of America

1. Introduction

Ischemic heart disease is the world's leading cause of mortality and also causes widespread morbidity and limitation of life-style. Coronary artery disease (CAD) is the predominant cause of ischemic heart disease and generally results from fixed coronary artery obstruction that limits myocardial oxygen delivery relative to demand. Mortality associated with CAD is relatively high and was estimated at more than 1¼ million deaths in industrialized countries in 2001 (Lopez et al., 2006). Of note, CAD is projected to remain the primary basis of mortality at least through year 2030 (Mathers & Loncar, 2006). The impact of CAD on quality of life is even more impressive. The symptom that most commonly limits life-style in patients with CAD is angina pectoris. Angina pectoris is a symptom characterized by (1) substernal chest discomfort that is (2) predictably provoked by exertion or emotional stress, (3) lasts up to 20 minutes after the triggering activity is stopped, and (4) is relieved within minutes by nitroglycerin or rest. If all of these criteria are met, the symptom is called "typical angina pectoris"; if only 2 are met, the symptom is called "atypical angina". If one or none are met, the symptom probably is non-cardiac in origin (Diamond et al., 1983). Typical angina has several different causes but predominantly results from CAD. Indeed, the presence of typical angina predicts CAD with a likelihood of 90%, while the association of atypical angina with CAD is reported to be 50%. CAD with ischemia also can cause other symptoms, such as abnormal chest sensations that do not meet the criteria for angina, dizziness, palpitation, dyspnea, etc.

Angina pectoris is the presenting symptom in 50% of those with CAD (O'Rourke, 2010). Most often, this symptom is "stable", i.e., after its onset, it occurs at a relatively predictable workload, frequency and severity. By convention, stable angina manifests little change in these characteristics over 2 weeks, though some variation can be expected if change occurs in myocardial oxygen demand, physical stress or ambient temperature (Braunwald et al., 1994). In general, stable angina correlates with the stability or quiescence of an atherosclerotic plaque. Almost 20% of acute myocardial infarctions (MI) are preceded by chronic stable angina (Thom et al., 2006). This symptom must be distinguished from the less frequent "unstable angina", considered to occur when angina first is manifest ("new onset angina"), or when angina-like discomfort is present at rest (i.e., without the activity/

emotional stress trigger of typical angina), or when angina severity and frequency progress relatively rapidly. Most importantly, patients with unstable angina can be divided into low, intermediate or high short term risk of death or nonfatal MI (Gibbons et al., 1999). Patients at high and intermediate risk often have coronary artery plaques that have recently ruptured. Their risk of death is intermediate between that of patients with acute MI and patients with stable angina. Stable angina pectoris (hereafter denoted as "angina") is common and disabling, affecting 30,000 to 40,000 per 1 million people in Europe and United States (Julian, 1997). As of 2006, approximately 10.2 million patients had angina in the United States. Angina often seriously limits routine daily activities and frequently leads to premature retirement from work (Julian, 1997). Despite availability and application of multiple anti-anginal drugs and mechanical therapy, angina remains very common in patients with known CAD, affecting 30 to 50% of such individuals (Gehi et al., 2008). One in 3 patients with stable angina will have more than one episode per week. Epidemiologically, self reported angina substantially increases the risk of coronary events compared to its absence; this risk increases even more when angina is associated with exercise induced ischemia (Gehi et al., 2008). Regardless of the negative impact of angina on quality of life, in one study almost half of general practitioners considered angina in their patients to be optimally controlled in the face of persistent weekly symptoms (Beltrame et al., 2009).

This chapter will review therapies currently available and in development for relief of acute episodes of angina and, more importantly, for prevention of this symptom in its chronic stable form (Table 1). Because, angina from CAD develops from myocardial oxygen supply-demand imbalance, therapy for patients with CAD and angina is targeted to restore this balance. Indeed, the United States Food and Drug Administration will not approve a therapy for angina unless both the symptoms and the underlying ischemia are relieved in pre-approval testing because of concerns for patient safety if this symptomatic warning of ischemia is masked and the inciting activity continues. The major determinants of myocardial oxygen demand are heart rate (Fox et al., 2007; Heusch, 2008), systolic blood pressure and contractility. Indeed, experimentally, a twofold increase in any of these determinants of oxygen consumption requires approximately 50% increase in coronary blood flow if ischemia is to be avoided (Libby et al., 2008). The primary determinants of myocardial oxygen supply are coronary artery patency, perfusion pressure, arterial oxygen content and duration of diastole, when coronary flow occurs. Because of the high resting oxygen extraction by myocardial tissue, increase in myocardial oxygen consumption is primarily compensated by proportional increases in coronary flow and oxygen delivery.

In patients with CAD, comprehensive management focuses not only on prevention and relief of the symptom but also on prevention of other sequelae common in patients with angina, including myocardial infarction, heart failure and death. Importantly, however, most antianginal therapies, pharmacological and mechanical, have **not** been assessed for their impact on adverse outcomes in patients with chronic stable angina. Management of patients with angina include life style modifications to prevent symptoms as well as to minimize known risk factors for adverse events, medications to prevent angina or to relieve acute episodes, medications to relieve risk factors (cholesterol-lowering agents, antihypertensive drugs, etc.), medications known to prevent other sequelae of CAD (e.g., anti-platelet drugs, certain angiotensin converting enzyme inhibitors) and revascularization or other mechanical therapy to relieve angina if it is inadequately managed with drugs alone.

Anti-Anginal Therapy	**Primary Pharmacological Effects**	**Putative Anti-ischemic Mechanism**
Pharmacological Therapies		
Nitrates	Smooth muscle relaxation, vasodilatation (venodilation> arteriolardilation)	↓↓preload, ↓afterload, (↓ myocardial oxygen demand), ↑oxygen supply
Calcium Channel Blockers	Smooth muscle relaxation (all), ↓inotropy (some), ↓chronotropy (some), ?improved endothelial function	↓preload, ↓afterload, ↓ inotropy with ↓ contractility(some) (↓demand), ↑oxygen supply
Beta adrenergic blockers	↓chronotropy, ↓inotropy,	↓blood pressure ↓demand, ↑oxygen supply
Miscellaneous		
a. Direct metabolic enhancers		
1. Ranolazine	Inhibits fatty acid oxydation thus improving cfficicncy of oxydative metabolism, Na-channel inhibition thus decreasing calcium overload	Improved cellular metabolism
2. Trimetazidine	Inhibits palmitoyl-carnitine oxidation, inhibit fatty acid oxydation	Improved cellular metabolism
b. Novel unloading or HR lowering drugs		
1. Ivabradine	Inhibits I_f current, reduces HR, preserves LV inotropy and lusitropy, does not affect coronary vasomotion	↓ myocardial oxygen demand, ↑oxygen supply
2. Nicorandil	Opens ATP sensitive K channels, vasodilator,	↓preload, ↓afterload, (↓demand)

Anti-Anginal Therapy	Primary Pharmacological Effects	Putative Anti-ischemic Mechanism
	promotes endothelial NO synthase, reduces calcium toxicity	
3. Fasudil	Rho-kinase inhibitor, coronary vasodilatation/anti-spasmodic	↑oxygen supply
Mechanical Interventions	**Known effects**	
a. Revascularization		
1. Coronary artery bypass grafting 2. Coronary angio-plasty/stenting	Relieves mechanical obstructions to coronary arteries	↑oxygen supply
b. Enhanced external counterpulsation (EECP)	Alters hemodynamics to improve coronary perfusion	↑oxygen supply, ↓ myocardial oxygen demand
c. Spinal cord stimulation	Decreases pain and sympathetic tone	↑oxygen supply,↓ myocardial oxygen demand
d. Carotid sinus stimulation	Increases parasympathetic tone	↑oxygen supply,↓ myocardial oxygen demand
Biological Therapy	**Putative Actions**	
1. Transmyocardial laser revascularization	direct perfusion of myocardium, angiogenesis, placebo or myocardial denervation	↑oxygen supply
2. Angiogenic gene therapy	angiogenesis	↑oxygen supply

HR=heart rate, K=potassium, LV=left ventricle, NO=nitric oxide

Table 1. Antianginal anti-ischemic therapies, proven and putative

Therapies shown to be effective in relieving acute episodes are limited to rapid onset, short acting nitrates and, though seldom used today, carotid sinus or spinal cord stimulation, all reviewed in this chapter. Prevention of angina can be achieved with a variety of drugs, though those most frequently employed today are beta blockers, calcium channel blockers and long acting nitrates. These and the other newer drugs now available will also be reviewed below. The various mechanical options, including coronary artery bypass grafting surgery, percutaneous coronary angioplasty, enhanced external counterpulsation, and laser-mediated angiogenesis, will be summarized. Finally, the current status of approaches that are not yet established but which hold promise for benefit and are under intensive study, including angiogenesis stimulated by growth factors directly or by gene insertions, and stem cell therapy, will be reviewed. Table 1 summarizes various approaches, pharmacological, mechanical and biological, now available or in relatively late stages of development.

2. Pharmacological therapy

2.1 Nitrates

Nitrates have been the staple of treatment for acute episodes of angina pectoris for almost 150 years, since the description of the effect of amyl nitrate for this condition in 1867 (Brunton, 1867). Indeed, such use of amyl nitrate was included in the Lillian Hellman play, "The Little Foxes", set just after the Civil War. Though the use of amyl nitrate has declined to application largely for diagnostic hemodynamic profiling for other conditions (e.g., idiopathic hypertrophic subaortic stenosis) other nitrates and, most particularly nitroglycerin, introduced by Murrell for this purpose in 1878 (Murrell, 1879), have gained enduring use, both for treatment of acute episodes and for prophylaxis.

2.1.1 Pharmacological effects

Like all anti-anginal anti-ischemic drugs, nitrates act to improve the imbalance of myocardial oxygen supply and demand that underlies angina (Grayson et al., 1967). Nitrates are believed to induce vasodilatation by interacting with sulfhydryl groups on nitrate receptors on cell membranes (Goldstein, 1979). The prototype nitrate, nitroglycerin, combines with sulfhydryls within smooth muscle cells, where the resulting molecule is biotransformed to an active form, S-nitrosothiol, by mitochondrial aldehyde dehydrogenase (Abrams, 1980). This short-lived compound activates intracellular guanylate cyclase to produce cyclic guanosine monophosphate. This molecule directly initiates smooth muscle relaxation to cause vasodilatation by decreasing myocytic intracellular calcium, either by inhibition of calcium ion entry or by promotion of calcium exit (Ignarro et al., 1981). This pharmacological effect renders nitroglycerin a potent vasodilator. Experimental studies suggest that nitroglycerin's action as a venodilator may exceed that as an arterial and arteriolar dilator, though the drug acts on both sides of the circulation. It has been suggested that reduction in left ventricular (LV) preload, resulting from venous dilatation, is the primary basis for the drug-induced reduction in myocardial oxygen demand and, perhaps, the increase in myocardial oxygen supply observed with nitroglycerin and, thus, may be the primary basis for its anti-anginal anti-ischemic effect (Goldstein, 1979). However, reduction in LV outflow impedance due its arterial and arteriolar effects likely also is involved.

Experimental evidence suggests that nitrates also may act directly to increase myocardial oxygen supply by dilatation of coronary arteries and arterioles. Conversion to nitric oxide, a deficiency of which is the putative basis of "endothelial dysfunction" observed in many patients with CAD (Parker & Parker, 1998), provides potential for vasodilatation and enhancement of coronary blood flow. However, the practical importance of this effect is unclear, since the calcified state of many atherosclerotic coronary arteries is likely to limit potential for arterial dilatation. Experimental evidence also suggests nitroglycerin may preferentially affect collateral vessels within the myocardium to increase flow to ischemic regions. Finally, as a result of preload reduction, nitroglycerin reduces LV diastolic pressure potentially enhancing perfusion pressure during diastole when most coronary flow occurs. This effect is apparent primarily in the subendocardium, where flow is particularly vulnerable, though little change in total myocardial perfusion appears to be associated with this effect (Bottcher et al., 2002). Finally, in experimental studies, nitroglycerin has antithrombogenic action, apparently mediated via stimulation of guanylate cyclase in platelets (Munzel et al., 2002). This effect would tend to minimize platelet aggregation. The clinical importance of this change, particularly for angina, is not known.

Irrespective of the underlying mechanisms, nitrates have been well demonstrated to increase exercise tolerance in patients with ischemic heart disease from CAD, while reducing ischemia as measured by increased time to ST segment depression during exercise in patients with chronic stable angina (Ben-Dor & Battler, 2007). Nitrates have additive effect when they are combined with beta-blockers or calcium channel blockers (Gibbons et al., 2003).

2.1.2 Clinical application

Nitroglycerin preparations are available as sublingual tablets, buccal spray and ointment (both in immediately available and prolonged release ["patch"] forms), the latter for prophylaxis rather than for treatment of acute episodes. Nitroglycerin tablets lose potency when exposed to light and, hence, are stored in dark containers. The sublingual preparation is the treatment of choice for acute episodes of angina because this mode of administration enables absorption without first pass metabolism in the liver, resulting rapidly in therapeutic concentrations in the circulation. (Buccal spray has a similar advantage.) From drug levels in the plasma, the half-lives of the compounds differ markedly, nitroglycerin having a half-life of 2-3 min, isosorbide dinitrate (ISDN) 20-30 min and isosorbide mononitrate (ISMN) 4-5 h (Olsson & Allgen, 1992). The beneficial clinical effect of nitroglycerin has a half-life of 30 minutes; its hemodynamic effects are seen even after 2 hours (Goldstein & Epstein, 1973).

Metabolism to inactive forms occurs in the liver. The usual dose of nitroglycerin for relief of an acute angina episode is 0.4 mg by the sublingual route, though smaller (and larger) doses are effective in some patients. Nitroglycerin spray dispenses 0.4 mg metered, aerosolized doses, which are better absorbed in patients with dry mucous membranes. There is evidence to show that when used in sublingual form, nitroglycerin is an effective antianginal and anti-ischemic agent that can abort an attack of established angina and, when taken prophylactically, prolong exercise tolerance (Aronow, 1973; Detry & Bruce, 1971; Goldstein et al., 1971). If symptoms persist after a single dose, additional doses can be given, usually at 5 minute intervals, though lack of relief with as much as 1.2 mg in a 15 minute interval suggests an acute coronary syndrome and should lead to emergency evaluation. Several long acting forms of nitrates have been developed. Their pharmacokinetics are such that they are not used for relief of acute angina episodes, but their persistence in the circulation and at active cellular sites can provide effective prophylaxis against angina. The most commonly employed are topical nitroglycerin ointment or nitroglycerin adherent to patches, oral ISDN and oral ISMN.

Topical cutaneous administration of nitroglycerin is possible either with an ointment or a polymer patch impregnated with the drug. Nitroglycerin ointment usually is applied in 0.5 - 2 inch doses, containing 15 mg of nitroglycerin per inch. The drug is effective for about 6 hours by this route. Absorption can be impeded if skin perfusion is minimized by hypotension or impaired cardiac output. Nitroglycerin patches release the drug at a rate of 0.1 to 0.8 mg/hour (depending on patch size) and are effective for approximately 12 to 18 hours. Tolerance generally is absent if the patch is used for no more than 12 to 14 hours

daily. Oral ISDN has relatively low bioavailability, undergoing rapid hepatic metabolism. It is usually administered in a dose of 30 mg 3 to 4 times daily. The antianginal effect lasts for 6 hours after the first dose, with decreased effect with each successive dose. Nitrate tolerance develops when it is administered four times daily. A dosing schedule permitting intermittent 10-12 hour nitrate free intervals helps to prevent tolerance.
ISMN is the active metabolite of ISDN. When administered orally, it doesn't undergo first pass metabolism and provides effective management of chronic stable angina. Steady state plasma concentration is achieved within 2 hours and its effect lasts for at least 8 hours. Tolerance is not reported when ISMN is administered once daily, but tolerance is common with twice daily dosing. A sustained release preparation is available in a dosage range from 30 to 240 mg daily. Nitroglycerin can also be used as an intravenous preparation with titration to symptoms and blood pressure. Though not strictly relevant for relief of chronic stable angina, this form has been used for patients with frequent ("unstable") angina at rest and requiring hospitalization (Frishman, 1985). It has also been used during acute coronary syndromes and has been effective in reducing ischemia during acute myocardial infarction (Borer et al., 1975) as well as in improving hemodynamics and reducing symptoms in heart failure, with or without infarction (Frishman, 1985).

2.1.3 Adverse effects

Most common adverse effects of nitrates and, specifically, of nitroglycerin, include headache, hypotension and flushing. These effects are due to vasodilatation. Methemoglobinemia is rare but reported after nitrate administration, most commonly after high doses of the intravenous form. Tolerance is reported with all forms of nitroglycerin. Tolerance to antianginal effects develops rapidly in humans during long-term, 4 times daily therapy with ISDN and continuous therapy with nitroglycerin patches (Crean et al., 1984; James et al., 1985; Parker & Fung, 1984; Reichek et al., 1984). The putative mechanism of tolerance is drug-induced generation of superoxide anions in the affected vessels, leading to impaired biotransformation and decreased responsiveness to nitric oxide (Gori & Parker, 2004). Tolerance can be best avoided by providing a nitrate free period, optimally of 10 to12 hours. Development of tolerance is rarely a problem when nitroglycerin sublingual tablets are taken intermittently, either for relief of an acute symptom or for short-term prophylaxis before activities predictably associated with angina. Some studies have shown that angiotensin receptor blockers may prevent nitrate tolerance (Hirai et al., 2003). Patients can develop rebound symptoms after abruptly stopping nitrates. With the recent increase in the use of sildenafil, a phosphodiesterase inhibitor, the dangers of interaction with nitrates have been highlighted, leading to proscription of this combination to prevent severe and potentially lethal hypotension.

2.2 Calcium channel blockers

Calcium Channel Blockers (CCB) bind to and inhibit L-type calcium channels, reducing calcium influx into cells. Intracellular calcium deprivation relaxes smooth muscle cells, causing vasodilatation in the peripheral and coronary beds and, in normal coronary arteries and perhaps diseased arteries, increased coronary blood flow. The 2 major subdivisions of CCBs are dihydropyridines (DHP) like nifedipine, amlodipine, felodipine, and nicardipine, and non-dihydropyridines which include verapamil and diltiazem.

2.2.1 Pharmacological effects

CCBs' main effect on angina is lowering myocardial oxygen demand by peripheral vascular smooth muscle relaxation. The result is to reduce blood pressure and impedance to LV outflow, in turn reducing myocardial wall tension, myocardial work load and oxygen consumption. However, they may cause dilatation of coronary arteries, as well, and thus may increase coronary blood flow/ myocardial perfusion. CCBs have been shown to be specifically and particularly effective in vasospastic angina pectoris (including "Prinzmetal's angina") and may be useful in effort-induced angina in part by relieving vasospasm associated with fixed obstructive lesions in some patients. In addition to vascular smooth muscle relaxation, the non-dihydropyridines also cause blockade of calcium entry into myocytes, leading to negative chronotropic effects due to action on the sinoatrial and atrioventricular nodal cells, and negative inotropic effects leading to depressed contractility due to action on ventricular myocytes.

Experimentally, calcium plays an integral role in the process of atherogenesis. Hence, it has been theorized that CCBs are anti-atherogenic. Some studies have shown that CCBs reduce the progression of atherosclerosis as measured by carotid intima-media thickness but there has been no difference in coronary atherosclerosis. The ENCORE I trial demonstrated that nifedipine improved coronary endothelial function in the most constricted segment (Azancot, 2003) and the ENCORE II study showed that nifedipine improved coronary endothelial function but had no effect on plaque volume (Luscher et al., 2009). The NICOLE study showed no effect of CCBs on reduction of angiographic progression of CAD (Dens et al., 2003). Thus, clinical studies to date provide equivocal evidence of anti-atherogenesis but stronger support for improvement of endothelial function.

2.2.2 Clinical application

From multiple trials, CCBs decrease the frequency of angina, reduce the need for nitrates, extend treadmill walking time, and improve ischemic ST-segment changes on exercise testing and electrocardiographic monitoring (Gibbons et al., 2003; Heidenreich et al., 1999; Nissen et al., 2004; Rice et al., 1990). Amlodipine, in particular, may have some independent action in relieving diastolic dysfunction other than by a reduction in blood pressure (Tapp et al., 2010), potentially improving myocardial oxygen supply by enhancing perfusion pressure. CCBs are used in patients who cannot tolerate β-blockers or in combination with other anti-ischemic agents for additive benefit. Though clearly effective antianginal agents, CCBs have not been found to modify the natural progression of CAD and have no effect on cardiovascular or all cause mortality in patients with CAD. DHP tend to cause reflex tachycardia because of lowering of blood pressure; this effect can be blunted by concomitant use of β-blockers. If clinically needed, verapamil or diltiazem may be used with caution to lower heart rate or slow atrioventricular (AV) conduction further when ventricular function is preserved. In a case control study among enrollees of the Group Health Cooperative of Puget Sound, a link was reported between short-acting nifedipine and coronary events when the drug was used as primary therapy for hypertension (Psaty et al., 1995). However, short-acting nifedipine never has been approved by the FDA for use for this indication (i.e., its use was "off label"), and its application for this purpose by the Puget Sound group was an act of highly questionable judgment. Meta-analysis by Furberg et al showed that nifedipine is associated with dose related increase in mortality in patients with CAD, a study which included patients with acute coronary syndromes (ACS) (Furberg et al., 1995). However, the only trial included in the meta-analysis that involved patients with stable angina was the International Nifedipine trial on Antiatherosclerotic Therapy (INTACT), which showed that patients on nifedipine had retardation of atherosclerotic disease by angiogram, though clinical symptoms were not reported (Lichtlen et al., 1990). A Coronary Disease Trial Investigating Outcome with Nifedipine gastrointestinal therapeutic system (ACTION) study reported that, in patients with stable angina and hypertension, long-acting nifedipine was acceptably safe (no increased incidence of myocardial infarction, heart failure or death), but there was no evidence of improvement in mortality or other major cardiac endpoints and no reduction in refractory angina in already maximally medically treated patients (Poole-Wilson et al., 2004; Sierra & Coca, 2008). In addition to vasodilatation, verapamil acts in part through its negative inotropic effect. Diltiazem has greater vasodilatory actions than verapamil. Both verapamil and diltiazem are contraindicated in patients with uncompensated heart failure because of their negative inotropic effects, whereas amlodipine and felodipine are relatively safe when LV dysfunction is present, particularly if compensated clinically (Sierra & Coca, 2008). Use of non-dihydropyridines after complex myocardial infarctions should be avoided, as well, because of the possibility of HF.

Although CCBs are effective anti-ischemic agents, they do not improve mortality in patients with ACS. DHP can also cause reflex tachycardia which can be deleterious in acute ischemia by increasing myocardial oxygen demand. In addition, DHP-induced hypotension may detrimentally lower coronary perfusion pressure. A meta-analysis of trials of CCBs and long acting nitrates did not show any difference in clinical outcomes between these types of agents (Heidenreich et al., 1999). Nifedipine is a potent, long-acting vasodilator that has proved highly efficacious in relieving angina caused by coronary vasospasm. In vivo, it exerts no myocardial depressant effects and has no antiarrhythmic properties. Nifedipine is available in doses of 10-30 mg given 3 times daily and in sustained release preparations in doses of 60 to 120 mg that can be administered once daily. Onset of action is 20 minutes after administration and half life is 2-5 hours. Steady state concentrations are reached in 48 hours. Immediate release formulation is not recommended for hypertension because of concerns of sudden hemodynamic compromise but it is still approved for coronary spasm and management of angina. Treatment with nifedipine can safely be combined with administration of a β receptor blocking agent.

Verapamil is usually started with 40 mg three times daily and titrated to a maximum dose of 480 mg daily. Sustained release preparations are available and can be given in doses of 120 mg daily to 480 mg daily. Onset of action of verapamil is in 30 minutes; elimination half life is 3-7 hours. Diltiazem is available in doses of 30-90 mg given up to four times daily. A sustained release or long-acting form usually is administered at a starting dose of 120 mg daily and can be increased to 360 mg daily. Its onset of action is within 30-60 minutes and it has a half life of 3-7 hours. It can take up to 2 weeks to achieve maximal effect of diltiazem.

2.2.3 Adverse effects

Common side effects of headache, dizziness, flushing and edema (particularly with DHP) are due to vasodilatation. Verapamil and diltiazem can interact with other negative chronotropic or negative inotropic agents to produce substantial bradycardia, conduction disturbances or clinically overt heart failure. CCBs may also suppress lower esophageal sphincter contraction and worsen gastroesophageal reflux. Particularly with verapamil and, to a lesser extent with diltiazem, bowel motility can be importantly reduced, causing constipation, a particularly frequent complaint in relatively elderly patients given these drugs. CCBs inhibit the CYPA4 enzyme in the liver and, therefore, may raise levels of statins and other drugs, resulting in adverse effects of the drugs so affected (Furberg et al., 1978). By blocking the microsomal enzymes, the liver enzymes that metabolize CCBs, cimetidine and grapefruit juice may raise blood CCB concentrations. Since magnesium is a calcium antagonist, magnesium supplements may enhance the actions of CCBs, particularly nifedipine.

2.3 Beta-blockers

Adrenergic receptors are G-protein-coupled molecules stimulated by circulating catecholamines. These receptors are broadly classified into α and β groups. Effects of β-receptors are mediated by adenyl cyclase. β-receptors are further classified into β1 and β2 subtypes. β1 stimulation results in increased chronotropy, inotropy, automaticity, release of renin from juxtaglomerular cells and lipolysis. β2 effects include relaxation of bronchial, vascular and other smooth muscle, with dilatation of peripheral, coronary, and carotid arteries, and promotion of glycogenolysis and gluconeogenesis. β-blockers are effective in preventing angina because they lower heart rate, reduce blood pressure, and reduce contractility, thereby reducing myocardial oxygen demand (Gibbons et al., 2003). However, of these effects, current data indicate that the most important is reduction in heart rate, the primary determinant of myocardial oxygen demand (Andrews et al., 1993; Borer et al., 2003; Daly et al., 2010). Most antianginal effects of β-blockers result from β1 inhibition. Also, because of the heart rate reduction, β-blockers can enhance myocardial oxygen supply by prolonging diastole, when coronary perfusion occurs. However, by blocking β2 receptors that can mediate coronary vasodilatation, some β-blockers can allow unopposed α-adrenergic stimulation, leading to coronary vasoconstriction and mitigating the potentially beneficial effects of prolongation of diastole. β-blockers also have negative lusitropic (relaxation) effects on the myocardium, minimizing the rate at which LV pressure falls during diastole and, thus, minimizing the increase in perfusion pressure that otherwise might be expected during prolonged diastole that drives coronary flow.

2.3.1 Pharmacological effects

Some β-blockers are partial agonists, manifesting intrinsic sympathomimetic activity, blunting secondary preventive benefits (Freemantle et al., 1999). These generally are not used for angina prevention. Some newer β-blockers, such as labetalol, carvedilol, and bucindolol, also have partial α1-adrenergic blocking effects, causing vasodilatation. Others have antiarrhythmic effects – propranolol, metoprolol, and carvedilol have effects similar to "class I" (sodium-channel blockade) antiarrhythmics, while sotalol has a "class III" (potassium channel blockade) effect. Further, experimentally, carvedilol and its metabolites have antioxidant and antiproliferative properties that inhibit apoptosis. Most β-blockers are well absorbed. β-blockers that are lipid-soluble, such as propranolol and metoprolol, have short half-lives because they are metabolized by the liver. Hydrophilic β-blockers such as atenolol and nadolol are eliminated through kidney and have longer half-lives.

Atenolol is usually started with a dose of 50 mg daily and can be titrated to a suggested maximal dose of 200 mg daily. Metoprolol can be started with 50-100 mg daily and titrated for heart rate and blood pressure. When used to prevent angina, β-blockers generally are titrated to a resting heart rate of 50–60 bpm and an exercise heart rate 75% of the rate that precipitates ischemia. In patients with severe angina, target heart rates of 50 bpm are sometimes used if neither symptoms (fatigue, lightheadedness) nor atrioventricular block supervenes.

2.3.2 Clinical application

β-blockers have been primary therapeutics for angina management since early after their development (Hoekenga & Abrams, 1984); indeed, slowing heart rate to prevent angina was the primary reason for their development, for which a Nobel Prize was awarded. Many β-blockers have been studied in chronic stable angina (Furberg et al., 1978; Jackson et al., 1978). β-blockers have been shown to reduce mortality in patients with relatively recent MI, primary angioplasty for ST elevation MI and CHF with LV dysfunction. However, no randomized trials ever have been performed to assess the effects of β-blockers on natural history outcomes in patients only with stable angina. Hence β-blockers are titrated for maximal symptom benefit with least adverse effects. No differences have been shown in antianginal effects of different beta blockers when they are titrated to similar heart rate reductions. β-blockers can be combined with nitrates, CCBs and other antianginals to enhance symptom relief.

2.3.3 Adverse effects

Absolute contraindications to β-blockers are severe bradycardia with or without conduction system disease, severe asthma or peripheral vascular disease with rest ischemia, depression, and acute decompensated heart failure (HF). β-blockers may cause dyslipidemia (increase in triglycerides and decrease in high-density lipoprotein cholesterol). The most common adverse effect is fatigue, a common complaint of patients receiving these agents. Mild depression, lack of motivation and erectile dysfunction have been well reported. β-blockers may blunt the tachycardic response to hypoglycemia in diabetics; worsening of hypoglycemia in diabetics on oral agents or insulin has been reported. β-blockers enhance insulin resistance, possibly accounting for the hyperglycemia. Patients with cocaine-induced coronary vasoconstriction may also react adversely when given β-blockers, with hypertension and seizures. Similarly, since β-adrenergic receptors may be up-regulated when patients are treated with β-blockers, these agents should not be abruptly discontinued, lest rebound vasoconstriction precipitate unstable angina or even MI or death (Miller et al., 1975; Psaty et al., 1990). Patients with asthma, claudication, or HF whose symptoms increase with β-blockers should be appropriately monitored and reevaluated for possible substitution with CCBs.

2.4 Ranolazine

Ranolazine is a piperazine derivative that has been shown to prevent stable angina pectoris. This agent was approved by FDA in 2006 for use in combination with other antianginals when angina is not adequately controlled with established therapies.

2.4.1 Pharmacological effects

The pharmacological effects most likely to underlie ranolazine's antianginal action are not fully elucidated. Several such effects have been suggested. Ranolazine has been shown to alter myocyte metabolism to favor oxidation of glucose over fatty acid by partial fatty acid oxidation (p-FOX) (Clarke et al., 1996). Less oxygen is required to metabolize glucose than fatty acids; consequently, ranolazine may improve efficiency of oxidative metabolism, allowing more mechanical activity for a given oxygen supply. However, in formal clinical testing, though time to angina was increased with ranolazine versus placebo, no evidence was found that cardiac workload at angina was increased when angina occurred, thus casting doubt on improved metabolic efficiency as the underlying cause of the drug's benefit. Experimentally, ranolazine reduces calcium overload in the ischemic myocyte through inhibition of the late sodium current (I_{Na}) (Antzelevitch et al., 2004; Belardinelli L, 2004). Excess intracellular sodium activates the sodium-calcium exchanger and can result in intracellular calcium overload via reverse transport of the sodium calcium exchanger. Ranolazine appears to minimize the intracellular consequences of myocardial ischemia by reducing excess late sodium ion influx, thereby reducing calcium overload (Chaitman & Sano, 2007). Indeed, the drug is now labeled to indicate that sodium channel inhibition is the most likely basis of its activity. However, the drug also has modest alpha- and β-blocking properties. Ranolazine is extensively metabolized by cytochrome P450 (mainly the 3A4 enzyme) and excreted mainly in urine, predominantly as metabolites (Abdallah & Jerling, 2005; Chu N, 2003). The elimination half life in healthy individuals is 5.3 to 8.9 hours which is significantly increased in severe renal impairment (Jerling & Abdallah, 2005).

2.4.2 Clinical application

Ranolazine has been investigated in Monotherapy Assessment of Ranolazine in Stable Angina (MARISA) trial, in which the drug was found to be well tolerated and effective in increasing exercise duration and time to ST segment depression in a dose dependent manner (Chaitman, 2002). In the Combination Assessment of Ranolazine in Stable Angina (CARISA) study, ranolazine was compared to placebo on a background of treatment with either atenolol 50 mg daily, amlodipine 5 mg daily, or diltiazem 180 mg daily. Ranolazine was effective in increasing exercise duration and mean time to onset of angina compared to placebo. There was also reduction in the frequency of angina as well as nitroglycerin use compared to placebo. In this trial, a higher dose of ranolazine (1000 mg twice daily) provided no extra benefit compared to the lower dose (750 mg twice daily) (Chaitman et al., 2004). In the Efficacy of Ranolazine in Chronic Angina (ERICA) trial, ranolazine was compared to a placebo on a background of amlodipine 10 mg daily. Again, ranolazine resulted in lower frequency of angina and nitroglycerin consumption and similar frequency of adverse effects (Stone et al., 2006). In the Metabolic Efficiency with Ranolazine for Less Ischemia in Non-ST Elevation (MERLIN-TIMI-36) trial, 6560 patients with acute coronary syndromes were randomized within 48 hours of symptom onset, to intravenous ranolazine or a placebo, in addition to standard therapy. Ranolazine was administered as a bolus of 200 mg over 1 hour and then continued as an infusion for 12 to 96 hours, followed by 1000 mg twice daily orally. After a median follow-up of 348 days, there was no difference in all-cause mortality, sudden cardiac death, or frequency of symptomatic arrhythmias between ranolazine and placebo. Though the trial failed to support ranolazine as a means of improving natural history in patients with CAD, it demonstrated the overall favorable safety profile of ranolazine, crucial for its FDA approval given prior concerns about drug-induced syncope and ECG QT prolongation with possible "pro-arrhythmia", while supporting its effectiveness in reducing angina (Morrow et al., 2007).

2.4.3 Adverse effects

Ranolazine is fairly well tolerated. Adverse effects (primarily dizziness, nausea, asthenia and constipation) appear to be dose related. Thus, in clinical trials, fewer than 8% of patients discontinued ranolazine due to adverse effects; three quarters of these withdrawals occurred at the 1500 mg twice daily dose. Consequently, the approved starting dose is 500 mg twice daily, with possible up titration to 750 mg twice daily and 1000 mg twice daily if lower doses do not adequately prevent angina (Chaitman et al., 2004). An extended release (ER) oral preparation is also available. Ketoconazole and diltiazem can increase ranolazine plasma concentrations; ranolazine increases digoxin plasma concentration (Jerling & Abdallah, 2005; Chaitman et al., 2004). Ranolazine prolongs QTc interval in a dose related manner but, as noted above, MERLIN-TIMI 36 failed to demonstrate excessive sudden death with the drug (Scirica et al., 2007), nor were these suggested in earlier, shorter trials.

2.5 Ivabradine

The principle of heart rate slowing for prevention of angina is well established based on pathophysiological studies and clinical assessments of heart rate lowering drugs (Daly et al., 2010). Indeed, heart rate is the major determinant of myocardial oxygen demand and its increase is a precipating factor for ischemia or angina (Andrews et al., 1993; Borer et al., 2003; Daly et al., 2010; Fox et al., 2007; Heusch, 2008; Tardif et al., 2005). Heart rate also predicts outcome in epidemiologic studies of patients with CAD, as well as those with heart failure, hypertension, and, indeed, in unselected free living populations without apparent heart disease (Daly et al., 2010; Diaz et al., 2005; Fox et al., 2007; Fox et al., 2008; Fox et al., 2008; Tardif et al., 2009). For example, the Coronary Artery Surgery Study (CASS) registry showed after a 14 year follow-up that cardiovascular and overall mortality was directly related to heart rate at entry into the study (Diaz et al., 2005). Similar results were seen in the placebo group of the prospective BEAUTIFUL [morBidity-mortality EvAlUaTion of the *If* inhibitor ivabradine in patients with coronary disease and left-ventricULar dysfunction] trial and in a retrospective assessment of the Treating to New Targets [TNT] study (Fox et al., 2008; Ho et al., 2010).

2.5.1 Pharmacological effects

As heart rate increases progressively myocardial oxygen demand increases (increase in myocardial work) and myocardial blood flow (and with it, potential myocardial oxygen supply) decreases because of reduction in the duration of diastole, when coronary flow occurs. When a threshold value is reached at which demand is greater than supply, ischemia results, often causing angina. Thus, Andrews et al showed that heart rate is a predictor of coronary ischemia in patients with stable CAD (Andrews et al., 1993). Ivabradine selectively inhibits the inward sodium–potassium I_f current, a relatively low amplitude primary modifier of the rate of spontaneous depolarization of the sino-atrial (SA) node myocytes (discovered in 1979 by DiFrancesco, et al (Brown et al., 1979; DiFrancesco & Camm, 2004)). Spontaneous depolarization, itself, is a function of other calcium and potassium currents. Ivabradine has no other known pharmacological actions on normal cardiovascular physiology. Therefore, it is considered a pure heart rate slowing drug (Thollon et al., 1994). Resting heart rate lowering by ivabradine is comparable to that achieved with β-blockers and is greater than that associated with CCBs (Pine et al., 1982; Tardif et al., 2005) for equal antianginal effect. The heart rate reduction is dose dependent (Borer et al., 2003; Thollon et al., 1994). Ivabradine is a selective and specific I_f inhibitor; it has no inotropic effect, no effect on relaxation (luisotropy), no impact on AV nodal conduction and no coronary vasoconstriction. Thus, ivabradine diminishes myocardial oxygen demand, increases myocardial oxygen supply, maintains contractile force, preserves ventricular relaxation and allows coronary vasodilatation. The drug improves coronary perfusion and maintains cardiac performance better than alternative equieffective anti-anginal drug therapy.

2.5.2 Clinical application

The first placebo controlled trial of ivabradine for angina prevention (Borer et al., 2003) showed that increasing doses progressively reduced heart rate at rest and during exercise. With these changes, there was progressive increase in time to limiting angina and time to 1mm ST depression on bicycle exercise; the drug also reduced the number of diary-reported weekly angina episodes (Borer et al., 2003). The INITIATIVE (the INternatIonal TrIAl on the Treatment of angina with IVabradinE vs. atenolol) study compared ivabradine with atenolol ; ivabradine was non-inferior to the beta blocker in increasing treadmill exercise tolerance and preventing angina at doses selected to cause heart rate reduction approximately equivalent to that achieved with atenolol (Tardif et al., 2005). Indeed, ivabradine nominally improved exercise parameters to a greater extent than atenolol, though these differences did not reach statistical significance. Ivabradine also reduced spontaneous angina episodes compared with baseline and was again equivalent to atenolol in this effect (Tardif et al., 2005). Importantly, when the specific increment in exercise duration was assessed as a function of heart rate reduction ("anti-anginal efficiency") ivabradine was markedly and significantly more efficient than atenolol. When compared with amlodipine, ivabradine was non-inferior in improving exercise tolerance and preventing angina, and increasing time to 1 mm ST depression on exercise (Ruzyllo et al., 2007). Though some concern initially was raised about the combination of ivabradine and beta blockers because of the potential for profound heart rate lowering, the ASSOCIATE (Efficacy of ivabradine, a new selective I(f) inhibitor, compared with atenolol in patients with chronic stable angina) trial of ivabradine versus placebo on a background of atenolol (Tardif et al., 2009) confirmed the experimental findings that ivabradine effect is « use dependent », i.e., the drug has its greatest rate-reducing effect at relatively high heart rates and has progessively less impact on heart rate as the pretherapy value decreases; more importantly, symptomatic bradycardia was rare with the combination, though significant antianginal efficacy was demonstrated with the combination compared with atenolol alone. When all clinical studies are considered, ivabradine has demonstrated consistent antianginal efficacy across all subpopulations, with reductions of 51% to 70% in the frequency of angina attacks (Tendera et al., 2009).

Almost uniquely among antianginal drugs, ivabradine has been demonstrated to exert a benefit on natural history end-points/cardiac events. Thus, in BEAUTIFUL, Fox et al showed that, among patients with chronic stable CAD, LV ejection fraction <40% and heart rate ≥70 bpm before therapy, heart rate reduction with ivabradine markedly and significantly reduced the incidence of fatal or non-fatal myocardial infarction, as well as the incidence of revascularization and non-MI acute coronary syndrome (Fox et al., 2008). In the BEAUTIFUL angina substudy (Fox et al, 2009) ivabradine not only reduced the frequency of angina, but it reduced the primary end-points of death, non-fatal myocardial infarction (both end-points similarly affected) or hospitalization for heart failure and improved quality of life. Among all patients in the subgroup (as well as those with pre-therapy heart rate ≥70 bpm), all cause mortality fell 10% (and 13%), fatal or non-fatal myocardial infarction incidence fell 42% (and 73%); hospitalization for heart failure and coronary revascularization fell 30% and 59% respectively (Fox et al., 2009). Though the BEAUTIFUL angina substudy was a "post-hoc" assessment that cannot be considered definitive, nonetheless, it strongly suggests that, for patients with angina, for whom ivabradine is already approved for marketing throughout Europe and other parts of the world, heart rate slowing with this drug has additional benefits, beyond angina prevention, in reducing major coronary events. In this regard, ivabradine is almost unique among all currently available anti-anginal anti-ischemic pharmacological agents. Though not specifically related to angina, the SHIFT (the Systolic Heart Failure Treatment with the I_f Inhibitor Ivabradine Trial) study in patients with moderately severe to severe systolic heart failure demonstrated the usefulness of ivabradine in reducing mortality or hospitalization for HF (Bohm et al., 2010; Swedberg et al., 2010), irrespective of the etiology of HF. Since the study population of more than 6500 patients predominantly involved patients with ischemic etiology, SHIFT, together with BEAUTIFUL and the various antianginal trials, demonstrated the benefit of pure heart rate reduction by ivabradine in patients with CAD in all its manifestations.

2.5.3 Adverse effects

Ivabradine is safe in combination with β-blockers and causes only a relatively small excess risk of symptomatic or dose-limiting bradycardia. The drug is well tolerated; the primary side effect is relatively infrequent transient and reversible "phosphenes" (flashing scotomata), that are sufficient to cause cessation of therapy in less than 1% of patients (Fox et al., 2008). This symptom is attributed to blockade of the retinal h channels, similar to the SA nodal f channels, by ivabradine.

2.6 Nicorandil

Nicorandil is a coronary and peripheral vasodilator which reduces LV preload and afterload. It also affects potassium channels involved in ischemic preconditioning and, thus, is suggested to have cardioprotective effects. The drug has been used in Europe for angina relief in patients with angina already receiving "conventional' antianginal drugs.

2.6.1 Pharmacological effects

Nicorandil is structurally a nicotinamide ester derivative. It enhances potassium ion conductance by opening adenosine triphosphate (ATP)-sensitive potassium channels, in turn activating the enzyme guanylate cyclase. Nicorandil also has a nitrate moiety and promotes expression of endothelial NO synthase, thus sharing nitrate smooth muscle relaxing properties. Consequently, the drug enhances dilatation of arterial, venous and epicardial coronary arteries, resulting in reduced preload, afterload and myocardial oxygen demand while possibly increasing myocardial oxygen supply (Jahangir et al., 2001). Nicorandil may be associated with improved myocardial function during ischemia-reperfusion, cardioprotective action during ischemia, shortened action potential duration, and prevention of intracellular calcium toxicity (Jahangir & Terzic, 2005; Jahangir et al., 2001; John et al., 2003; Zingman et al., 2007).

2.6.2 Clinical application

Nicorandil has antianginal efficacy similar to that of β-blockers, nitrates and calcium channels blockers. In the Impact Of Nicorandil in Angina (IONA) randomized trial, nicorandil 20mg twice daily showed a 17% relative risk reduction (Hazard ratio of 0.83,

P=0.014) in hospitalization for chest pain, MI, and cardiac death when added to standard antianginal therapy (Ford, 2002). However, the result was driven by effects of nicorandil on "hospital admission for cardiac chest pain", and the risk reduction for cardiac death or non-fatal MI during 1.6 years of treatment was non significant. Thus the value of the treatment has been disputed (Fox et al., 2006). Several small randomized trials have shown that Nicorandil prolongs the time to onset of ST-segment depression and exercise tolerance during treadmill exercise testing in patients with stable angina (Di Somma et al., 1993; Meeter et al., 1992; Raftery et al., 1993). Markham et al also have shown that nicorandil prolongs time to the onset of angina, time to 1 mm ST depression, improves exercise duration and reverses ischemia-related impairment in regional wall motion during exercise (Markham et al., 2000). In a multicenter, randomized trial (197 patients) comparing it to isosorbide mononitrate, nicorandil was found to be both safe and effective in preventing angina (Doring, 1992). A dose of 10–40 mg twice daily controls symptoms in 70%–80% of patients with chronic stable angina; the effect of a single administration is maintained for about 12 hours (Meeter et al., 1992).

2.6.3 Adverse effects

In the IONA trial, the drop out-rates were about 10%, mainly due to headache in the nicorandil group. Nicorandil is not yet approved for use in the United States, but is widely available for angina therapy in Europe and other countries.

2.7 Fasudil

Fasudil is a Rho-kinase inhibitor and a vasodilator. Rho-kinase has been identified as one of the effectors of the small GTP-binding protein, Rho. The Rho/Rho-kinase pathway plays an important role in various cellular functions including vascular smooth muscle cell contraction, actin cytoskeleton integrity and gene expression. As a Rho-kinase inhibitor, fasudil has been utilized in cerebral vasospasm, pulmonary hypertension and, recently, in angina.

2.7.1 Pharmacological effects

The Rho molecules are small GTP-binding proteins that mediate intracellular signaling by activation of G-protein-coupled receptors and growth factor receptors. The Rho/Rho-kinase signaling pathway is known to be involved in the pathogenesis of coronary artery spasm (Shimokawa & Takeshita, 2005). Rho molecules are known to modulate Ca^{2+}-sensitization of vascular smooth muscle cells and may act by inhibiting myosin phosphatase activity (Fukata et al., 2001). As a Rho-kinase inhibitor, fasudil is a vasodilator.

2.7.2 Clinical application

Fasudil can increase coronary artery diameter to an extent greater than that achievable with nitroglycerin in patients with documented vasospasm (Otsuka et al., 2008). Vasospastic angina precipitated by acetylcholine can be prevented by intracoronary infusion of fasudil (Mohri et al., 2003). When used as monotherapy, fasudil doses ranging from 5 mg three times daily to 40 mg three times daily have increased maximum exercise time and time to the onset of ST segment depression compared with baseline. Fasudil is well tolerated, with minimal effects on blood pressure and heart rate at rest or during exercise (Shimokawa et al., 2002). In a double blind, placebo controlled randomized clinical trial of 84 patients with chronic stable angina, both placebo and fasudil increased exercise time on treadmill testing compared to baseline, but the difference between active drug and placebo was not statistically significant, though time to onset of ischemic ST segment depression during exercise was significantly prolonged compared to placebo (Vicari et al., 2005). Fasudil is not yet approved for use in United States. An intravenous formulation is approved in Japan to prevent cerebral vasospasm after subarachnoid hemorrhage.

2.7.3 Adverse effects

Vicari et al reported adverse effects in 41 patients and compared them to those reported with placebo. Overall incidence of adverse effects were similar in the 2 groups. The common organ systems reported to be involved were skin, subcutaneous tissue and the vascular system. Common disorders reported (incidence <20%) were allergic dermatitis, bruising, diaphoresis, facial erythema, facial flushing, hypotension or hypertension and a Raynaud-like phenomenon. The majority of adverse events were classified as mild to moderate. No deaths were reported (Vicari et al., 2005).

2.8 Trimetazidine

Trimetazidine (1-[2,3,4-trimethoxybenzyl] piperazine dihydrochloride) is a prototype of a group of antianginal agents thought to act by affecting myocardial metabolism directly.

2.8.1 Pharmacological effects

As for most if not all antianginal drugs, the mechanism of action of trimetazidine is not fully clear. The proposed mechanism is direct enhancement of myocardial energy metabolism, resulting in cytoprotective effects (Harpey, 1989; Kay et al., 1995). Fantini et al showed that in isolated rat heart mitochondria, trimetazidine has an inhibitory effect on palmitoyl-carnitine oxidation, with no significant effect on pyruvate oxidation (Fantini et al., 1994). This suggests that trimetazidine inhibits fatty acid oxidation in the heart. It has been shown that high fatty acid oxidation rates are detrimental in the setting of ischemia because of inhibition of the more energy efficient glucose oxidation, resulting in exacerbation of ischemic injury and a decrease in cardiac efficiency during reperfusion. Kantor et al demonstrated that trimetazidine suppresses fatty acid oxidation secondary to inhibition of long-chain 3-ketoacyl CoA thiolase, resulting in an increase in glucose oxidation. As a result, switching energy substrate preference from fatty acid oxidation to glucose oxidation may explain the antianginal properties of trimetazidine (Kantor et al., 2000). Unlike several other antianginals, trimetazidine has no effect on vascular smooth muscle and thus has been termed a "cellular anti-ischemic agent".

2.8.2 Clinical application

The European Collaborative Working Group has demonstrated that trimetazidine is equivalent to propranolol in its antianginal efficiency, but is devoid of measurable hemodynamic effects (Detry et al., 1994). Similar results were reported in comparison with nifedipine (Dalla-Volta et al., 1990). Additive antianginal effects were observed when trimetazidine was combined with diltiazem (Levy, 1995; Manchanda & Krishnaswami, 1997), while the benefits of combination with metoprolol were demonstrated in the TRIMPOL II (Szwed et al., 2001) trial.

2.8.3 Adverse effects

Trimetazidine is relatively safe and is very well tolerated; there are few known drug interactions. Because of its safety profile, compliance has been quite good. In one uncontrolled trial, 2.4% of patients had adverse events during an 8-week treatment period. Nausea was the most frequent adverse event (0.4%) (Makolkin, 2003).

3. Non-pharmacological therapy

Despite maximized pharmacological therapy and life style modification, many patients with CAD continue to suffer from angina, including so-called "refractory angina", which is defined as Canadian Cardiovascular Society (CCS) class III or IV angina with marked limitation during ordinary physical activity or inability to perform ordinary physical activity without discomfort (Gowda et al., 2005). Patients with refractory angina typically experience poor general health status, psychological distress, impaired role functioning, activity restriction, and inability to manage their living situation (Brorsson et al., 2002; Erixson, 1997; McGillion et al., 2007). Refractory angina is debilitating and its treatment is challenging. In the past several decades, a number of nonpharmacological treatments have been developed to help resolve this problem. These therapies will be outlined in this section.

3.1 Mechanical therapy

3.1.2 Revascularization

Coronary angiography and possible revascularization should be considered in patients with refractory angina. Revascularization includes percutaneous coronary interventions (PCI) and coronary artery bypass graft surgery.

3.1.2.1 Percutaneous coronary intervention

PCI, initially involving balloon angioplasty and later generally comprising balloon angioplasty plus stent placement to support and maintain the new channel, was developed for the relief of angina in patients refractory to medication. This remains one of the few data-supported applications of the technique.

3.1.2.1.1 Evidence

A comparison of balloon angioplasty with pharmacological therapy in treating patients with single vessel CAD (ACME) showed that angioplasty resulted in a greater proportion of patients free of angina at 6 months and greater improvement in treadmill exercise duration than did pharmacological therapy (Parisi et al., 1992). This study predated the routine use of stents and manifested a high rate (20%) of PCI failure but nonetheless supported the superiority of mechanical angioplasty to drug therapy alone for angina prevention. The multicenter Randomized Intervention Treatment of Angina (RITA) 2 trial was one of the largest trials prospectively assessing the impact of balloon angioplasty vs medical therapy on angina. Angina was of relatively mild severity (CCS 0-2) in 80 % of patients (Chamberlain, 1997). Angina frequency, exercise time and quality of life all improved in both groups. However, the subgroup of patients with CCS≥2 derived significantly greater symptom-relieving benefit from PCI than from pharmacological therapy during a 1 year follow-up interval. By 3 years, this advantage was lost, though interpretation of this finding is confounded by a relatively high (23%) crossover rate of medically treated patients to PCI. The Atorvastatin versus Revascularization Treatment (AVERT) trial assessed patients with angina CCS class 0-2. In this study, half the PCI group received stents as well as balloon angioplasty (Pitt et al., 1999). Patients in the PCI group evidenced greater improvement than those receiving pharmacological therapy. Bucher et al conducted a systematic review of 6 trials from 1979 through1998, including a total of 1904 patients with stable single vessel CAD and normal LV function (4). Balloon angioplasty was associated with a significant improvement in angina compared with pharmacological therapy alone. There was no difference of mortality or myocardial infarction between PCI and drug therapy (Bucher et al., 2000). Recently, 2 trials, MASS (Medicine, Angioplasty or Surgery Study) II (Hueb et al., 2004) and COURAGE (Clinical Outcomes utilizing Revascularization and Aggressive Drug Therapy) (Boden et al., 2007) compared PCI versus pharmacological therapy in stable CAD. MASS-II included 611 patients; after 1 year of follow up, 79% of patients in PCI group, 88% of patients in surgery group and 46% in medical therapy group were free of angina, though no difference was found in mortality rates among the groups. COURAGE compared initial PCI with "optimal medical management". At baseline, 43% of patients either did not have symptoms or had Class 1 angina. After 5 years follow up, 74% of patients in the PCI group and 72% patients in the medical therapy group were free of angina. By this time, one-third of patients had crossed over from medical therapy to PCI group. No evidence of benefit was found in terms of mortality or major morbidity when the groups were analyzed according to intention to treat.

3.1.2.1.2 Conclusion

The decision to perform PCI for symptom relief in patients with angina remains complex and needs to be individualized based on analysis of goals and risks. The relevant trials performed to date have important limitations for extrapolation to current decisions including the possible impact of recent improvements in PCI techniques, changes in pharmacology and alterations in the populations at risk, in part because of drug therapy that can modify atherosclerosis. Most trials show that PCI results in greater symptom relief and better exercise tolerance than drug therapy but suggest that this advantage is of relatively limited duration, requiring adjunctive or additional therapy to maintain anti-anginal benefits. However, for patients with angina refractory to pharmacological therapy, current evidence clearly supports PCI as an appropriate therapy for symptom improvement. Nonetheless, because of the rapidly changing landscape of therapy noted above, the appropriate approach to achieve optimal symptom prevention is a moving target, and more studies would be useful.

3.1.2.2 Coronary artery bypass grafting (CABG) surgery

CABG is an important therapeutic modality for millions of patients with CAD. Surgery has evolved over the more than 4 decades since its introduction, both in terms of duration of benefit (open arteries) and in reduction of peri-operative complications.

3.1.2.2.1 Evidence

Early trials included the European Coronary Surgery Study (ECSS) (Varnauskas, 1988), Veterans Cooperative Study (Detre, 1984) and Coronary Artery Surgery Study (CASS) (Killip, 1983). These studies were designed to assess the benefits of CABG for survival and prevention of major morbidity, but provided information about angina prevention, as well. In each of these studies, CABG was compared with medical therapy in patients with stable CAD and angina. Yusuf et al conducted a meta-analysis of earlier surgery trials which included a total of 2649 patients in which outcomes were evaluated at 5 and 10 years (Yusuf et al., 1994). CABG improved survival compared with pharmacological therapy. Importantly, though, CABG also produced greater freedom from symptoms and less use of antianginal medications than pharmacological therapy during a 5 year follow-up. Not surprisingly, benefits were greatest among those with the most severe disease at randomization, those with left main or multivessel disease and those with one or two vessel disease involving the proximal left anterior descending artery. Survival benefits were greater among patients with at least moderately subnormal LV ejection fraction than among those with normal LV performance. Bypass Angioplasty Revascularization Investment (BARI) trial was the largest (1829 patients) randomized study comparing balloon angioplasty versus CABG in symptomatic multivessel CAD (Alderman, 1996). After 10 years of follow up, angina rates in the two groups were similar. There were higher subsequent revascularization rates in balloon angioplasty group than in those who were randomized to CABG. Also, as noted above, MASS-II showed that 88% of patients in surgery group, 79% of patients in PCI group and 46% in medical therapy group were free of angina at pre-specified follow-up (Hueb et al., 2004). Bravata et al did a meta-analysis of 23 trials which included a total of 9963 patients, indicating that angina was relieved at 5 years in 79% of PCI patients and 84% of CABG patients (Bravata et al., 2007). Data also indicate that approximately 80-90% patients who are symptomatic on medical therapy become symptom free following CABG. This benefit has been shown to extend even to low-risk patients in whom mortality benefit with surgery has not been shown (Yusuf et al., 1994).

3.1.2.2.2 Conclusion

Both CABG and PCI are effective in relieving angina but CABG achieves this benefit with less need for repeat procedures than does PCI. In addition, though not specifically relevant to angina relief, several subsets of patients with chronic stable CAD can anticipate survival benefit from CABG; no parallel data are available for PCI. However, many of the relevant data were obtained with techniques and devices that have been superseded in this rapidly developing area. Thus, more data with the most up-to date techniques would be useful, on a background of the most modern pharmacological therapy to beneficially alter CAD progression. Nonetheless, as suggested by data from matched cohorts from the New York State coronary surgery database (Hannan et al., 2005), even as PCI techniques develop, CABG remains superior in terms of survival but the effects of newer approaches on angina remain to be defined.

3.1.3 Enhanced External Counterpulsation

Enhanced External Counterpulsation (EECP) is a non-invasive treatment that has been studied and employed with variable success for more than 30 years (Amin et al., 2010). EECP is carried out by placing compressible cuffs around the calves and lower and upper thighs, inflating them sequentially during diastole and deflating them simultaneously at the onset of systole. Throughout this process, the patient is connected to an electrocardiogram (ECG) and a finger plethysmograph. The R wave of the ECG is used to gate inflation and deflation. Treatment typically involves 35 sessions, each lasting 1 hour, undertaken over a 7-week interval (Sinvhal et al., 2003). EECP is believed to improve coronary perfusion pressure through diastolic augmentation while decreasing cardiac workload by reducing aortic impedance during systole.

3.1.3.1 Evidence

EECP is generally considered acceptably safe and is without specific contraindications. The few adverse effects associated with EECP generally are related to the physical characteristics of the equipment and its application, e.g., leg and back pain, abrasion of skin, bruising, blistering, edema and paresthesia (Arora et al., 1999). The effectiveness of EECP for refractory angina has been investigated in several studies over the last two decades. In the only published randomized clinical trial (Arora et al., 1999), the Multicenter Study of Enhanced External Counterpulsation (MUST-EECP), which involved 139 patients with angina and documented CAD, patients were randomised to either 35 h of active counterpulsation (300 mm Hg maximal cuff pressure) or inactive counterpulsation (75 mm Hg maximal cuff pressure) over a 4–7 week-period. Exercise duration increased in both groups to a similar degree ($p > 0.3$) and nitroglycerin use did not differ between groups ($P>0.7$). However, time to ≥1-mm ST segment depression (exercise-induced ischemia) increased significantly from baseline in active counterpulsation compared with inactive counterpulsation ($p = 0.01$). More active counterpulsation patients saw a decrease and fewer experienced an increase in angina episodes as compared with inactive counterpulsation patients ($p < 0.05$). The investigators concluded that EECP reduced angina and extended time to exercise-induced *ischemia* in patients with symptomatic *CAD*. Treatment was relatively well tolerated and was free of limiting side effects in most patients. The limitations of this trial include fairly stringent patient selection criteria precluding simple extrapolation of the data, the preponderance of patients with only Class I or II symptoms, and the lack of data about natural history outcomes. Also, there were more withdrawals due to adverse effects in active EECP group than in the control group.

To further assess EECP effects on both exercise tolerance and cardiac function, Urano et al (Urano et al., 2001) examined 12 stable patients with CAD and evidence of exercise-induced myocardial ischemia despite conventional medical or surgical therapies. These investigators found that, compared with baseline values, EECP improved all exercise test parameters, reduced exercise-induced reversible perfusion defects by thallium scintigraphy, and improved diastolic filling and LV end-diastolic pressure. These hemodynamic improvements were associated with decreased plasma brain natriuretic peptide levels. The investigators concluded that EECP definitely was effective in patients with CAD.

To clarify the mechanism underlying EECP benefits, Shechter et al (Shechter et al., 2003) investigated the influence of short-term EECP on vascular endothelial function in patients with CAD. They used high-resolution ultrasound to assesse endothelium-dependent brachial artery flow-mediated dilation (FMD) and endothelium-independent nitroglycerin-mediated vasodilation before and after EECP therapy. EECP resulted in significant improvement in post-intervention FMD but no significant effect on nitroglycerin-induced vasodilation. EECP significantly reduced angina as assessed by mean daily sublingual nitrate consumption and mean CCS angina class. The investigators concluded that EECP improved vascular endothelial function and angina in patients with CAD and refractory angina pectoris, suggesting a causal relation.

Few studies have evaluated the long-term effects of EECP. Loh et al (Loh et al., 2008) used the International EECP Patient Registry (IEPR-1) that enrolled consecutive patients treated with EECP in more than 100 centers; follow-up duration was 3 years. These investigators found that immediately post-EECP, the proportion of patients with severe angina (CCS III/IV) was reduced from 89% to 25% ($p<0.001$). The benefit was sustained in 74% during follow-up. This is the longest follow-up from IEPR-1 to date and tends to confirm the safety and immediate benefits of EECP as well as suggesting that sustained symptomatic and quality of life benefit can be achieved in most patients for up to 3 years. However, this observational study lacked a control group, weakening the conclusions. Further, the results are impaired by patient selection and survival bias. Other non- randomized studies (Barsheshet et al., 2008; Holubkov et al., 2002; Shechter et al., 2003; Urano et al., 2001) have been difficult to interpret. All assessments need to be treated with considerable caution due to selection bias and absence of blinding (McKenna et al., 2009).

3.1.3.2 Conclusion

With its development, it was hoped that EECP would be a viable adjunct for patients with CAD patients and angina inadequately responsive to medication and revascularization. To date, results from well-designed clinical trials are relatively few. However, these data provide a suggestion of no more than limited clinical effectiveness. Issues of adverse effects and cost-effectiveness have limited application of EECP therapy. Finally, evaluation in a truly refractory population with predominantly Class III/IV patients has not been undertaken. The ACC/AHA 2002 guideline update for the management of patients with chronic stable angina assigns EECP therapy a level of evidence of Class IIB (the usefulness/ efficacy is less well established by evidence/opinion). This suggests there may be some benefit, but additional clinical trial data are needed before EECP can be recommended definitively (Gibbons et al., 2003). EECP was not mentioned in the 2007 Chronic Angina Focused Update of the ACC/AHA 2002 Guidelines for the Management of Patients with Chronic Stable Angina (Fraker et al., 2007). Thus, additional data from randomized controlled trials are needed with regards to exercise tolerance, angina frequency and nitroglycerin use, ischemia reduction and, if possible, long term benefit on quality of life, as well as mortality or major morbid cardiovascular events.

3.1.4 Carotid Sinus Nerve Stimulation

Fifty years ago, carotid sinus nerve stimulation (CSNS) to slow heart rate and, to a lesser extent, to lower blood pressure was conceived (Lown & Levine, 1961) as an alternative treatment for refractory angina. Stimulation of the carotid sinus nerves reflexly reduces the frequency of sympathetic efferent impulses which, in turn, results in reduction in arterial pressure, myocardial contractility, and heart rate; as a consequence, myocardial oxygen demand is diminished and angina is relieved. Small, non-randomized studies demonstrated that CSNS relieved angina and allowed patients to perform more exercise without developing angina (Braunwald et al., 1967; Epstein et al., 1969; Rotem, 1974). However, due to the need for invasive implantation of the stimulator using the somewhat crude methods of the time, CSNS never was broadly applied. Nonetheless, it proved the principle that angina relief could be achieved directly by altering certain hemodynamic variables.

3.1.5 Spinal Cord Stimulation

Spinal cord stimulation (SCS), also called dorsal column stimulation or neurostimulation, is a neuromodulation therapy to alleviate pain by electrically activating pain-inhibiting neuronal circuits in the dorsal horn and inducing paresthesia that masks the original pain sensations. Local anesthesia is used during SCS implantation, via an incision at the level of thoracic vertebrae 6-8, an electrode is inserted into the epidural space and guided via X-ray monitoring up to the level of the thoracic 1-2 vertebrae. Its location is adjusted until the patient experiences paresthesiae within the area of the anginal pain. An extension wire is then tunneled subcutaneously via an incision to the left flank, where it is connected to a subcutaneous pulse-generator below the left costal arch. The stimulation intensity is then fine-tuned post-operatively. The patient can regulate the strength of the actual stimulation using a remote control (Borjesson et al., 2008). SCS has been successfully reported to relieve pain in a number of chronic conditions including neuropathic pain and peripheral vascular disease (Kemler et al., 2000; Kumar et al., 2007; Lee & Pilitsis, 2006). Since the late 1980s, SCS has been used to treat patients with chronic refractory angina who are not responsive to conventional medical therapy and revascularization (Murphy & Giles, 1987). Although the underlying mechanism is not fully elucidated, it has been proposed that SCS exerts beneficial effects by decreasing pain and sympathetic tone, yielding reductions in myocardial oxygen consumption and improved myocardial microcirculatory blood flow (Latif et al., 2001).

3.1.5.1 Evidence

Published evidence supports SCS as effective and acceptably safe for patients with refractory angina who are unresponsive to medical and surgical intervention (Bondesson et al., 2008; de Vries et al., 2007; Diedrichs et al., 2005; Dyer et al., 2008; Eddicks et al., 2007; Lapenna et al., 2006; McNab et al., 2006). Recently, a meta-analysis of 7 randomized controlled trials involving 270 patients (Taylor et al., 2009) found benefits similar to those of CABG and percutaneous myocardial laser revascularization (PMR). Compared to the control, there was some evidence of improvement in all outcomes following SCS implantation with significant gains observed in pooled exercise capacity and health related quality of life. However, the trials were small and varied considerably in quality. The healthcare costs of SCS appeared to be lower than CABG at 2-years follow up. One particular challenge of SCS evaluation is the difficulty in patient blinding, as the therapy produces paresthesia in the area of the pain if SCS is effective. In addition, the implantation procedure might produce a placebo effect, but sham operations are ethically difficult to justify (Van Zundert, 2007). Further high quality trials and cost effectiveness evidence is needed before SCS can be accepted as a routine treatment for refractory angina.

3.1.5.2 Conclusion

SCS has been used for treatment of refractory angina in Europe for 20 years. In the European Society of Cardiology guidelines on management of angina (Fox et al., 2006), SCS is accepted as a "well established method" for the management of refractory angina. Patients experience a favorable analgesic effect and positive effects on symptoms from SCS, though long-term effects are unknown. The ACC/AHA guidelines for the management of patients with chronic stable angina (Fraker et al., 2007; Gibbons et al., 2003) provided a class II b recommendation, suggesting that SCS should only be used in patients who cannot be managed adequately by medical therapy and who are not candidates for revascularization.

3.1.6 Transmyocardial revascularization

Transmyocardial revascularization (TMR) applies high-energy laser beams to create non-transmural endomyocardial channels. These channels can be generated surgically, using an epicardial approach, or percutaneously (PMR), via catheter, an endocardial approach. The basis for angina prevention with TMR is unclear. The initial hypothesis was that the channels provided oxygenated blood from the LV to directly perfuse the myocardium; support for this mechanism is not compelling; more recently, it has been proposed that clinical improvement may be secondary to angiogenesis, placebo effect, or myocardial denervation (Huikeshoven et al., 2002). TMR also has been combined with administration of angiogenic growth factors and/or angiogenic gene vectors introduced via the channels to stimulate angiogenesis (see Biological Therapy, below).

3.1.6.1 Evidence

Since its initial application in association with CABG in 1983, surgical TMR has been considered an alternative for patients with refractory angina who were not amenable to conventional revascularization (Smith et al., 1995). However, though several preliminary studies demonstrated a decrease in angina severity in most patients (Cooley et al., 1996; Horvath et al., 1996), subsequent randomized controlled trials (RCT) have reported contradictory results (Aaberge et al., 2000; Burkhoff et al., 1999; Campbell et al., 2001; Jones et al., 1999; March, 1999; van der Sloot et al., 2004). Briones et al (Briones et al., 2009) conducted a Cochrane systematic review to assess the efficacy and safety of TMR versus optimized drug therapy in alleviating angina and improving survival and heart function. The 7 RCTs included in the review involved 1137 patients of whom 559 were randomized to TMR. Overall, 43.8% of patients in the treatment group decreased two angina classes, compared to 14.8% in the control group (95% confidence interval 3.43 to 6.25). Mortality analyzed on an intention-to-treat basis was similar in both groups at 30 days (4.0% in the TMR group vs. 3.5% in the control group) and at one year (12.2% in the TMR group vs. 11.9% in the control group). However, the per protocol 30-day mortality was 6.8% in the TMR group compared to 0.8% in the control group (OR 3.76 [95% CI, 1.63 to 8.66]). The authors concluded that evidence is insufficient to support the presumption that clinical benefits of TMR outweigh the potential risks. Importantly, the observed improvement in angina was not measured using blinded methods and is therefore subject to significant potential bias, and there was no difference in survival.

PMR is less invasive than TMR, utilizing a fiberoptic catheter inserted through a femoral artery under conscious sedation to carry the laser energy to the endocardial surface. Laser firing is synchronized during systole to create a series of nontransmural channels in targeted regions (Oesterle et al., 1998). Recently McGillion et al (McGillion et al., 2010) conducted a meta-analysis to assess the effectiveness of PMR versus optimized drug therapy for reducing angina and improving health-related quality of life (HRQL), and exercise performance. Seven RCT trials, involving 1,213 participants, were included. At 12-month follow-up, the PMR group had more than 2 CCS class symptom reductions as well as improvements in HRQL, disease perception and physical limitations. However, PMR had no significant impact on all-cause mortality. In the secondary analyses, in which the data were from a single trial that employed a higher-dose laser group, the result showed no significant overall impact of PMR across outcomes.

3.1.6.2 Conclusion

When applied in carefully selected patients with refractory angina, TMR can provide durable reduction in self-reported angina and improvement in quality of life compared to drug treatment alone. However, evidence of improvement in exercise tolerance, the "objectification" of angina, is less strong, and impact on survival has not been demonstrated. For PMR, evidence is insufficient to demonstrate efficacy for angina prevention (and, therefore, of benefit to risk relation). Long-term outcomes of PMR are not clear. PMR devices have not been approved by the FDA due to lack of adequate evidence of efficacy in their use. ACC/AHA guidelines (Eagle et al., 2004; Gibbons et al., 2003) recommend TMR as a Class IIa procedure, stating that TMR alone or in combination with CABG is reasonable in patients with angina refractory to medical therapy who are not candidates for PCI or CABG but does not recommend PMR, noting that it should still be considered experimental.

3.2 Biological therapy

3.2.1 Angiogenic gene therapy

Angiogenesis is the biological process involving formation of new blood vessels from pre-existing vessels under physiological or pathological conditions. In patients with chronic CAD, angiogenesis in response to repeated myocardial ischemia can provide collateral blood flow to muscle distal to sites of coronary stenoses. Theoretically, stimulation of angiogenesis presents an attractive approach for the treatment of CAD. Attempts at therapeutic angiogenesis have employed molecules (growth factors) shown experimentally to improve jeopardized blood supply, thereby relieving myocardial ischemia, improving regional and global LV performance, lessening angina, and improving clinical outcomes (Simons & Ware, 2003). A number of growth factors have been demonstrated to stimulate blood vessel growth in humans and are the focus of recent angiogenic gene therapy studies. These include several fibroblast growth factors (FGFs), vascular endothelial growth factors (VEGFs) and granulocyte/macrophage colony stimulating factor (GM-CSF) (Zachary & Morgan, 2011).

3.2.1.1 Evidence

How to effectively and safely deliver growth factors to the target tissue remains a major problem in therapeutic angiogenesis trials. The accepted consensus is that effective angiogenic intervention will require the presence of the therapeutic agent at the desired site of action for as long as four to six weeks. In early experience, delivery of growth factors was achieved either by systemic infusion or intracoronary infusion, but results were disappointing, perhaps because of short residence time of the infused proteins in target tissues. Repeated administration or the use of sustained release polymers may prove more effective, but remains to be tested. Introduction of angiogenic genes into the myocardium offers a theoretical alternative approach to delivery that might obviate the need for repeated administrations of short-lived proteins, and avoid the potential risks of short-term systemic exposure to relatively high concentrations of proteins (Simons et al., 2000). Introduction of angiogenic genes with both plasmid and adenoviral vectors has been associated with improvements in heart function and perfusion in different animal models of myocardial ischaemia (Hammond & McKirnan, 2001). Several clinical gene therapy trials of angiogenic growth factors have been conducted using either plasmid or adenoviral vectors. Effects of intramyocardially delivered plasmid VEGF were assessed in two randomised, double-blinded, placebo-controlled trials, EUROINJECT-ONE (Kastrup et al., 2005) and NORTHERN (Stewart et al., 2009) involving, respectively, 80 and 93 patients with severe stable ischemic heart disease (CCS III/IV). Neither trial demonstrated alteration in the primary end point, change in myocardial perfusion, by therapy, despite the use of a high plasmid dose (2 mg) in the NORTHERN study. There was a trend toward improvement in exercise treadmill time and angina reduction, but again no significant differences were observed. Another RCT, REVASC (Stewart et al., 2006) employed an adenoviral vector (AdVEGF121) delivered into the myocardium at surgery in 67 patients with refractory angina. In this study, a statistically significant increase in the primary end point, time to 1 mm ST-segment depression on treadmill exercise, was observed at 26 weeks in the active treatment group. Another RCT, KAT (Hedman et al., 2003), compared AdVEGF165 with either plasmid VEGF or placebo for effect on myocardial perfusion in 103 patients. In this trial, the vectors were administered by intracoronary injection at angioplasty. There was no significant difference in the rates of restenosis between treatment groups at 6 months, but myocardial perfusion improved in the AdVEGF165 group compared with plasmid VEGF. In an 8-year follow-up study of the KAT trial, the incidence of major adverse cardiovascular events, cancer or diabetes did not differ between the treatment groups (Hedman et al., 2009). A series of AGENT trials investigated the safety and efficacy of intracoronary injections of an adenoviral-encoded FGF-4 gene. The AGENT-1 trial (Grines et al., 2002) enrolled 79 patients and found a trend toward improved exercise time at four weeks in treatment group compared to the placebo group; when only patients with baseline exercise time ≤10 minutes were considered, exercise time increased significantly. The subsequent AGENT-2 trial of 52 patients with AdFGF-4 found a nonsignificant reduction in the size of the ischemic defect on perfusion imaging between treatment and placebo (Kapur & Rade, 2008). However, two large double-blind phase III trials of Ad-FGF4 (AGENT-3 and AGENT-4) were negative for their primary end point although a post-hoc analysis suggested a benefit in a certain population of middle aged women (Henry et al., 2007).

3.2.1.2 Conclusion

Though therapeutic angiogenesis theoretically is an attractive option for improving the quality of life in chronic ischemic heart disease, no large clinical trial yet has shown substantial clinical benefit. However, efforts are ongoing to improve delivery and expression and biological efficacy of the angiogenic genes (Zachary & Morgan, 2011).

3.2.2 Stem cell therapy

Hematopoietic stem cells are bone marrow-derived cells capable of differentiating into a variety of cell types. Such cells may be obtained directly from the bone marrow or, using apheresis techniques, from peripheral blood, usually after stimulation with granulocyte-colony stimulating factor (G-CSF). Cardiac stem cell therapy has been evaluated clinically during the past 10 years. Many clinical trials have been conducted on treatment for heart failure (Menasche et al., 2008; Stamm et al., 2007) and acute MI (Martin-Rendon et al., 2008) but the study of stem cell therapy for refractory angina is in early stages of development. The mechanisms of potential benefit remain uncertain. The initial hypothesis of transdifferentiation into cardiomyocytes no longer is generally accepted (Murry et al., 2004). The currently favored hypothesis is that increased angiogenesis is stimulated by angiogenic growth factors released by bone marrow cells, particularly by the CD34+ fraction (Menasche, 2011).

3.2.2.1 Evidence

Losordo et al (Losordo et al., 2007) showed the efficacy of intramyocardial transplantation of autologous G-CSF-mobilized peripheral blood CD34+ stem cells for prevention of angina. Twenty-four patients with CCS class III or IV angina who were undergoing optimized medical treatment and who were not candidates for mechanical revascularization were enrolled in a double-blind, randomized (3:1), placebo-controlled dose-escalating study. CD34+ progenitors were collected following GCSF-induced cell mobilization and apheresis.

Electromechanical mapping was performed to identify ischemic but viable regions of myocardium for injection of cells (versus saline). The intramyocardial injection of cells or saline did not result in cardiac enzyme elevation, perforation, or pericardial effusion. Neither ventricular tachycardia nor ventricular fibrillation occurred during the administration of G-CSF or intramyocardial injections. Efficacy parameters including angina frequency, nitroglycerin usage, exercise time, and CCS class showed trends that favored CD34+ cell-treated patients versus placebo-treated controls. A phase II b study in a larger population is currently under way.
A recent RCT of intracoronary infusion with autologous bone marrow CD34+ stem cells involved 112 patients with intractable angina (Wang et al., 2010). No myocardial infarction or other major adverse event was observed during the procedure. Investigators found significantly greater reduction in angina frequency by diary at 3 and 6 months after active treatment than after control. Other efficacy parameters, such as nitroglycerin use, exercise time and the CCS class, also were improved by active treatment versus control, as was myocardial perfusion imaging assessment of ischemia.

3.2.2.2 Conclusion

Stem cell therapy is an investigational technique that has reduced angina frequency and severity by several measures in small populations with refractory angina. However, additional studies are required to determine the magnitude, consistency and durability of anti-anginal benefit, as well as the long-term safety of this approach for treatment of patients with angina due to CAD.

4. Acknowledgment

Dr. Borer's research is supported in part by grants from The Howard Gilman Foundation, New York, NY,_The Schiavone Family Foundation, White House Station, N.J., The Charles and Jean Brunie Foundation, Bronxville, N.Y., The American Cardiovascular Research Foundation, New York, N.Y., The Irving A. Hansen Foundation, New York, N.Y., The Mary A.H. Rumsey Foundation, New York, N.Y., The Messinger Family Foundation, New York, N.Y., The Daniel and Elaine Sargent Charitable Trust, New York, N.Y., and by much appreciated gifts from Donna and William Acquavella, New York, N.Y.,and Clyde and Diana Brownstone, New York, NY. In addition, he is a paid consultant to Servier Laboratoires, Neuilly sur Seine, France, manufacturer of ivabradine, in the course of which he has performed and advised on antianginal drug studies. His work on this manuscript was not supported by Servier.

5. References

Aaberge, L., Nordstrand, K.,Dragsund, M., et al. (2000). Transmyocardial revascularization with CO2 laser in patients with refractory angina pectoris. Clinical results from the Norwegian randomized trial. *J Am Coll Cardiol,* 35, 5, (Apr), pp. 1170-7.

Abdallah, H. & Jerling, M. (2005). Effect of hepatic impairment on the multiple-dose pharmacokinetics of ranolazine sustained-release tablets. *J Clin Pharmacol,* 45, 7, (Jul), pp. 802-9.

Abrams, J. (1980). Nitroglycerin and long-acting nitrates. *N Engl J Med,* 302, 22, (May), pp. 1234-7.

Alderman, E. L., Andrews, K., Bost, J., et al. (1996). Comparison of coronary bypass surgery with angioplasty in patients with multivessel disease. The Bypass Angioplasty Revascularization Investigation (BARI) Investigators. *N Engl J Med*, 335, 4, (Jul), pp. 217-25.

Amin, F.,Al Hajeri, A.,Civelek, B., et al. (2010). Enhanced external counterpulsation for chronic angina pectoris. *Cochrane Database Syst Rev*, 2, CD007219.

Andrews, T. C.,Fenton, T.,Toyosaki, N., et al. (1993). Subsets of ambulatory myocardial ischemia based on heart rate activity. Circadian distribution and response to anti-ischemic medication. The Angina and Silent Ischemia Study Group (ASIS). *Circulation*, 88, 1, (Jul), pp. 92-100.

Antzelevitch, C.,Belardinelli, L.,Wu, L., et al. (2004). Electrophysiologic properties and antiarrhythmic actions of a novel antianginal agent. *J Cardiovasc Pharmacol Ther*, 9 Suppl 1, (Sep), pp. S65-83.

Aronow, W. S. (1973). Management of stable angina. *N Engl J Med*, 289, 10, (Sep 6), pp. 516-20.

Arora, R. R.,Chou, T. M.,Jain, D., et al. (1999). The multicenter study of enhanced external counterpulsation (MUST-EECP): effect of EECP on exercise-induced myocardial ischemia and anginal episodes. *J Am Coll Cardiol*, 33, 7, (Jun), pp. 1833-40.

Azancot, I., Balbi, M., Bonnier, J.J.R.M., et al. (2003). Effect of nifedipine and cerivastatin on coronary endothelial function in patients with coronary artery disease: the ENCORE I Study (Evaluation of Nifedipine and Cerivastatin On Recovery of coronary Endothelial function). *Circulation*, 107, 3, (Jan), pp. 422-8.

Barsheshet, A.,Hod, H.,Shechter, M., et al. (2008). The effects of external counter pulsation therapy on circulating endothelial progenitor cells in patients with angina pectoris. *Cardiology*, 110, 3, pp. 160-6.

Belardinelli L, A. C., Fraser H (2004). Inhibition of late (sustained/persistent) sodium current: a potential drug target to reduce intracellular sodium-dependent calcium overload and its detrimenta leffects on cardiomyocyte function. *Eur Heart J*, 6(suppl 1), pp. 13-17.

Beltrame, J. F.,Weekes, A. J.,Morgan, C., et al. (2009). The prevalence of weekly angina among patients with chronic stable angina in primary care practices: The Coronary Artery Disease in General Practice (CADENCE) Study. *Arch Intern Med*, 169, 16, (Sep), pp. 1491-9.

Ben-Dor, I. & Battler, A. (2007). Treatment of stable angina. *Heart*, 93, 7, (Jul), pp. 868-74.

Boden, W. E.,O'Rourke, R. A.,Teo, K. K., et al. (2007). Optimal medical therapy with or without PCI for stable coronary disease. *N Engl J Med*, 356, 15, (Apr), pp. 1503-16.

Bohm, M.,Swedberg, K.,Komajda, M., et al. (2010). Heart rate as a risk factor in chronic heart failure (SHIFT): the association between heart rate and outcomes in a randomised placebo-controlled trial. *Lancet*, 376, 9744, (Sep), pp. 886-94.

Bondesson, S.,Pettersson, T.,Erdling, A., et al. (2008). Comparison of patients undergoing enhanced external counterpulsation and spinal cord stimulation for refractory angina pectoris. *Coron Artery Dis*, 19, 8, (Dec), pp. 627-34.

Borer, J. S.,Fox, K.,Jaillon, P., et al. (2003). Antianginal and antiischemic effects of ivabradine, an I(f) inhibitor, in stable angina: a randomized, double-blind, multicentered, placebo-controlled trial. *Circulation*, 107, 6, (Feb), pp. 817-23.

Borer, J. S.,Redwood, D. R.,Levitt, B., et al. (1975). Reduction in myocardial ischemia with nitroglycerin or nitroglycerin plus phenylephrine administered during acute myocardial infarction. *N Engl J Med,* 293, 20, (Nov), pp. 1008-12.

Borjesson, M.,Andrell, P.,Lundberg, D., et al. (2008). Spinal cord stimulation in severe angina pectoris--a systematic review based on the Swedish Council on Technology assessment in health care report on long-standing pain. *Pain,* 140, 3, (Dec), pp. 501-8.

Bottcher, M.,Madsen, M. M.,Randsbaek, F., et al. (2002). Effect of oral nitroglycerin and cold stress on myocardial perfusion in areas subtended by stenosed and nonstenosed coronary arteries. *Am J Cardiol,* 89, 9, (May), pp. 1019-24.

Braunwald, E.,Epstein, S. E.,Glick, G., et al. (1967). Relief of angina pectoris by electrical stimulation of the carotid-sinus nerves. *N Engl J Med,* 277, 24, (Dec), pp. 1278-83.

Braunwald, E.,Jones, R. H.,Mark, D. B., et al. (1994). Diagnosing and managing unstable angina. Agency for Health Care Policy and Research. *Circulation,* 90, 1, (Jul), pp. 613-22.

Bravata, D. M.,Gienger, A. L.,McDonald, K. M., et al. (2007). Systematic review: the comparative effectiveness of percutaneous coronary interventions and coronary artery bypass graft surgery. *Ann Intern Med,* 147, 10, (Nov), pp. 703-16.

Briones, E.,Lacalle, J. R. & Marin, I. (2009). Transmyocardial laser revascularization versus medical therapy for refractory angina. *Cochrane Database Syst Rev,* 1, CD003712.

Brorsson, B.,Bernstein, S. J.,Brook, R. H., et al. (2002). Quality of life of patients with chronic stable angina before and four years after coronary revascularisation compared with a normal population. *Heart,* 87, 2, (Feb), pp. 140-5.

Brown, H. F.,DiFrancesco, D. & Noble, S. J. (1979). How does adrenaline accelerate the heart? *Nature,* 280, 5719, (Jul), pp. 235-6.

Brunton, T. L. (1867). On the use of nitrite of amyl in angina pectoris. *Lancet,* 2, pp. 97-98

Bucher, H. C.,Hengstler, P.,Schindler, C., et al. (2000). Percutaneous transluminal coronary angioplasty versus medical treatment for non-acute coronary heart disease: meta-analysis of randomised controlled trials. *BMJ,* 321, 7253, (Jul), pp. 73-7.

Burkhoff, D.,Schmidt, S.,Schulman, S. P., et al. (1999). Transmyocardial laser revascularisation compared with continued medical therapy for treatment of refractory angina pectoris: a prospective randomised trial. ATLANTIC Investigators. Angina Treatments-Lasers and Normal Therapies in Comparison. *Lancet,* 354, 9182, (Sep), pp. 885-90.

Campbell, H. E.,Tait, S.,Buxton, M. J., et al. (2001). A UK trial-based cost--utility analysis of transmyocardial laser revascularization compared to continued medical therapy for treatment of refractory angina pectoris. *Eur J Cardiothorac Surg,* 20, 2, (Aug), pp. 312-8.

Chaitman, B. R. (2002). Measuring antianginal drug efficacy using exercise testing for chronic angina: improved exercise performance with ranolazine, a pFOX inhibitor. *Curr Probl Cardiol,* 27, 12, (Dec), pp. 527-55.

Chaitman, B. R.,Pepine, C. J.,Parker, J. O., et al. (2004). Effects of ranolazine with atenolol, amlodipine, or diltiazem on exercise tolerance and angina frequency in patients with severe chronic angina: a randomized controlled trial. *JAMA,* 291, 3, (Jan), pp. 309-16.

Chaitman, B. R. & Sano, J. (2007). Novel therapeutic approaches to treating chronic angina in the setting of chronic ischemic heart disease. *Clin Cardiol,* 30, 2 Suppl 1, (Feb), pp. I25-30.

Chamberlain, D. A., Fox, K.A., Henderson, R.A., Julian, D.G., Parker, J.S., Pocock, S.J. (1997). Coronary angioplasty versus medical therapy for angina: the second Randomised Intervention Treatment of Angina (RITA-2) trial. RITA-2 trial participants. *Lancet,* 350, 9076, (Aug), pp. 461-8.

Chu N, S. D., Sun HL (2003). In vitro metabolism of ranolazine. *Drug Metab Rev,* 35, Supp.2 (abst no. 363), 182.

Clarke, B.,Wyatt, K. M. & McCormack, J. G. (1996). Ranolazine increases active pyruvate dehydrogenase in perfused normoxic rat hearts: evidence for an indirect mechanism. *J Mol Cell Cardiol,* 28, 2, (Feb), 341-50.

Cooley, D. A.,Frazier, O. H.,Kadipasaoglu, K. A., et al. (1996). Transmyocardial laser revascularization: clinical experience with twelve-month follow-up. *J Thorac Cardiovasc Surg,* 111, 4, (Apr), pp. 791-7.

Crean, P. A.,Ribeiro, P.,Crea, F., et al. (1984). Failure of transdermal nitroglycerin to improve chronic stable angina: a randomized, placebo-controlled, double-blind, double crossover trial. *Am Heart J,* 108, 6, (Dec), pp. 1494-500.

Dalla-Volta, S.,Maraglino, G.,Della-Valentina, P., et al. (1990). Comparison of trimetazidine with nifedipine in effort angina: a double-blind, crossover study. *Cardiovasc Drugs Ther,* 4 Suppl 4, (Aug), pp. 853-9.

Daly, C. A.,Clemens, F.,Sendon, J. L., et al. (2010). Inadequate control of heart rate in patients with stable angina: results from the European heart survey. *Postgrad Med J,* 86, 1014, (Apr), pp. 212-7.

de Vries, J.,Dejongste, M. J.,Durenkamp, A., et al. (2007). The sustained benefits of long-term neurostimulation in patients with refractory chest pain and normal coronary arteries. *Eur J Pain,* 11, 3, (Apr), pp. 360-5.

Dens, J. A.,Desmet, W. J.,Coussement, P., et al. (2003). Long term effects of nisoldipine on the progression of coronary atherosclerosis and the occurrence of clinical events: the NICOLE study. *Heart,* 89, 8, (Aug), pp. 887-92.

Detre, K. M., Peduzzi, P., Takaro, T. (1984). Eleven-year survival in the Veterans Administration randomized trial of coronary bypass surgery for stable angina. The Veterans Administration Coronary Artery Bypass Surgery Cooperative Study Group. *N Engl J Med,* 311, 21, (Nov), pp. 1333-9.

Detry, J. M. & Bruce, R. A. (1971). Effects of nitroglycerin on "maximal" oxygen intake and exercise electrocardiogram in coronary heart disease. *Circulation,* 43, 1, (Jan), pp. 155-63.

Detry, J. M.,Sellier, P.,Pennaforte, S., et al. (1994). Trimetazidine: a new concept in the treatment of angina. Comparison with propranolol in patients with stable angina. Trimetazidine European Multicenter Study Group. *Br J Clin Pharmacol,* 37, 3, (Mar), pp. 279-88.

Di Somma, S.,Liguori, V.,Petitto, M., et al. (1993). A double-blind comparison of nicorandil and metoprolol in stable effort angina pectoris. *Cardiovasc Drugs Ther,* 7, 1, (Feb), pp. 119-23.

Diamond, G. A.,Staniloff, H. M.,Forrester, J. S., et al. (1983). Computer-assisted diagnosis in the noninvasive evaluation of patients with suspected coronary artery disease. *J Am Coll Cardiol,* 1, 2 Pt 1, (Feb), pp. 444-55.

Diaz, A.,Bourassa, M. G.,Guertin, M. C., et al. (2005). Long-term prognostic value of resting heart rate in patients with suspected or proven coronary artery disease. *Eur Heart J,* 26, 10, (May), pp. 967-74.

Diedrichs, H.,Zobel, C.,Theissen, P., et al. (2005). Symptomatic relief precedes improvement of myocardial blood flow in patients under spinal cord stimulation. *Curr Control Trials Cardiovasc Med,* 6, 1, (May), pp. 7.

DiFrancesco, D. & Camm, J. A. (2004). Heart rate lowering by specific and selective I(f) current inhibition with ivabradine: a new therapeutic perspective in cardiovascular disease. *Drugs,* 64, 16, pp. 1757-65.

Doring, G. (1992). Antianginal and anti-ischemic efficacy of nicorandil in comparison with isosorbide-5-mononitrate and isosorbide dinitrate: results from two multicenter, double-blind, randomized studies with stable coronary heart disease patients. *J Cardiovasc Pharmacol,* 20 Suppl 3, pp. S74-81.

Dyer, M. T.,Goldsmith, K. A.,Khan, S. N., et al. (2008). Clinical and cost-effectiveness analysis of an open label, single-centre, randomised trial of spinal cord stimulation (SCS) versus percutaneous myocardial laser revascularisation (PMR) in patients with refractory angina pectoris: The SPiRiT trial. *Trials,* 30, 9, (Jun), pp. 40.

Eagle, K. A.,Guyton, R. A.,Davidoff, R., et al. (2004). ACC/AHA 2004 guideline update for coronary artery bypass graft surgery: summary article: a report of the American College of Cardiology/American Heart Association Task Force on Practice Guidelines (Committee to Update the 1999 Guidelines for Coronary Artery Bypass Graft Surgery). *Circulation,* 110, 9, (Aug), pp. 1168-76.

Eddicks, S.,Maier-Hauff, K.,Schenk, M., et al. (2007). Thoracic spinal cord stimulation improves functional status and relieves symptoms in patients with refractory angina pectoris: the first placebo-controlled randomised study. *Heart,* 93, 5, (May), pp. 585-90.

Epstein, S. E.,Beiser, G. D.,Goldstein, R. E., et al. (1969). Treatment of angina pectoris by electrical stimulation of the carotid-sinus nerves. *N Engl J Med,* 280, 18, (May), pp. 971-8.

Erixson, G., Jerlock, M., Dahlberg, K. (1997). Experience of living with angina pectoris. *Nurs Sci Res Nordic Countries,* 17, pp. 34-38.

Fantini, E.,Demaison, L.,Sentex, E., et al. (1994). Some biochemical aspects of the protective effect of trimetazidine on rat cardiomyocytes during hypoxia and reoxygenation. *J Mol Cell Cardiol,* 26, 8, (Aug), pp. 949-58.

Ford, I., Dargie, H.J., Fox, K.M., Hillis, W.S. (2002). Effect of nicorandil on coronary events in patients with stable angina: the Impact Of Nicorandil in Angina (IONA) randomised trial. *Lancet,* 359, 9314, (Apr), 1269-75.

Fox, K.,Borer, J. S.,Camm, A. J., et al. (2007). Resting heart rate in cardiovascular disease. *J Am Coll Cardiol,* 50, 9, (Aug), 823-30.

Fox, K.,Ford, I.,Steg, P. G., et al. (2008). Ivabradine for patients with stable coronary artery disease and left-ventricular systolic dysfunction (BEAUTIFUL): a randomised, double-blind, placebo-controlled trial. *Lancet,* 372, 9641, (Sep), 807-16.

Fox, K.,Ford, I.,Steg, P. G., et al. (2008). Heart rate as a prognostic risk factor in patients with coronary artery disease and left-ventricular systolic dysfunction (BEAUTIFUL): a subgroup analysis of a randomised controlled trial. *Lancet,* 372, 9641, (Sep), pp. 817-21.

Fox, K.,Ford, I.,Steg, P. G., et al. (2009). Relationship between ivabradine treatment and cardiovascular outcomes in patients with stable coronary artery disease and left ventricular systolic dysfunction with limiting angina: a subgroup analysis of the randomized, controlled BEAUTIFUL trial. *Eur Heart J,* 30, 19, (Oct), pp. 2337-45.

Fox, K.,Garcia, M. A.,Ardissino, D., et al. (2006). Guidelines on the management of stable angina pectoris: executive summary: The Task Force on the Management of Stable Angina Pectoris of the European Society of Cardiology. *Eur Heart J,* 27, 11, (Jun), pp. 1341-81.

Fraker, T. D., Jr.,Fihn, S. D.,Gibbons, R. J., et al. (2007). 2007 chronic angina focused update of the ACC/AHA 2002 guidelines for the management of patients with chronic stable angina: a report of the American College of Cardiology/American Heart Association Task Force on Practice Guidelines Writing Group to develop the focused update of the 2002 guidelines for the management of patients with chronic stable angina. *J Am Coll Cardiol,* 50, 23, (Dec), pp. 2264-74.

Freemantle, N.,Cleland, J.,Young, P., et al. (1999). beta Blockade after myocardial infarction: systematic review and meta regression analysis. *BMJ,* 318, 7200, (Jun), pp. 1730-7.

Frishman, W. H. (1985). Pharmacology of the nitrates in angina pectoris. *Am J Cardiol,* 56, 17, (Dec), pp. 8I-13I.

Fukata, Y.,Amano, M. & Kaibuchi, K. (2001). Rho-Rho-kinase pathway in smooth muscle contraction and cytoskeletal reorganization of non-muscle cells. *Trends Pharmacol Sci,* 22, 1, (Jan), pp. 32-9.

Furberg, B.,Dahlqvist, A.,Raak, A., et al. (1978). Comparison of the new beta-adrenoceptor antagonist, nadolol, and propranolol in the treatment of angina pectoris. *Curr Med Res Opin,* 5, 5, pp. 388-93.

Furberg, C. D.,Psaty, B. M. & Meyer, J. V. (1995). Nifedipine. Dose-related increase in mortality in patients with coronary heart disease. *Circulation,* 92, 5, (Sep), pp. 1326-31.

Gehi, A. K.,Ali, S.,Na, B., et al. (2008). Inducible ischemia and the risk of recurrent cardiovascular events in outpatients with stable coronary heart disease: the heart and soul study. *Arch Intern Med,* 168, 13, (Jul), 1423-8.

Gibbons, R. J.,Abrams, J.,Chatterjee, K., et al. (2003). ACC/AHA 2002 guideline update for the management of patients with chronic stable angina--summary article: a report of the American College of Cardiology/American Heart Association Task Force on practice guidelines (Committee on the Management of Patients With Chronic Stable Angina). *J Am Coll Cardiol,* 41, 1, (Jan 1), pp. 159-68.

Gibbons, R. J.,Chatterjee, K.,Daley, J., et al. (1999). ACC/AHA/ACP-ASIM guidelines for the management of patients with chronic stable angina: a report of the American College of Cardiology/American Heart Association Task Force on Practice Guidelines (Committee on Management of Patients With Chronic Stable Angina). *J Am Coll Cardiol,* 33, 7, (Jun), pp. 2092-197.

Goldstein, R. E., Bennett, E.D., Leech, G.L. (1979). Effects of glyceryl trinitrate on echocardiographic left ventricular dimensions during exercise in the upright position. *Br Heart J,* 42, 3, (Sep), pp. 245-254.

Goldstein, R. E. & Epstein, S. E. (1973). Editorial: Nitrates in the prophylactic treatment of angina pectoris. *Circulation,* 48, 5, (Nov), pp. 917-20.

Goldstein, R. E.,Rosing, D. R.,Redwood, D. R., et al. (1971). Clinical and circulatory effects of isosorbide dinitrate. Comparison with nitroglycerin. *Circulation,* 43, 5, (May), pp. 629-40.

Gori, T. & Parker, J. D. (2004). Long-term therapy with organic nitrates: the pros and cons of nitric oxide replacement therapy. *J Am Coll Cardiol,* 44, 3, (Aug), pp. 632-4.

Gowda, R. M.,Khan, I. A.,Punukollu, G., et al. (2005). Treatment of refractory angina pectoris. *Int J Cardiol,* 101, 1, (May), pp. 1-7.

Grayson, J.,Irvine, M. & Parratt, J. R. (1967). The effects of amyl nitrite inhalation on myocardial blood flow and metabolic heat production. *Br J Pharmacol Chemother,* 30, 3, (Aug), pp. 488-96.

Grines, C. L.,Watkins, M. W.,Helmer, G., et al. (2002). Angiogenic Gene Therapy (AGENT) trial in patients with stable angina pectoris. *Circulation,* 105, 11, (Mar), pp. 1291-7.

Hammond, H. K. & McKirnan, M. D. (2001). Angiogenic gene therapy for heart disease: a review of animal studies and clinical trials. *Cardiovasc Res,* 49, 3, (Feb), pp. 561-7.

Hannan, E. L.,Racz, M. J.,Walford, G., et al. (2005). Long-term outcomes of coronary-artery bypass grafting versus stent implantation. *N Engl J Med,* 352, 21, (May), pp. 2174-83.

Harpey, C., Clauser, P., Labrid, C., et al. (1989). Trimetazidine, a cellular anti-ischemic agent. *Cardiovasc Drug Rev,* 6, pp. 292-312.

Hedman, M.,Hartikainen, J.,Syvanne, M., et al. (2003). Safety and feasibility of catheter-based local intracoronary vascular endothelial growth factor gene transfer in the prevention of postangioplasty and in-stent restenosis and in the treatment of chronic myocardial ischemia: phase II results of the Kuopio Angiogenesis Trial (KAT). *Circulation,* 107, 21, (Jun), pp. 2677-83.

Hedman, M.,Muona, K.,Hedman, A., et al. (2009). Eight-year safety follow-up of coronary artery disease patients after local intracoronary VEGF gene transfer. *Gene Ther,* 16, 5, (May), pp. 629-34.

Heidenreich, P. A.,McDonald, K. M.,Hastie, T., et al. (1999). Meta-analysis of trials comparing beta-blockers, calcium antagonists, and nitrates for stable angina. *JAMA,* 281, 20, (May), pp. 1927-36.

Henry, T. D.,Grines, C. L.,Watkins, M. W., et al. (2007). Effects of Ad5FGF-4 in patients with angina: an analysis of pooled data from the AGENT-3 and AGENT-4 trials. *J Am Coll Cardiol,* 50, 11, (Sep), pp. 1038-46.

Heusch, G. (2008). Heart rate in the pathophysiology of coronary blood flow and myocardial ischaemia: benefit from selective bradycardic agents. *Br J Pharmacol,* 153, 8, (Apr), pp. 1589-601.

Hirai, N.,Kawano, H.,Yasue, H., et al. (2003). Attenuation of nitrate tolerance and oxidative stress by an angiotensin II receptor blocker in patients with coronary spastic angina. *Circulation,* 108, 12, (Sep), pp. 1446-50.

Ho, J. E.,Bittner, V.,Demicco, D. A., et al. (2010). Usefulness of heart rate at rest as a predictor of mortality, hospitalization for heart failure, myocardial infarction, and stroke in patients with stable coronary heart disease (Data from the Treating to New Targets [TNT] trial). *Am J Cardiol,* 105, 7, (Apr), pp. 905-11.

Hoekenga, D. & Abrams, J. (1984). Rational medical therapy for stable angina pectoris. *Am J Med,* 76, 2, (Feb), pp. 309-14.

Holubkov, R.,Kennard, E. D.,Foris, J. M., et al. (2002). Comparison of patients undergoing enhanced external counterpulsation and percutaneous coronary intervention for stable angina pectoris. *Am J Cardiol,* 89, 10, (May), pp. 1182-6.

Horvath, K. A.,Mannting, F.,Cummings, N., et al. (1996). Transmyocardial laser revascularization: operative techniques and clinical results at two years. *J Thorac Cardiovasc Surg,* 111, 5, (May), pp. 1047-53.

Hueb, W.,Soares, P. R.,Gersh, B. J., et al. (2004). The medicine, angioplasty, or surgery study (MASS-II): a randomized, controlled clinical trial of three therapeutic strategies for multivessel coronary artery disease: one-year results. *J Am Coll Cardiol,* 43, 10, (May), pp. 1743-51.

Huikeshoven, M.,Beek, J. F.,van der Sloot, J. A., et al. (2002). 35 years of experimental research in transmyocardial revascularization: what have we learned? *Ann Thorac Surg,* 74, 3, (Sep), pp. 956-70.

Ignarro, L. J.,Lippton, H.,Edwards, J. C., et al. (1981). Mechanism of vascular smooth muscle relaxation by organic nitrates, nitrites, nitroprusside and nitric oxide: evidence for the involvement of S-nitrosothiols as active intermediates. *J Pharmacol Exp Ther,* 218, 3, (Sep), pp. 739-49.

Jackson, G.,Harry, J. D.,Robinson, C., et al. (1978). Comparison of atenolol with propranolol in the treatment of angina pectoris with special reference to once daily administration of atenolol. *Br Heart J,* 40, 9, (Sep), pp. 998-1004.

Jahangir, A. & Terzic, A. (2005). K(ATP) channel therapeutics at the bedside. *J Mol Cell Cardiol,* 39, 1, (Jul), pp. 99-112.

Jahangir, A.,Terzic, A. & Shen, W. K. (2001). Potassium channel openers: therapeutic potential in cardiology and medicine. *Expert Opin Pharmacother,* 2, 12, (Dec), pp. 1995-2010.

James, M. A.,Walker, P. R.,Papouchado, M., et al. (1985). Efficacy of transdermal glyceryl trinitrate in the treatment of chronic stable angina pectoris. *Br Heart J,* 53, 6, (Jun), pp. 631-5.

Jerling, M. & Abdallah, H. (2005). Effect of renal impairment on multiple-dose pharmacokinetics of extended-release ranolazine. *Clin Pharmacol Ther,* 78, 3, (Sep), pp. 288-97.

John, S. A.,Weiss, J. N.,Xie, L. H., et al. (2003). Molecular mechanism for ATP-dependent closure of the K+ channel Kir6.2. *J Physiol,* 552, Pt 1, (Oct), pp. 23-34.

Jones, J. W.,Schmidt, S. E.,Richman, B. W., et al. (1999). Holmium:YAG laser transmyocardial revascularization relieves angina and improves functional status. *Ann Thorac Surg,* 67, 6, (Jun), pp. 1596-601.

Julian, D. G., Bertrand, M.E., Hjalmarson, A. et al (1997). Management of stable angina pectoris. Recommendations of the Task Force of the European Society of Cardiology. *Eur Heart J,* 18, 3, (Mar), pp. 394-413.

Kantor, P. F.,Lucien, A.,Kozak, R., et al. (2000). The antianginal drug trimetazidine shifts cardiac energy metabolism from fatty acid oxidation to glucose oxidation by

inhibiting mitochondrial long-chain 3-ketoacyl coenzyme A thiolase. *Circ Res,* 86, 5, (Mar), pp. 580-8.
Kapur, N. K. & Rade, J. J. (2008). Fibroblast growth factor 4 gene therapy for chronic ischemic heart disease. *Trends Cardiovasc Med,* 18, 4, (May), pp. 133-41.
Kastrup, J.,Jorgensen, E.,Ruck, A., et al. (2005). Direct intramyocardial plasmid vascular endothelial growth factor-A165 gene therapy in patients with stable severe angina pectoris A randomized double-blind placebo-controlled study: the Euroinject One trial. *J Am Coll Cardiol,* 45, 7, (Apr), pp. 982-8.
Kay, L.,Finelli, C.,Aussedat, J., et al. (1995). Improvement of long-term preservation of the isolated arrested rat heart by trimetazidine: effects on the energy state and mitochondrial function. *Am J Cardiol,* 76, 6, (Aug), pp. 45B-49B.
Kemler, M. A.,Barendse, G. A.,van Kleef, M., et al. (2000). Spinal cord stimulation in patients with chronic reflex sympathetic dystrophy. *N Engl J Med,* 343, 9, (Aug), pp. 618-24.
Killip, T., Fisher, L.D., Mock, M.B. (1983). Coronary artery surgery study (CASS): a randomized trial of coronary artery bypass surgery. Quality of life in patients randomly assigned to treatment groups. *Circulation,* 68, 5, (Nov), pp. 951-60.
Kumar, K.,Taylor, R. S.,Jacques, L., et al. (2007). Spinal cord stimulation versus conventional medical management for neuropathic pain: a multicentre randomised controlled trial in patients with failed back surgery syndrome. *Pain,* 132, 1-2, (Nov), pp. 179-88.
Lapenna, E.,Rapati, D.,Cardano, P., et al. (2006). Spinal cord stimulation for patients with refractory angina and previous coronary surgery. *Ann Thorac Surg,* 82, 5, (Nov), pp. 1704-8.
Latif, O. A.,Nedeljkovic, S. S. & Stevenson, L. W. (2001). Spinal cord stimulation for chronic intractable angina pectoris: a unified theory on its mechanism. *Clin Cardiol,* 24, 8, (Aug), pp. 533-41.
Lee, A. W. & Pilitsis, J. G. (2006). Spinal cord stimulation: indications and outcomes. *Neurosurg Focus,* 21, 6, pp. E3.
Levy, S. (1995). Combination therapy of trimetazidine with diltiazem in patients with coronary artery disease. Group of South of France Investigators. *Am J Cardiol,* 76, 6, (Aug), pp. 12B-16B.
Libby, P., Bonow, R., Mann, DL, Zipes DP (2008). *Braunwald's heart disease : a textbook of cardiovascular medicine,* Saunders, an imprint of Elsevier Inc. 978-1-4160-4106-1.
Lichtlen, P. R.,Hugenholtz, P. G.,Rafflenbeul, W., et al. (1990). Retardation of angiographic progression of coronary artery disease by nifedipine. Results of the International Nifedipine Trial on Antiatherosclerotic Therapy (INTACT). INTACT Group Investigators. *Lancet,* 335, 8698, (May), pp. 1109-13.
Loh, P. H.,Cleland, J. G.,Louis, A. A., et al. (2008). Enhanced external counterpulsation in the treatment of chronic refractory angina: a long-term follow-up outcome from the International Enhanced External Counterpulsation Patient Registry. *Clin Cardiol,* 31, 4, (Apr), pp. 159-64.
Lopez, A. D.,Mathers, C. D.,Ezzati, M., et al. (2006). Global and regional burden of disease and risk factors, 2001: systematic analysis of population health data. *Lancet,* 367, 9524, (May), pp. 1747-57.

Losordo, D. W.,Schatz, R. A.,White, C. J., et al. (2007). Intramyocardial transplantation of autologous CD34+ stem cells for intractable angina: a phase I/IIa double-blind, randomized controlled trial. *Circulation,* 115, 25, (Jun), pp. 3165-72.

Lown, B. & Levine, S. A. (1961). The carotid sinus. Clinical value of its stimulation. *Circulation,* 23, (May), pp. 766-89.

Luscher, T. F.,Pieper, M.,Tendera, M., et al. (2009). A randomized placebo-controlled study on the effect of nifedipine on coronary endothelial function and plaque formation in patients with coronary artery disease: the ENCORE II study. *Eur Heart J,* 30, 13, (Jul), pp. 1590-7.

Makolkin, V. I., Osadchii, K.K. (2003). Efficacy and tolerabiligy of trimetazidine in the treatment of stable effort angina (TRIUMPH Study in Russia). *Kardologiia,* 43, 6, pp. 18-22.

Manchanda, S. C. & Krishnaswami, S. (1997). Combination treatment with trimetazidine and diltiazem in stable angina pectoris. *Heart,* 78, 4, (Oct), pp. 353-7.

March, R. J. (1999). Transmyocardial laser revascularization with the CO2 laser: one year results of a randomized, controlled trial. *Semin Thorac Cardiovasc Surg,* 11, 1, (Jan), pp. 12-8.

Markham, A.,Plosker, G. L. & Goa, K. L. (2000). Nicorandil. An updated review of its use in ischaemic heart disease with emphasis on its cardioprotective effects. *Drugs,* 60, 4, (Oct), pp. 955-74.

Martin-Rendon, E.,Brunskill, S. J.,Hyde, C. J., et al. (2008). Autologous bone marrow stem cells to treat acute myocardial infarction: a systematic review. *Eur Heart J,* 29, 15, (Aug), pp. 1807-18.

Mathers, C. D. & Loncar, D. (2006). Projections of global mortality and burden of disease from 2002 to 2030. *PLoS Med,* 3, 11, (Nov), pp. e442.

McGillion, M.,Cook, A.,Victor, J. C., et al. (2010). Effectiveness of percutaneous laser revascularization therapy for refractory angina. *Vasc Health Risk Manag,* 6, pp. 735-47.

McGillion, M.,Watt-Watson, J.,LeFort, S., et al. (2007). Positive shifts in the perceived meaning of cardiac pain following a psychoeducation program for chronic stable angina. *Can J Nurs Res,* 39, 2, (Jun), pp. 48-65.

McKenna, C.,McDaid, C.,Suekarran, S., et al. (2009). Enhanced external counterpulsation for the treatment of stable angina and heart failure: a systematic review and economic analysis. *Health Technol Assess,* 13, 24, (Apr), iii-iv, ix-xi, 1-90.

McNab, D.,Khan, S. N.,Sharples, L. D., et al. (2006). An open label, single-centre, randomized trial of spinal cord stimulation vs. percutaneous myocardial laser revascularization in patients with refractory angina pectoris: the SPiRiT trial. *Eur Heart J,* 27, 9, (May), pp. 1048-53.

Meeter, K.,Kelder, J. C.,Tijssen, J. G., et al. (1992). Efficacy of nicorandil versus propranolol in mild stable angina pectoris of effort: a long-term, double-blind, randomized study. *J Cardiovasc Pharmacol,* 20 Suppl 3, pp. S59-66.

Menasche, P. (2011). Cardiac cell therapy: Lessons from clinical trials. *J Mol Cell Cardiol,* 50, 2, (Feb), pp. 258-65.

Menasche, P.,Alfieri, O.,Janssens, S., et al. (2008). The Myoblast Autologous Grafting in Ischemic Cardiomyopathy (MAGIC) trial: first randomized placebo-controlled study of myoblast transplantation. *Circulation,* 117, 9, (Mar), pp. 1189-200.

Miller, R. R.,Olson, H. G.,Amsterdam, E. A., et al. (1975). Propranolol-withdrawal rebound phenomenon. Exacerbation of coronary events after abrupt cessation of antianginal therapy. *N Engl J Med,* 293, 9, (Aug), pp. 416-8

Mohri, M.,Shimokawa, H.,Hirakawa, Y., et al. (2003). Rho-kinase inhibition with intracoronary fasudil prevents myocardial ischemia in patients with coronary microvascular spasm. *J Am Coll Cardiol,* 41, 1, (Jan), pp. 15-9.

Morrow, D. A.,Scirica, B. M.,Karwatowska-Prokopczuk, E., et al. (2007). Effects of ranolazine on recurrent cardiovascular events in patients with non-ST-elevation acute coronary syndromes: the MERLIN-TIMI 36 randomized trial. *JAMA,* 297, 16, (Apr), pp. 1775-83.

Munzel, T.,Mulsch, A. & Kleschyov, A. (2002). Mechanisms underlying nitroglycerin-induced superoxide production in platelets: some insight, more questions. *Circulation,* 106, 2, (Jul), pp. 170-2.

Murphy, D. F. & Giles, K. E. (1987). Dorsal column stimulation for pain relief from intractable angina pectoris. *Pain,* 28, 3, (Mar), pp. 365-8.

Murrell, W. (1879). Nitroglycerin as a remedy for angina pectoris. *Lancet,* 1, 80-81, pp. 113-115,

Murry, C. E.,Soonpaa, M. H.,Reinecke, H., et al. (2004). Haematopoietic stem cells do not transdifferentiate into cardiac myocytes in myocardial infarcts. *Nature,* 428, 6983, (Apr), pp. 664-8.

Nissen, S. E.,Tuzcu, E. M.,Libby, P., et al. (2004). Effect of antihypertensive agents on cardiovascular events in patients with coronary disease and normal blood pressure: the CAMELOT study: a randomized controlled trial. *JAMA,* 292, 18, (Nov), pp. 2217-25.

O'Rourke, R. A. (2010). Alternative strategies for the management of chronic stable angina. *Curr Probl Cardiol,* 35, 8, (Aug), pp. 384-446.

Oesterle, S. N.,Reifart, N. J.,Meier, B., et al. (1998). Initial results of laser-based percutaneous myocardial revascularization for angina pectoris. *Am J Cardiol,* 82, 5, (Sep), pp. 659-62.

Olsson, G. & Allgen, J. (1992). Prophylactic nitrate therapy in angina pectoris--is there an optimal treatment regimen? *Br J Clin Pharmacol,* 34 Suppl 1, pp. 19S-23S.

Otsuka, T.,Ibuki, C.,Suzuki, T., et al. (2008). Administration of the Rho-kinase inhibitor, fasudil, following nitroglycerin additionally dilates the site of coronary spasm in patients with vasospastic angina. *Coron Artery Dis,* 19, 2, (Mar), pp. 105-10.

Parisi, A. F.,Folland, E. D. & Hartigan, P. (1992). A comparison of angioplasty with medical therapy in the treatment of single-vessel coronary artery disease. Veterans Affairs ACME Investigators. *N Engl J Med,* 326, 1, (Jan), pp. 10-6.

Parker, J. D. & Parker, J. O. (1998). Nitrate therapy for stable angina pectoris. *N Engl J Med,* 338, 8, (Feb), pp. 520-31.

Parker, J. O. & Fung, H. L. (1984). Transdermal nitroglycerin in angina pectoris. *Am J Cardiol,* 54, 6, (Sep), pp. 471-6.

Pine, M. B.,Citron, P. D.,Bailly, D. J., et al. (1982). Verapamil versus placebo in relieving stable angina pectoris. *Circulation,* 65, 1, (Jan), pp. 17-22.

Pitt, B.,Waters, D.,Brown, W. V., et al. (1999). Aggressive lipid-lowering therapy compared with angioplasty in stable coronary artery disease. Atorvastatin versus Revascularization Treatment Investigators. *N Engl J Med,* 341, 2, (Jul), pp. 70-6.

Poole-Wilson, P. A.,Lubsen, J.,Kirwan, B. A., et al. (2004). Effect of long-acting nifedipine on mortality and cardiovascular morbidity in patients with stable angina requiring treatment (ACTION trial): randomised controlled trial. *Lancet,* 364, 9437, (Sep), pp. 849-57.

Psaty, B. M.,Heckbert, S. R.,Koepsell, T. D., et al. (1995). The risk of myocardial infarction associated with antihypertensive drug therapies. *JAMA,* 274, 8, (Aug), pp. 620-5.

Psaty, B. M.,Koepsell, T. D.,Wagner, E. H., et al. (1990). The relative risk of incident coronary heart disease associated with recently stopping the use of beta-blockers. *JAMA,* 263, 12, (Mar), pp. 1653-7.

Raftery, E. B.,Lahiri, A.,Hughes, L. O., et al. (1993). A double-blind comparison of a beta-blocker and a potassium channel opener in exercise induced angina. *Eur Heart J,* 14 Suppl B, (Jul), pp. 35-9.

Reichek, N.,Priest, C.,Zimrin, D., et al. (1984). Antianginal effects of nitroglycerin patches. *Am J Cardiol,* 54, 1, (Jul), pp. 1-7.

Rice, K. R.,Gervino, E.,Jarisch, W. R., et al. (1990). Effects of nifedipine on myocardial perfusion during exercise in chronic stable angina pectoris. *Am J Cardiol,* 65, 16, (May), pp. 1097-101.

Rotem, C. E. (1974). Carotid sinus nerve stimulation in the management of intractable angina pectoris: four-year follow-up. *Can Med Assoc J,* 110, 3, (Feb), pp. 285-8.

Ruzyllo, W.,Tendera, M.,Ford, I., et al. (2007). Antianginal efficacy and safety of ivabradine compared with amlodipine in patients with stable effort angina pectoris: a 3-month randomised, double-blind, multicentre, noninferiority trial. *Drugs,* 67, 3, pp. 393-405.

Scirica, B. M.,Morrow, D. A.,Hod, H., et al. (2007). Effect of ranolazine, an antianginal agent with novel electrophysiological properties, on the incidence of arrhythmias in patients with non ST-segment elevation acute coronary syndrome: results from the Metabolic Efficiency With Ranolazine for Less Ischemia in Non ST-Elevation Acute Coronary Syndrome Thrombolysis in Myocardial Infarction 36 (MERLIN-TIMI 36) randomized controlled trial. *Circulation,* 116, 15, (Oct), pp. 1647-52.

Shechter, M.,Matetzky, S.,Feinberg, M. S., et al. (2003). External counterpulsation therapy improves endothelial function in patients with refractory angina pectoris. *J Am Coll Cardiol,* 42, 12, (Dec), pp. 2090-5.

Shimokawa, H.,Hiramori, K.,Iinuma, H., et al. (2002). Anti-anginal effect of fasudil, a Rho-kinase inhibitor, in patients with stable effort angina: a multicenter study. *J Cardiovasc Pharmacol,* 40, 5, (Nov), pp. 751-61.

Shimokawa, H. & Takeshita, A. (2005). Rho-kinase is an important therapeutic target in cardiovascular medicine. *Arterioscler Thromb Vasc Biol,* 25, 9, (Sep), pp. 1767-75.

Sierra, C. & Coca, A. (2008). The ACTION study: nifedipine in patients with symptomatic stable angina and hypertension. *Expert Rev Cardiovasc Ther,* 6, 8, (Sep), pp. 1055-62.

Simons, M.,Bonow, R. O.,Chronos, N. A., et al. (2000). Clinical trials in coronary angiogenesis: issues, problems, consensus: An expert panel summary. *Circulation,* 102, 11, (Sep), pp. E73-86.

Simons, M. & Ware, J. A. (2003). Therapeutic angiogenesis in cardiovascular disease. *Nat Rev Drug Discov,* 2, 11, (Nov), pp. 863-71.

Sinvhal, R. M.,Gowda, R. M. & Khan, I. A. (2003). Enhanced external counterpulsation for refractory angina pectoris. *Heart,* 89, 8, (Aug), pp. 830-3.

Smith, J. A.,Dunning, J. J.,Parry, A. J., et al. (1995). Transmyocardial laser revascularization. *J Card Surg,* 10, 5, (Sep), pp. 569-72.

Stamm, C.,Kleine, H. D.,Choi, Y. H., et al. (2007). Intramyocardial delivery of CD133+ bone marrow cells and coronary artery bypass grafting for chronic ischemic heart disease: safety and efficacy studies. *J Thorac Cardiovasc Surg,* 133, 3, (Mar), pp. 717-25.

Stewart, D. J.,Hilton, J. D.,Arnold, J. M., et al. (2006). Angiogenic gene therapy in patients with nonrevascularizable ischemic heart disease: a phase 2 randomized, controlled trial of AdVEGF(121) (AdVEGF121) versus maximum medical treatment. *Gene Ther,* 13, 21, (Nov), pp. 1503-11.

Stewart, D. J.,Kutryk, M. J.,Fitchett, D., et al. (2009). VEGF gene therapy fails to improve perfusion of ischemic myocardium in patients with advanced coronary disease: results of the NORTHERN trial. *Mol Ther,* 17, 6, (Jun), pp. 1109-15.

Stone, P. H.,Gratsiansky, N. A.,Blokhin, A., et al. (2006). Antianginal efficacy of ranolazine when added to treatment with amlodipine: the ERICA (Efficacy of Ranolazine in Chronic Angina) trial. *J Am Coll Cardiol,* 48, 3, (Aug), pp. 566-75.

Swedberg, K.,Komajda, M.,Bohm, M., et al. (2010). Ivabradine and outcomes in chronic heart failure (SHIFT): a randomised placebo-controlled study. *Lancet,* 376, 9744, (Sep), pp. 875-85.

Szwed, H.,Sadowski, Z.,Elikowski, W., et al. (2001). Combination treatment in stable effort angina using trimetazidine and metoprolol: results of a randomized, double-blind, multicentre study (TRIMPOL II). TRIMetazidine in POLand. *Eur Heart J,* 22, 24, (Dec), pp. 2267-74.

Tapp, R. J.,Sharp, A.,Stanton, A. V., et al. (2010). Differential effects of antihypertensive treatment on left ventricular diastolic function: an ASCOT (Anglo-Scandinavian Cardiac Outcomes Trial) substudy. *J Am Coll Cardiol,* 55, 17, (Apr), pp. 1875-81.

Tardif, J. C.,Ford, I.,Tendera, M., et al. (2005). Efficacy of ivabradine, a new selective I(f) inhibitor, compared with atenolol in patients with chronic stable angina. *Eur Heart J,* 26, 23, (Dec), pp. 2529-36.

Tardif, J. C.,Ponikowski, P. & Kahan, T. (2009). Efficacy of the I(f) current inhibitor ivabradine in patients with chronic stable angina receiving beta-blocker therapy: a 4-month, randomized, placebo-controlled trial. *Eur Heart J,* 30, 5, (Mar), pp. 540-8.

Taylor, R. S.,De Vries, J.,Buchser, E., et al. (2009). Spinal cord stimulation in the treatment of refractory angina: systematic review and meta-analysis of randomised controlled trials. *BMC Cardiovasc Disord,* 9, (Mar), pp. 13.

Tendera, M.,Borer, J. S. & Tardif, J. C. (2009). Efficacy of I(f) inhibition with ivabradine in different subpopulations with stable angina pectoris. *Cardiology,* 114, 2, (May), pp. 116-25.

Thollon, C.,Cambarrat, C.,Vian, J., et al. (1994). Electrophysiological effects of S 16257, a novel sino-atrial node modulator, on rabbit and guinea-pig cardiac preparations: comparison with UL-FS 49. *Br J Pharmacol,* 112, 1, (May), pp. 37-42.

Thom, T.,Haase, N.,Rosamond, W., et al. (2006). Heart disease and stroke statistics--2006 update: a report from the American Heart Association Statistics Committee and Stroke Statistics Subcommittee. *Circulation,* 113, 6, (Feb), pp. e85-151.

Urano, H.,Ikeda, H.,Ueno, T., et al. (2001). Enhanced external counterpulsation improves exercise tolerance, reduces exercise-induced myocardial ischemia and improves left ventricular diastolic filling in patients with coronary artery disease. *J Am Coll Cardiol*, 37, 1, (Jan), pp. 93-9.

van der Sloot, J. A.,Huikeshoven, M.,Tukkie, R., et al. (2004). Transmyocardial revascularization using an XeCl excimer laser: results of a randomized trial. *Ann Thorac Surg*, 78, 3, (Sep), pp. 875-81.

Van Zundert, J. (2007). Clinical research in interventional pain management techniques: the clinician's point of view. *Pain Pract*, 7, 3, (Sep), pp. 221-9.

Varnauskas, E. (1988). Twelve-year follow-up of survival in the randomized European Coronary Surgery Study. *N Engl J Med*, 319, 6, (Aug), pp. 332-7.

Vicari, R. M.,Chaitman, B.,Keefe, D., et al. (2005). Efficacy and safety of fasudil in patients with stable angina: a double-blind, placebo-controlled, phase 2 trial. *J Am Coll Cardiol*, 46, 10, (Nov), pp. 1803-11.

Wang, S.,Cui, J.,Peng, W., et al. (2010). Intracoronary autologous CD34+ stem cell therapy for intractable angina. *Cardiology*, 117, 2, pp. 140-7.

Yusuf, S.,Zucker, D.,Peduzzi, P., et al. (1994). Effect of coronary artery bypass graft surgery on survival: overview of 10-year results from randomised trials by the Coronary Artery Bypass Graft Surgery Trialists Collaboration. *Lancet*, 344, 8922, (Aug), pp. 563-70.

Zachary, I. & Morgan, R. D. (2011). Therapeutic angiogenesis for cardiovascular disease: biological context, challenges, prospects. *Heart*, 97, 3, (Feb), pp. 181-9.

Zingman, L. V.,Alekseev, A. E.,Hodgson-Zingman, D. M., et al. (2007). ATP-sensitive potassium channels: metabolic sensing and cardioprotection. *J Appl Physiol*, 103, 5, (Nov), pp. 1888-93.

5

Beta-Blockers and Coronary Flow Reserve

Maurizio Galderisi
Director of Unit of Post-myocardial infarction Follow-up
Director of Laboratory of Echocardiography
Cardioangiology with CCU
Department of Clinical and Experimental Medicine
Federico II University Hospital, Naples
Italy

1. Introduction

The knowledge of the impact of beta-blockers on Coronary Flow Reserve (CFR) is based on experimental and clinical studies which used invasive methods (mainly Doppler Flow Wire, DFW) and non-invasive tools including scintigraphic (mainly Positron Emission Tomography, PET), magnetic resonance and Doppler ultrasound imaging.
Beta-blockers have a large therapeutic indication in the treatment of coronary artery disease, due to their anti-ischemic and anti-arrhythmic effect. The anti-ischemic effect is based on the oxygen sparing mechanism with a reduction in rate-pressure product. Changes in coronary hemodynamics associated with the administration of beta-blockers have been extensively studied. These drugs may affect CFR by modifying either resting or maximal coronary blood flow (CBF) or even both. When assessing the impact of beta-blockers on CFR it is important to distinguish the effects exerted by first-and second generation beta-blockers from those due the mechanisms of third generation beta-blockers, which are provided of vasodilating action.

2. First and second generation beta-blockers and coronary flow reserve

Animal and human experiments have shown that first- and second generation beta-blockers (propranolol, practolol metoprolol, atenolol) induce a reduction of CBF at rest (1-7), which has been mainly attributed to coronary vasoconstriction (8,9). Both non selective (propranolol) and selective (atenolol) beta-blocking agents have shown a gradual vasoconstriction, i.e., a decrease in coronary artery diameter by approximately 20-25%, over 20 min after their acute administration, an effect which is overcome by nitrates (3). An alternative mechanisms for explaining the reduction of CBF at rest is provided by the reduction of myocardial oxygen demand since these drugs lower blood pressure and heart rate with variable degree (4,5). After acute injection, beta-blockers decrease myocardial contractility and work, leading to a reduction of resting CBF (5).
The effects of first and second generation beta-blockers on maximal CBF are more controversial. A clinical study assessing the effects of non-selective beta-blocker propranolol

(0.1 mg/kg i.v.) after cold pressure test (CPT), a stimulus completely mediated to the endothelial function ("reactive hyperemia") suggests that this drug leads to enhanced coronary vascular resistance during hyperemia, due to unopposed alpha-adrenergic vasomotor tone (6). The oral administration of the cardio-selective atenolol produces similar action in hypertensive patients without coronary artery stenosis, inducing even a reduction of CFR and raising the suspicion that it may worsen coronary microvascular function (7). On the other hand, in patients with coronary artery disease the acute intravenous administration of the selective beta-blocker metoprolol (5 mg) has shown an increase of pharmacologically induced (adenosine) CBF velocities and post-ischemic coronary flow velocity reserve (CFVR) measured by the means of DFW (5). Boettcher and coworker have reported similar results, with an increase in PET-derived CFR after 50 mg oral metoprolol, achieved by an increase in maximal CBF which is further enhanced by a decrease in resting CBF (6).

Based on these experiences, the controversial influence of first- and second-generation beta-blocking agents on CFR has to be acknowledged. It can be explained by taking into account the interaction of the pharmacological effects on CBF at rest, generally reduced under the action of these categories of beta-blockers, and after maximal hyperemia, when minimal coronary resistance can be increased (mainly by non selective beta-adrenergic antagonists and by selective atenolol) or reduced (by some selective beta-blockers such as metoprolol).

3. Third generation Beta-blockers (with vasodilating action) and Coronary Flow Reserve

The third generation beta-blockers have the common characteristic to combine a vasodilating action to the classic beta-blocking properties. The association of these two effects is particularly pronounced in carvedilol and nebivolol, which have earned important positions in the therapy of chronic heart failure, with a recognized positive influence on left ventricular (LV) function and prognosis (10-13). The influence of these two drugs on CFR has been tested in the clinical setting. The improvement of coronary microvascular function obtainable by both carvedilol (14-17) and nebivolol (7,18-21) could be at least one of the substrates underlying the improvement in LV function due to both these drugs. Except for the experience of Koepfli et al (14), where a significant drug-induced increase on PET-derived CFR was achieved only pooling 36 patients with coronary artery disease treated by either carvedilol or atenolol (12 week treatment), all the other clinical studies demonstrated a positive effect of carvedilol or nebivolol on CFR (**Table 1**) (22).

The beneficial action of carvedilol on CFVR was observed in three reports, including exclusively patients with idiopathic dilated cardiomyopathy, with a therapy time duration ranging between 1 month and 6 months (16-18). In these experiences, the increase of CFVR was mainly due to the increase of maximal CBF velocity, attributable to diminution of extravascular compressive forces and of LV filling pressure (5,6), to blunted heart rate response beneficially affecting the diastolic myocardial perfusion during hyperemia (6), to alpha-adrenergic blocking action and to improved endothelial function (23,24) possibly producing a better hyperemic microvascular vasodilation..

The studies performed by using nebivolol involved several clinical settings, such as patients with arterial hypertension (7,18,21), idiopathic dilated cardiomyopathy (19) and coronary artery disease (20). In particular, Togni et al (20) evaluated the acute effect of intracoronary administration of nebivolol, while the other studies evaluated the therapeutic effect of oral

Drug	Authors	Method for measuring CFR	Setting / therapy duration	Effect on CFR
Carvedilol, 20 mg/day	Sugioka K et al, JACC 2005	TTE, Aden 0.14 mg/Kg/min	12 IDCM pts, 3-6 months	2.6±0.9 (baseline) 3.5±0.7 (3 months) 3.7±0.6 (6 months)
Carvedilol 25-50 mg/day	Neglia D et al, Heart 2007	PET Dip 0.56 mg/Kg	16 IDCM pts, 6 months	1.67±0.63 (baseline) 2.58±1.04 (6 months)
Carvedilol 20 mg/day	Sugioka K et al, Am Heart J 2007	TTE, Aden 0.14 mg/Kg/min	18 IDCM pts, 1 month	CFR change = 1.3±0.6*
Nebivolol, 5 mg/day	Galderisi M et al, J Hypertens 2004	TTE, Dip 0.56 mg/kg	14 HTN pts, 4 weeks	1.89±0.31 (baseline) 2.12±0.33 (4 weeks)
Nebivolol, 5mg/day	Gullu H et al, Heart 2006	TTE, Dip 0.84 mg/Kg	30 HTN pts, 8 weeks	2.45±0.48 (baseline) 2.56±0.52 (8 weeks)
Nebivolol, 5 mg/day	Erdogan D et al, Heart 2007	TTE, Dip 0.56 mg/Kg	21 IDCM pts, 1 month	2.02±0.35 (baseline) 2.61±0.43 (1 month)
Nebivolol, 0.1 mg, 0.25 mg, 0.50 mg (intracoronary)	Togni M et al, Cardiovasc Drug Ther 2007	DFW, Aden 12-18 μg (intracoronary)	8 CAD pts, Acute effect	2.10±0.4 (baseline) 2.30±0.7 (0.1 mg) 2.60±0.9 (0.25 mg) 2.60±0.5 (0.50 mg)
Nebivolol 5 mg/day	Galderisi M et al, J Hypertens 2009	TTE, Dip 0.84 mg/Kg	20 HTN pts, 3 months	2.07±0.2 (baseline) 2.20±0.2 (3 months)

* CFR change in patients with improvement of LV ejection fraction ≥ 10%.
Aden = Adenosine, CAD = Coronary artery disease, DFW = Doppler flow wire, Dip = Dipyridamole, HTN = Hypertension IDCM = Idiopathic dilated cardiomyopathy, PET = Positron emission tomography, pts = Patients, TTE = Trans-thoracic echocardiography

Table 1. Main studies showing favourable effect of beta-blockers with vasodilator action on CFR in humans (Modified by Galderisi M et al, Ref # 21).

administration (5 mg daily) after 8 weeks (7) and 4 weeks (18,19) and 3 months (21). With the exception of the observation of Gullu (7), where the improvement of CFVR was exclusively due to the decrease of CBF velocities at rest, in the other 4 studies nebivolol increased significantly hyperemic CBF velocities (18-21). Coronary vasodilation due to either adenosine or dipyridamole is primarily endothelium independent but the increment in CBF may trigger further flow-induced vasodilation, which is endothelium dependent (25,26). Nebivolol has vasodilating properties with increasing endothelial NO release due to effects on the L-arginine/NO pathway that reduce peripheral vascular resistance (27). It is able not only to increase NO release but also to inhibit the synthesis of endothelin-1 (28), a mediator contributing to vascular resistance (29). Although these effects cannot be automatically applied to the coronary circulation of the studies which demonstrated the beneficial effects of nebivolol on CFVR – since they did not use any NO antagonist to target the mechanism of action - in our experience (18) dipyridamole-induced increase in rate-pressure product during pharmacological stress was similar before and during nebivolol therapy and could not explain alone the changes induces on CBF velocities. This highlights indirectly the possible beneficial effect of the drug on the endothelial function. A similar effect of nebivolol has been demonstrated in humans on brachial artery flow mediated dilation (30), a completely endothelium-dependent stimulus (31).

The increase of CFR induced by beta-blocking agents with vasodilating properties has potential clinical implications. This increase appears clearly beneficial in patients with coronary artery disease, where a better hyperemic CBF (increase of O_2 supply), combined with a reduction of rate-pressure product (decrease of O_2 demand), may be the cause underlying the anti-ischemic effect of these drugs. The increase of CFR might also indicate an improvement of coronary microvascular dysfunction, responsible of microvascular angina pectoris or silent ischemia in patients without epicardial artery stenosis (32). The improvement of coronary microvessel function could be even one of the mechanisms sustaining the improvement of LV function demonstrated by both carvedilol and nebivolol (33-40). Sugioka and coworkers (17) observed that CFVR improvement after carvedilol was greater in patients with LV ejection fraction increase $\geq 10\%$ (1.3 ± 0.6) than in those with election fraction increase $< 10\%$ (0.4 ± 0.5) ($p<0.01$). Data from our laboratory have shown a relation between the positive influence exerted by 3-month oral administration of nebivolol on CFVR and the reduction of non invasively determined LV filling pressure in uncomplicated arterial hypertension (21). Accordingly, the absence of a significant restoration of CFVR after short-term third-generation beta-blockers may imply a poor chance of improvement in LV function, while a great CFVR increase may indicate a higher chance of it. Therefore, one possible clinical implication is that changes of CFVR after short-term beta-blocking therapy is helpful to predict the response or the further improvement of LV function to treatment.

4. Conclusions

The impact of beta-blocking medications on coronary flow reserve is related to the specific characteristics of the drug. First- and second-generation beta-blockers significantly reduce coronary flow at rest (because of reduction of myocardial oxygen demand and vasoconstriction effects) while their action on the hyperemic coronary flow is variable. Third-generation beta-blockers induce a true amelioration of the maximal hyperemia of coronary blood flow which appears be possibly due to alpha-adrenergic blockade and to nitric oxide-mediated vasodilator action. These effects might have potential beneficial prognostic impact in the setting of patients where CFR reduction has a recognized independent, negative predictive value on outcome and mortality (41-43).

5. References

[1] Young MA, Vatner SE, Vatner SF. Alpa- and beta-adrenergic control of large coronary arteries in conscious dogs. Circ Res 1974;34:812-823.

[2] Marshall RJ, Parratt JR. Comparative effects of propranolol and practolol in the early stages of experimental canine myocardial infarction. *Br J Pharmacol* 1976;57:295-303.

[3] Lichtlen PR, Rafflenbeul W, Jost S, et al. Coronary vasomotion tone in large epicardial coronary arteries with special emphasis on beta-adrenergic vasomotion, effect of beta-blockade. Basic Res Cardiol 1990;85(Suppl 1):335-346.

[4] Hoffman JIE. Maximal coronary flow and the concept of coronary flow reserve. *Circulation* 1984;70:153-159.

[5] Billinger M, Seller C, Fleisch M, et al. Effect of beta-adrenergic blocking agents increase coronary flow reserve? *J Am Coll Cardiol* 2001;38:1866-1871.

[6] Bottcher M, Czernin J, Sun K, et al. Effects of β1 adrenergic blockade on myocardial blood flow and vasodilatory capacity. *J Nucl Med* 1997;38:442-446.

[7] Gullu H, Erdogan D, Caliskan M, et al. Different effects of atenolol and nebivolol on coronary flow reserve. *Heart* 2006;92:1690-1691.

[8] Strauer BE. The hypertensive heart. Effect of atenolol on the function, coronary hemodynamics and oxygen uptake of the left ventricle. *Dtsch Med Wochenschr* 1978;103:1785-1789.

[9] Kern MJ, Ganz P, Horowitz DJ, Gaspar J, et al. Potentiation of coronary vasoconstriction by beta-adrenergic blockade in patients with coronary artery disease. *Circulation* 1983;67:1178-1185.

[10] Dargie HJ. Effect of carvedilol on outcome after myocardial infarction in patients with left-ventricular dysfunction: the CAPRICORN randomised trial. *Lancet* 2001;357:1385-1390.

[11] Packer M, Coats AJ, Fowler MB, et al. Carvedilol Prospective Randomized Cumulative Survival Study Group. Effect of carvedilol on survival in severe chronic heart failure. *N Engl J Med* 2001;344:1651-1658.

[12] Poole-Wilson PA, Swedberg K, Cleland JG, et al. Carvedilol or Metoprolol European Trial Investigators. Comparison of carvedilol and metoprolol on clinical outcomes in patients with chronic heart failure in the Carvedilol Or Metoprolol European Trial (COMET): randomised controlled trial. *Lancet* 2003;362:7-13.

[13] Flather MD, Shibata MC, Coats AJ, et al. SENIORS Investigators. Randomized trial to determine the effect of nebivolol on mortality and cardiovascular hospital admission in elderly patients with heart failure (SENIORS). *Eur Heart J* 2005;26:215-225.

[14] Koepfli P, Wyss CA, Namdar M, et al. B-adrenergic blockade and myocardial perfusion in coronary artery disease: differential effects in stenotic versus remote myocardial segments. *J Nucl Med* 2004;45:1628-1631.

[15] Sugioka K, Hozumi T, Takemoto Y, et al. Early recovery of impaired coronary flow reserve by carvedilol therapy in patients with idiopathic dilated cardiomyopathy: a serial transthoracic Doppler echocardiographic study. *J Am Coll Cardiol* 2005;45:318-319.
[16] Neglia D, De Maria R, Masi S, et al. Effects of long-term treatment with carvedilol on myocardial blood flow in idiopathic dilated cardiomyopathy. *Heart* 2007;93:803-813.
[17] Sugioka K, Hozumi T, Takemoto Y, et al. Relation of early improvement in coronary flow reserve to late recovery of left ventricular function after beta-blocker therapy in patients with idiopathic dilated cardiomyopathy. *Am Heart J* 2007;153:1080e1-1080e6.
[18] Galderisi M, Cicala S, D'Errico A, et al. Nebivolol improves coronary flow reserve in hypertensive patients without coronary heart disease. *J Hypertens* 2004;22:2201-2208.
[19] Erdogan D, Gullu H, Caliskan M, et al. Nebivolol improves coronary flow reserve in patients with idiopathic dilated cardiomyopathy. *Heart* 2007;93:319-324.
[20] Togni M, Vigorito F, Windecker S, et al. Does the beta-Blocker Nebivolol Increase Coronary Flow Reserve? *Cardiovasc Drug Ther* 2007; Jan 26; [Epub ahead of print].
[21] Galderisi M, D'Errico A, Sidiropulos M, Innelli P, de Divitiis O, de Simone G. Nebivolol induces parallel improvement of left ventricular filling pressure and coronary flow reserve in uncomplicated arterial hypertension. *J Hypertens* 2009;27:2108-2115.
[22] Galderisi M, D'Errico A. Beta-blocker and coronary flow reserve. The importance of a vasodilatory action. *Drugs* 2008;68:579-580.
[23] Drexler H, Zeiber AM, Wollschlager H, et al. Flow dependent coronary artery dilation in humans, *Circulation* 1989;80:466-474.
[24] Lorenzoni R, Rosen SD, Camici PG. Effect of alpha1-adrenoceptor blockade on resting and hyperemic myocardial blood flow in normal humans. *Am J Physiol* 1996;271:H1302-H1306.
[25] Yue TL, Ruffolo RR jr, Feuerstein G. Antioxidant action of carvedilol: a potential role in treatment of heart failure. *Heart Fail Rev* 1999;4:39-51.
[26] Kuo L, Davis MJ, Chilian WH. Endothelium-dependent, flow induced dilation of isolated coronary arterioles. *Am J Physiol* 1990;259:H1063-H1070.
[27] Ignarro LJ, Byrns RE, Trinh K, et al. Nebivolol: a selective beta(1)-adrenergic receptor antagonist that relaxes vascular smooth muscle by nitric oxide- and cyclic GMP-dependent mechanisms. *Nitric Oxide* 2002;7:75-82.
[28] Brehm BR, Bertsch D, von Fallois J, et al. Beta-blockers of the third generation inhibit endothelin-1 liberation, mRNA production and proliferation of human coronary smooth muscle and endothelial cells. *J Cardiovasc Pharmacol* 2000;36:S401-S403.
[29] Mundhenke M, Schwartzkopff B, Köstering M, et al. Endogenous plasma endothelin concentrations and coronary circulation in patients with mild dilated cardiomyopathy. *Heart* 1999;81:278-284.

[30] Lekakis JP, Protogerou A, Papamichael C, et al. Effect of nebivolol and atenolol on brachial artery flow-mediated vasodilation in patients with coronary artery disease. *Cardiovasc Drugs Ther* 2005;19:277-281.

[31] Corretti MC, Anderson TJ, Benjamin EJ, et al. International Brachial Artery Reactivity Task Force. Guidelines for the ultrasound assessment of endothelial-dependent flow-mediated vasodilation of the brachial artery: a report of the International Brachial Artery Reactivity Task Force. *J Am Coll Cardiol* 2002;39:257-265.

[32] Zeiher AM, Krause T, Schächinger V, Minners J, Moser E. Impaired endothelium-dependent vasodilation of coronary resistance vessels is associated with exercise-induced myocardial ischemia. *Circulation* 1995;91:2345-2352.

[33] Olsen SL, Gilbert EM, Renlund DG, et al. Carvedilol improves left ventricular function and symptoms in chronic heart failure: a double-blind randomized study. *J Am Coll Cardiol* 1995;25:1225-1231.

[34] Australia/New Zealand Heart Failure Research Collaborative Group. Randomised, placebo-controlled trial of carvedilol in patients with congestive heart failure due to ischaemic heart disease. *Lancet* 1997; 349:375-380.

[35] Di Lenarda A, Sabbadini G, Salvatore L, et al. Long-term effects of carvedilol in idiopathic dilated cardiomyopathy with persistent left ventricular dysfunction despite chronic metoprolol. The Heart-Muscle Disease Study Group. *J Am Coll Cardiol* 1999;33:1926-1934.

[36] Palazzuoli A, Quatrini I, Vecchiato L, et al. Left ventricular diastolic function improvement by carvedilol therapy in advanced heart failure. *J Cardiovasc Pharmacol* 2005;45:563-568.

[37] Wisenbaugh T, Katz I, Davis J, et al. Long-term (3-month) effects of a new beta-blocker (nebivolol) on cardiac performance in dilated cardiomyopathy. *J Am Coll Cardiol* 1993;21:1094-1100.

[38] Nodari S, Metra M, Dei Cas L. Beta-blocker treatment of patients with diastolic heart failure and arterial hypertension. A prospective, randomized, comparison of the long-term effects of atenolol vs. nebivolol. *Eur J Heart Fail* 2003;5:621-627.

[39] Edes I, Gasior Z, Wita K. Effects of nebivolol on left ventricular function in elderly patients with chronic heart failure: results of the ENECA study. *Eur J Heart Fail* 2005;7:631-639.

[40] Ghio S, Magrini G, Serio A, et al. Effects of nebivolol in elderly heart failure patients with or without systolic left ventricular dysfunction: results of the SENIORS echocardiographic substudy. *Eur Heart J* 2006;27:506-507.

[41] Rigo F, Cortigiani L, Pasanisi E, et al. The additional prognostic value of coronary flow reserve on left anterior descending artery in patients with negative stress echo by wall motion criteria. A transthoracic vasodilator stress echocardiography study. *Am Heart J* 2006;151:124-130.

[42] Rigo F, Gherardi S, Galderisi M, et al. The independent prognostic value of contractile and coronary flow reserve determined by dipyridamole stress echocardiography in patients with idiopathic dilated cardiomyopathy. *Am J Cardiol* 2007;99:1154-1158.

[43] Cortigiani L, Rigo F, Gherardi S, et al. Additional prognostic value of coronary flow reserve in diabetic and non diabetic patients with negative dipyridamole stress echocardiography by wall motion criteria. *J Am Coll Cardiol* 2007;50:1354-1361.

6

The Role of Enhanced External Counterpulsation Therapy in the Management of Coronary Artery Disease

Ozlem Soran
University of Pittsburgh, Heart and Vascular Institute
USA

1. Introduction

Coronary artery disease (CAD) is a narrowing or blockage of the arteries and vessels that provide oxygen and nutrients to the heart. It is caused by atherosclerosis, an accumulation of fatty materials on the inner linings of arteries. According to the American Heart Association and American Stroke Association's 2010 publication on heart disease and stroke statistics, cardiovascular disease remains the leading cause of mortality in the United States in men and women of every major ethnic group. It accounts for nearly 1 million deaths per year as of 2006 and was responsible for one in almost three deaths in the United States in 2006. Approximately 17 million persons have a history of coronary artery disease and 8 million have suffered a myocardial infarction (American Heart Association 2010). Medication and invasive revascularization are the most common approaches for treating CAD. Invasive revascularization includes percutaneus coronary interventions (PCI: stent implantation or balloon angioplasty)and Coronary Bypass Surgery (CABG). Even though both treatment options are commonly used, it is important to note that neither of these approaches provides a cure. In other words, although the symptoms are eliminated or alleviated, the disease and its causes are still present after treatment. Both treatments target lesions that cause the obstructions however, CAD is a progressive disease. New treatment approaches are in need to prevent the disease from progressing and the symptoms from recurring. Enhanced External Counterpulsation (EECP) therapy with its different mode of action provides a new treatment modality in the management of CAD and complements the invasive revascularization (Fig. 1).

This chapter summarizes the current evidence to support the role of EECP therapy in CAD management and provides information on its mechanism of action.

2. What is EECP?

EECP therapy consists of a treatment bed attached to an air compressor unit which is attached to a computerized control console. Three sets of cuffs wrapped around the lower legs and the buttocks of the patient. It is a noninvasive outpatient therapy consisting of electrocardiography (ECG)-gated sequential leg compression, which produces hemodynamic effects similar to those of an intra-aortic balloon pump (IABP) (Fig. 2).

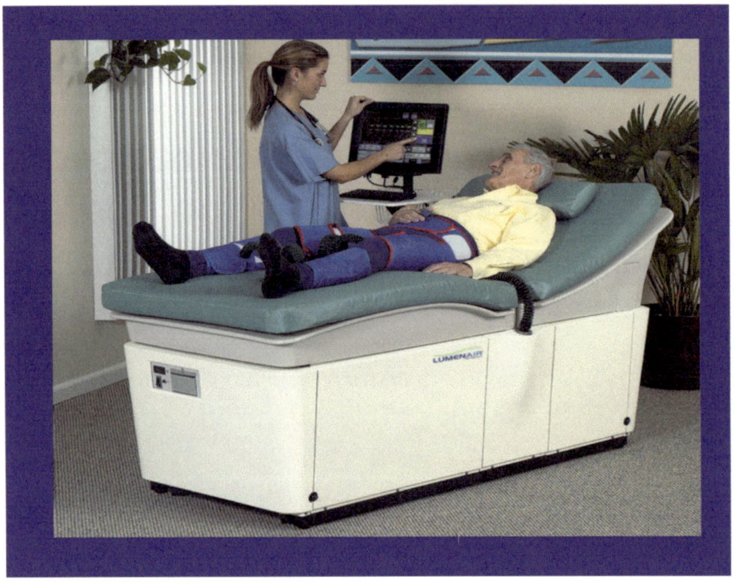

EECP Therapy: Consisting of a patient bed attached to an air compressor unit; computerized control consul; 3 sets of cuffs wrapped around the lower legs and the buttocks of the patient. (With permission from Vasomedical Inc., NY). EECP: Enhanced External Counterpulsation

Fig. 1. EECP Therapy

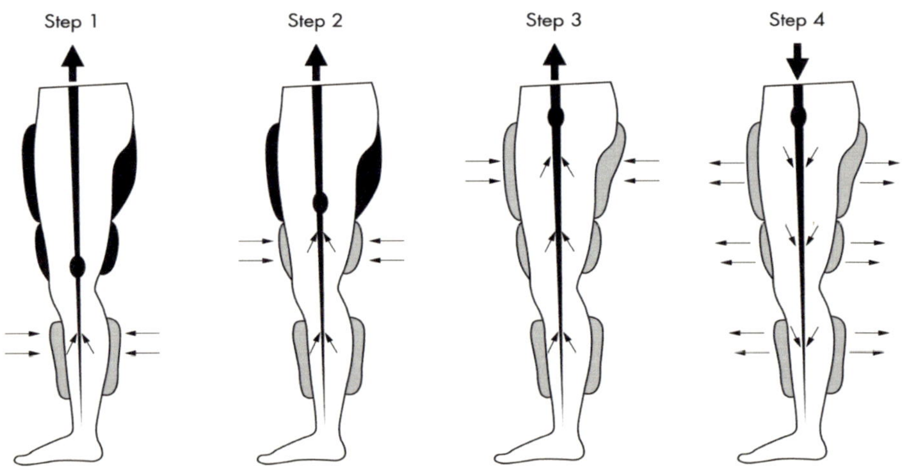

Three pairs of pneumatic cuffs are applied to the calves, lower thighs, and upper thighs. The cuffs are inflated sequentially during diastole, distal to proximal. The compression of the lower extremity vascular bed increases diastolic pressure and flow and increases venous return. The pressure is then released at the onset of systole. Inflation and deflation are timed according to the R wave on the patient's cardiac monitor. The pressures applied and the inflation-deflation timing can be altered by using the pressure waveforms and ECG on the EECP therapy monitor. (Adapted from Manchanda and Soran 2007)
ECG: Electrocardiogram; EECP: Enhanced External Counterpulsation

Fig. 2. Technique of EECP Therapy

However, unlike IABP therapy, EECP therapy also increases venous return (Manchanda and Soran 2007, Birtwell et al 1968). Cuffs resembling oversized blood pressure cuffs—on the calves and lower and upper thighs, including the buttocks—inflate rapidly and sequentially via computer interpreted ECG signals, starting from the calves and proceeding upward to the buttocks during the resting phase of each heartbeat (diastole). This creates a strong retrograde counterpulse in the arterial system, forcing freshly oxygenated blood toward the heart and coronary arteries while increasing the volume of venous blood return to the heart under increased pressure. Just before the next heartbeat, before systole, all three cuffs deflate simultaneously, significantly reducing the heart's workload. This is achieved because the vascular beds in the lower extremities are relatively empty when the cuffs are deflated; significantly lowering the resistance to blood ejected by the heart and reducing the amount of work the heart must do to pump oxygenated blood to the rest of the body. A finger plethysmogram is used throughout treatment to monitor diastolic and systolic pressure waveforms. The current EECP device can generate external cuff pressures as high as 220 to 300 mmHg. A typical therapy course consists of 35 treatments administered for 1 hour a day over 7 weeks.

2.1 Historical perspective

The concept of counterpulsation was introduced in the U.S. in 1953 when Kantrowitz first proposed that elevations of aortic diastolic pressure could improve coronary blood flow and could benefit patients with coronary insufficiency. Although subsequent studies suggested that counterpulsation would indeed benefit some patients with coronary insufficiency, the development of the necessary technology proved challenging. A group of devices that increased coronary blood flow, including flow assist devices and venoarterial bypass systems, proved effective in providing increased coronary blood flow but were unable to reduce the tension time index or work load of the heart. External cardiac massage, internal cardiac massage, veno-arterial bypass, implantable auxillary ventricules, intra-aortic balloon pumps, and cardiopulmonary bypass have all demonstrated hemodynamic benefits; however, their usefulness in clinical practice has been limited because of their inherent invasiveness.

In the mid 1960s, several groups began to explore a non-invasive method for producing the salutary physiologic effects of counterpulsation. First external countrepulation device introduced by Harvard investigators, consisted of a hydraulically driven unit with a pair of water -filled bladders that could be wrapped around the lower legs and thighs of the patient. (Birtwell et al, 1968) However, the external pressure could only be applied to a limited amount of tissue mass thereby producing suboptimal diastolic augmentation of coronary flow. Investigators did not give up on the idea and kept working on to improve the technology. Over the years air-driven EECP system consisting of three sets of balloons wrapped around the lower legs, thighs and upper thighs of the patient has been developed. Air pressure was applied sequentially from the lower legs to the thigh and upper thigh resulting in "milking" of oxygenated blood from the lower extremities toward the heart with greater efficiency. (Amsterdam et al.,1980; Zeng et al., 1983). It has been demonstrated that the sequential inclusion of the upper thigh provided a critical advantage to EECP, affecting a 44% increase in diastolic augmentation compared with studies using only the lower extremity cuffs. Subsequent modifications of the EECP prototype with microprocessors allowed for precise cuff inflation and deflation and gating with the electrocardiogram. The lower cuffs were inflated at the start of diastole as represented by the beginning of the T wave, while simultaneous deflation of all three chambers was triggered just prior to systole at the onset of the P wave. The retrograde flow provided by EECP increased both the volume and pressure of diastolic flow such that diastolic to systolic ratios exceeded 1.0-1.2. (Soran et al., 1999). In summary, it took 40 years for investigators to develop the enhanced technology that is being currently used. (Fig 1)

2.2 Acute hemodynamic effects of EECP therapy

Acute hemodynamic effects of EECP has been assessed through both noninvasive and invasive techniques.(Soran et al., 2001; Stys et al., 2001; Michaelset al.,2001; Lakshmi et al. 2002; Nichols et al., 2006; Taguchi et al., 2004).
Taguchi *et al*, assessed the hemodynamic effects of EECP and compared it with IABP in 39 patients with uncomplicated acute myocardial infarction who underwent successful balloon coronary angioplasty within 12 hours after onset of chest pain. The radial artery and subclavian vein were cannulated to measure right atrial pressure, pulmonary capillary wedge pressure (PCWP), cardiac index, and systemic vascular resistance. Radial artery pressure tracing was used to measure area under artery pressure curves in systolic and diastolic phases. Sixty minutes treatment was administered to the patients in the EECP group. All parameters were measured before EECP, at 15, 30, 45, and 60 minutes after starting EECP, and 60 minutes after stopping EECP. After starting IABP support, measurements were obtained at 15, 30, 45, and 60 minutes. There were no significant changes in heart rate in either group before, during, and after treatments. Right atrial pressure increased significantly at 15 and 30 minutes after starting EECP, and then decreased gradually. There was no significant increase in right atrial pressure at 45 and 60 minutes after starting EECP compared with baseline. Right atrial pressure did not change in the IABP group, and there was no significant difference between 2 groups, except at 15 minutes after starting treatment. In the EECP group the PCWP significantly increased at 15 and 30 minutes, and then decreased gradually, but no significant change was seen in IABP group. Between two groups, there were no significant differences at baseline and during treatment. However, 60 minutes after stopping treatment, PCWP was significantly lower in the EECP group. The cardiac index in EECP group increased significantly at 45 and 60 minutes compared with the baseline, but no significant change was noted in IABP group. The increase in cardiac index at 60 minutes in the EECP group was significantly greater than that in the IABP group. Mean values of the area under the arterial pressure curves during the diastolic phase increased significantly in both groups, and there was no significant difference between two groups at any measuring point. Mean values of the areas under the artery pressure curves during the systolic phase decreased significantly during treatment compared with baseline in the IABP group. No significant change was observed in the EECP group. In both groups, systemic vascular resistance decreased significantly during treatment compared with baseline, but no significant difference was seen between two groups. This study showed that the hemodynamic effects of EECP were similar to those of IABP for diastolic augmentation and systemic vascular resistance. However, right atrial pressure, PCWP, and cardiac index increased during EECP in contrast to IABP. These effects suggest that EECP increases venous return, raises cardiac preload, and increases cardiac output. (Taguchi et al., 2004; Michaels et al., 2009)

In another study, Taguchi et al., assessed the hemodynamic and neurohormonal changes during EECP. Sixty minutes of EECP therapy has been performed in patients with stable acute myocardial infarction who had undergone PCI. Right heart catheterization and neurohumoral parameters were assessed before, during 15, 30 and 60 minutes after EECP. Blood levels of atrial natriuretic peptide (ANP), brain (or B type) natriuretic peptide (BNP), renin, aldosterone, dopamine, and noradrenaline were assessed. Left ventricular ejection fraction and size were assessed invasively during the admission and between days 13 to 16. Cardiac index increased from 3.3±0.8 L/min before treatment to 4.1±0.8 L/min at 60 minutes (P<0.01). Right atrial pressure increased from 6.4±3.3 mmHg at baseline to 9.8±4.0 mmHg at 15 minutes (P<0.01), and PCWP increased from 8.9±4.0 mmHg to 12.6±5.3 mmHg (P<0.05). The blood levels of ANP increased from 54±42 pg/ml at baseline to 70±46 pg/ml at 60 minutes, which returned to baseline level 60 minutes after EECP treatment. The pretreatment concentrations of BNP, dopamine, noradrenaline, renin and aldosterone did not change during or after EECP treatment. Left ventricular end-diastolic pressure decreased from 18.6±1.6 mmHg during the acute stage to 13.8±6.4 mmHg during subacute follow-up, but there was no change in left ventricular ejection fraction or end-diastolic volume index. Blood concentrations of ANP increased at 15 minutes after initiation of EECP, which suggested that EECP treatment increased the volume of venous return, resulting in an increased atrial load. EECP significantly improved cardiac index with a significant increase in blood ANP concentration but without increase in heart rate or BNP. These findings suggest that there be an increased atrial preload without any significant change in ventricular preload.(Taguchi et al.,2004; Michaels et al., 2010)

Michaels et al., used an invasive approach to measure intracoronary, central aortic, and left ventricular pressure and intracoronary Doppler flow to assess the acute hemodynamic effects of EECP. Ten patients who were referred for cardiac catheterization (5 with suspected coronary artery disease, 3 with severe mitral regurgitation, and 2 with heart transplant patients) were included in the study. Key exclusion criteria included severe aortic insufficiency, decompensated heart failure, significant arrhythmia, systolic blood pressure more than 180 mmHg, and symptomatic peripheral arterial disease. EECP was performed at external cuff pressures ranging from 100 to 300 mmHg. At baseline and during EECP, simultaneous central aortic and intracoronary pressure, intracoronary Doppler flow velocity, and corrected thrombosis in Myocardial Infarction study (TIMI) frame count (CTFC) were measured. Peak aortic systolic pressure decreased 11% from 114 ±19 mmHg at baseline to 101±28 mmHg during EECP (P=0.02). These findings indicate that EECP acutely reduces ventricular afterload. Left ventricular end-diastolic pressure decreased during EECP (15±7 mmHg at baseline, 13±6 mmHg during EECP; P=0.17). Aortic diastolic pressure increased 92% from 71±10 mmHg to 136±22 mmHg (P<0.0001), and mean aortic pressure increased 16% from 88±10 mmHg to 102± 14 mmHg during EECP (P=0.0007), indicating significant. Intracoronary pressure was measured in an unobstructed epicardial coronary artery using the micromanometer-tipped 0.014-inch pressure wire. There was a 93% increase in intracoronary peak diastolic pressure (71±10 mmHg at baseline to 137±21 mmHg during EECP; P<0.0001;. (Michaels et al., 2002; Fig 3)

Mean pressure increased by 16% from 88±9 mmHg at baseline to 102±16 mmHg during EECP (P=0.006). EECP decreased peak systolic pressure by 15% from 116±20 mmHg at baseline to 99±26 mmHg during EECP (P=0.002). Planimetry of the intracoronary pressure tracings showed a 28% increase in diastolic pressure (42±9 mmHg·sec at baseline; 54±15 mmHg·sec during EECP; P=0.0003) and a 12% decrease in systolic pressure

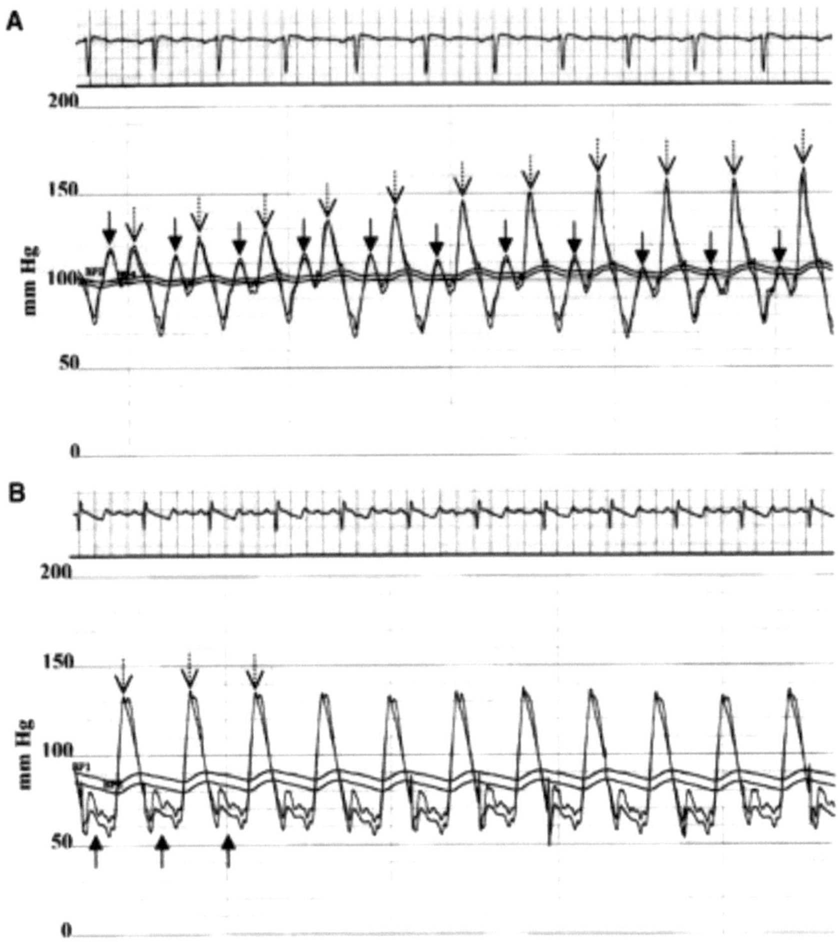

Representative simultaneous hemodynamic tracings of central aortic pressure from the coronary catheter and intracoronary pressure from the PressureWire. In tracings of both phasic and mean pressure (bottom) obtained at the beginning of EECP (A), there is a gradual increase in peak diastolic (dashed arrows) and mean pressure with a decrease in peak systolic pressure (solid arrows) attributable to systolic unloading as the inflation pressure is increased in the EECP device. In another patient, diastolic augmentation is demonstrated during EECP at a cuff pressure of 300 mm Hg (B). The intracoronary coronary pressure was 5 mm Hg lower than central aortic pressure, attributable to diffuse coronary atherosclerosis. The paper speed is 25 mm/sec. (With permission from Michaels AD,2002)

Fig. 3. Hemodynamic tracings of central aortic pressure

(33±6 mmHg·sec at baseline; 29±7 mmHg·sec during EECP; *P*=0.008). Intracoronary Doppler flow velocity was measured using a 0.014-inch FloWire (Fig 2). The average peak velocity increased 109% from 11±5 cm/s at baseline to 23 ±5 cm/s during EECP (*P*=0.001). The peak diastolic velocity increased 150% from 18±7 cm/s at baseline to 45±14 cm/s during EECP (*P*=0.0004). The diastolic-to-systolic velocity ratio increased 100% from 1.0±0.3 to 2.0±0.7 during EECP (*P*=0.003). There was no significant change in peak systolic velocity. The CTFC, another measure of coronary flow velocity, significantly decreased 28% from 37±18 at baseline to 27±13 during EECP (*P*=0.001). This study provides solid evidence of the increase

in directly measured aortic and coronary diastolic pressure and flow velocity from EECP. There is a significant reduction in left ventricular afterload and left ventricle work secondary to systolic unloading.
(Michaels et al., 2010)
Acute hemodynamic effects of EECP can be summarized as: (Fig 4)

1. Increased retrograde aortic blood flow; diastolic augmentation;
2. Increased coronary blood flow ; increased perfusion pressure;
3. Increased venous return;
4. Increased cardiac output;
5. Systolic unloading;
6. Decreased left ventricular workload

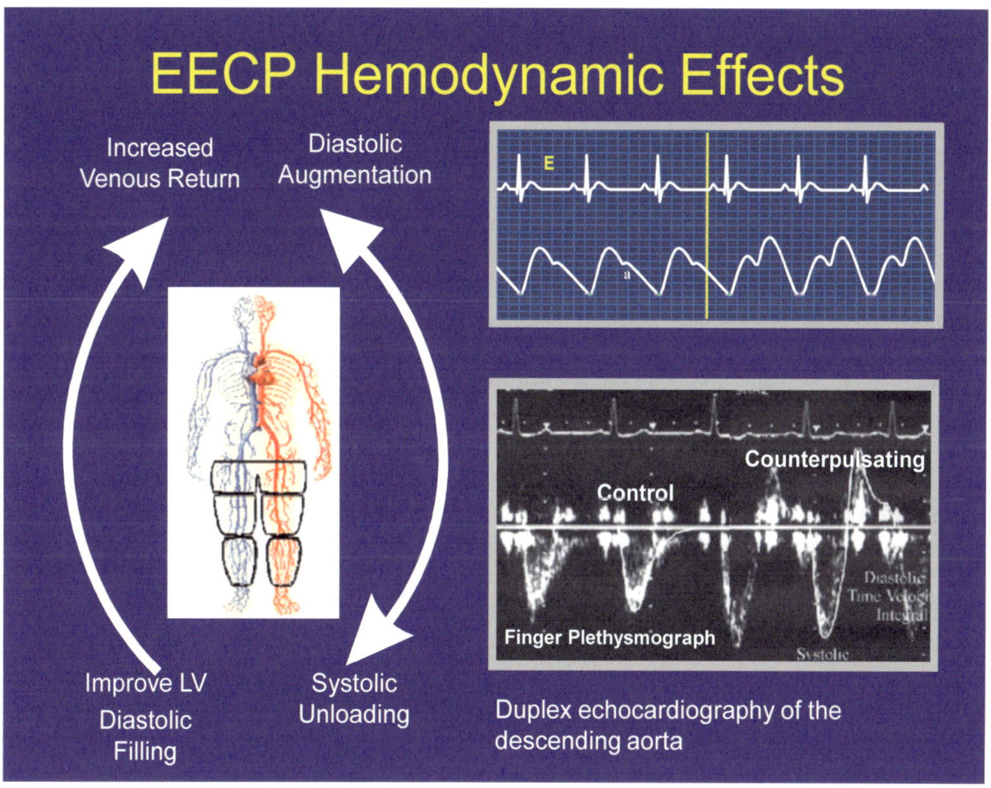

Right upper corner: Showing the ECG tracing and finger pletysmogram. As soon as the device turned on (yellow line) diastolic augmentation starts. Right lower corner: showing the diastolic augmentation by echocardiography. EECP: Enhanced External Counterpulsation; a: aortic notch (With permission from Dr Soran and Katz 1998)

Fig. 4. Acute hemodynamic effects of EECP Therapy

3. EECP therapy in CAD management

Several nonrandomized and randomized trials have demonstrated a consistently positive clinical response among patients with CAD treated with EECP (Lawson et al. 1992, Arora et al. 1999). Benefits associated with EECP therapy include reduction in angina and nitrate use, increased exercise tolerance, favorable psychosocial effects, and enhanced quality of life as well as prolongation of the time to exercise-induced ST-segment depression and an accompanying resolution of myocardial perfusion defects. Numerous clinical trials in the past two decades have shown EECP therapy to be safe and effective for patients with CAD, with a clinical response rate averaging 70% to 80%, which is sustained up to 5 years. (Lawson et al. 2000; Masuda et al. 2001; Stys et al. 2002; Pettersson et al.2006; Braverman, DL. 2009).

Most studies on EECP therapy cannot be double blind and lack good control groups because of technical limitations, drawbacks that have frequently raised questions regarding operator bias. However, the Multicenter Study of EECP (MUSTEECP), a randomized double-blinded placebo-controlled trial, did document a clinical benefit from EECP therapy in patients with chronic stable angina and positive exercise stress tests. In this study, 139 patients (mean age 63 years, range 35 years to 81 years) with angina pectoris (typical Canadian Cardiovascular Society (CCS) classes I, II, and III angina) and documented coronary ischemia were equally randomized to hemodynamically inactive counterpulsation with EECP versus active counterpulsation. Patients in the active EECP therapy group showed a statistically significant increase in time to exercise-induced ST-segment depression when compared with sham and baseline, and reported a statistically significant decrease in the frequency of angina episodes when compared with sham and baseline. Exercise duration increased significantly in both groups; however, the increase was greater in the active EECP group. Moreover, a MUST-EECP sub study demonstrated a significant improvement in quality-of life parameters in patients assigned to active treatment, and this improvement was sustained during a 12-month follow-up (Arora et al. 2002).

Tartaglia et al assessed the effect of EECP on exercise capacity and myocardial perfusion by comparing results of maximal exercise radionuclide testing pre- and post-EECP treatment. This prospective study included 25 patients with angina who had performed maximal symptom-limited exercise tolerance tests with Bruce protocol and radionuclide perfusion single-photon emission computed tomography (SPECT) study prior to and at completion of EECP treatment. After 35 h of EECP, 93% improved by at least one functional angina class. There is a significant improvement in their total treadmill times and a significant change in their peak double products, from 18,891 +/- 3,939 pre-EECP to 20,464 +/- 4,305 post-EECP exercise tolerance tests ($p < 0.03$). Pre EECP, 16 patients had ST-segment depression on their initial exercise tolerance tests. After EECP, 80% either no longer had ST depression or had a significant increase in their time to ST depression. The radionuclide perfusion scores also showed a significant reduction in ischemic segments. In this study, patients treated with EECP demonstrated a reduction in angina symptoms, improvement in exercise capacity, increase in time to ST-segment depression, and decrease in perfusion defects despite performing at a higher workload.

In another study, investigators evaluated the effects of EECP therapy on dobutamine stress-induced wall motion score among patients with angina pectoris. In this prospective study, 43% of patients with severe chronic angina pectoris and had a positive dobutamine stress echocardiogram had normal or reduced dobutamine induced wall motion abnormalities after EECP therapy. (Bagger et al., 2004)

British investigators assessed the immediate and long-term effect of EECP in treatment of chronic stable refractory angina. Sixty-one patients were treated with EECP and 58 completed a course of treatment. About 52% of patients suffered from CCS III and IV angina prior to EECP. Immediately post-EECP, angina improved by at least one CCS class in 86% and by two classes in 59%. At 1-year follow-up, sustained improvement in CCS was observed in 78% of the patients. The median weekly angina frequency and nitroglycerin use were significantly reduced immediately after EECP. In 48 patients, their mean exercise time improved significantly after EECP. Major-adverse events were rare. This study showed that for patients who fail to respond to conventional measures, a high proportion gain symptomatic benefit from EECP.

In 2006, Swedish investigators assess the long-term outcome of EECP treatment at a Scandinavian centre, in relieving angina in patients with chronic refractory angina pectoris. 55 patients were treated with EECP. CCS class, antianginal medication and adverse clinical events were collected prior to EECP, at the end of the treatment, and at six and 12 months after EECP treatment. Clinical signs and symptoms were recorded. EECP treatment significantly improved the CCS class in 79% of the patients with chronic angina pectoris. The reduction in CCS angina class was seen in patients with CCS class III and IV and persisted 12 months after EECP treatment. In accordance with the reduction in CCS classes there was a significant decrease in the weekly nitroglycerin usage. The results showed that EECP was a safe and effective treatment in CAD patients and the beneficial effects were sustained during a 12-months follow-up period. (Pettersson et al.,2006).

Same year, Italian investigators tested efficacy of EECP on symptoms, myocardial ischaemia and cardiac performance in patients with intractable angina, refractory to surgical and medical treatment. Twenty-five patients (mean age 65 years) with persistent ischaemia notwithstanding optimal medical therapy or after interventional or surgical procedure, received EECP sessions for 35 h. Each patient underwent dobutamine stress echocardiography before and after treatment. Eighty-four percent of patients showed an increase in at least one functional angina class. Thirty-six percent of patients had a reduction in the area of inducible ischaemia at dobutamine stress echocardiography after treatment. They concluded that EECP therapy was effective in relieving symptoms in patients with refractory angina and may reduce inducible ischaemia at dobutamine stress echocardiography, especially in patients with reduced systolic function and compromised segmental kinesis. (Novo et al., 2006)

Although randomized (including placebo-controlled) and nonrandomized studies have shown beneficial effects of EECP therapy, investigators saw the need to assess EECP's effectiveness in real-world settings, leading them to develop the International EECP Patient Registry (IEPR) under the management of the University of Pittsburgh (Michaels et al. 2004, Soran et al., 2010). More than 5000 patients were enrolled in phase I and another 2500 patients enrolled in phase II of the study, and more than 90 centers participated. Results from the IEPR and the EECP Clinical Consortium have demonstrated that the symptomatic benefit observed in controlled studies translates to the heterogeneous patient population seen in clinical practice. Moreover, follow-up data indicate that the clinical benefit may be maintained for up to 5 years in patients with a favorable initial clinical response (Lawson et al. 2000; Loh et al 2008)

Soran et al., compared the efficacy, repeat EECP and 6-months major adverse cardiovascular events (MACE: Death/CABG/PCI/MI) free survival rates for patients treated with EECP for angina management in Europe (EU) with the United States (US); 4658 were treated and followed in the US and 262 in EU. EU were younger (p<0.001) with a higher proportion of men. Previous revascularization rate was higher in US (p<0.001). EU had less diabetes, hypertension, hyperlipidemia, multivessel disease, Class IV angina, and higher rates of nitroglycerin usage (p<0.001). After a mean treatment course of 34 hours, both groups showed a significant reduction in the severity of angina (78% vs 76%). Discontinuation of nitroglycerin usage was similar in both groups (50%). MACE during the treatment period was low in both groups (<3%).Compliance with the treatment course was better in EU (p<0.001).

At 6-month follow up 66% of EU and 76% of US had maintained the improvement in angina class; survival rate was 99% in EU and 97% in US. MACE free survival rate was 92% in EU vs 90% in US. Repeat EECP rates at 6months follow up were significantly lower in EU (0.5% vs. 4%, p<0.01).Patients presenting for EECP treatment from EU and US populations showed very different baseline profiles. However, both cohorts achieved substantial reduction in angina with high event free survival rates at 6 months. (Soran et al., 2010)

EECP was suggested as a safe treatment option for selected symptomatic PCI candidates with obstructive CAD. Baseline characteristics and 1-year outcome in 2 cohorts of PCI candidates presenting with stable symptoms: 323 patients treated with EECP in the IEPR, and 448 NHLBI Dynamic Registry patients treated with elective PCI, were compared. Compared with patients receiving PCI, IEPR patients had a higher prevalence of many risk factors including prior PCI prior coronary artery bypass grafting, prior myocardial infarction, history of congestive heart failure, and history of diabetes. Left ventricular ejection fraction was lower among IEPR patients (mean 50.3% vs 59.2%, p <0.001). At 1 year, survival was comparable in the 2 cohorts (98.7% IEPR vs 96.8% PCI, P = NS), as were rates of coronary artery bypass grafting during follow-up (4.5% IEPR vs 5.7% PCI, P = NS). At 1 year, 43.7% of IEPR patients reported no anginal symptoms compared with 73.4% of Dynamic Registry patients (p <0.001). Rates of severe symptoms (CCS class III, IV, or unstable) at 1 year were 15.5% among IEPR patients and 9.5% in the Dynamic Registry (p = 0.02). PCI candidates suitable for and treated with EECP had 1-year major event rates comparable to patients receiving elective PCI. These results suggested that EECP, as a noninvasive treatment, could be used as a first -line treatment with invasive revascularization reserved for EECP failures, or high -risk patients. (Holubkov et al., 2002). **The results of this study warrant the initiation of a randomized controlled study to ascertain the efficacy of EECP combined with drug therapy as a first line treatment in selected patients with CAD.**

3.1 EECP therapy in CAD with left ventricular dysfunction

When providing EECP therapy to patients with heart failure, the initial researchers were concerned primarily that the increased venous return resulting from EECP therapy might precipitate pulmonary edema in angina patients with severe left ventricular dysfunction (SLVD).

Using outcomes data from 363 patients enrolled in the IEPR, Soran et al. (Soran et al. 2006, Soran et al. 2002) evaluated the safety and efficacy of EECP therapy in those with refractory angina pectoris and SLVD (ejection fraction [EF] < 35%). In this study patients' average duration of clinical CAD was nearly 13 years; 84% had multivessel disease and 93% were not candidates for further revascularization due to the extent and severity of disease, LV dysfunction, co-morbid conditions, previous interventions, or risk/benefit ratio. Angina was severe (class III/IV) in 93% of patients. There was a high prevalence of cardiac risk factors (i.e., 45% had DM, 85% had prior MI, ,78% had hyperlipidemia, 77% had a history of smoking and 82% had a family history of premature atherosclerotic cardiovascular disease). More than 50% reported quality of life as poor. On average, patients underwent an EECP treatment course of 32 hours, with 81% completing the course. Twelve percent discontinued due to a clinical event, and 7% stopped due to patient preference. Major adverse cardiovascular events that occurred over the course of EECP therapy were low (Death/ myocardial infarction [MI]/CABG/PCI<2%). After completion of treatment, there was a significant reduction in angina severity: 72% improved from severe angina to no or mild angina. Fifty-two percent of the patients stopped using nitroglycerin. There was also a significant increase in quality of life. At 2-year follow-up, angina reduction was maintained in 55% of patients, the survival rate was 83%, and event-free (death/MI/PCI/CABG)

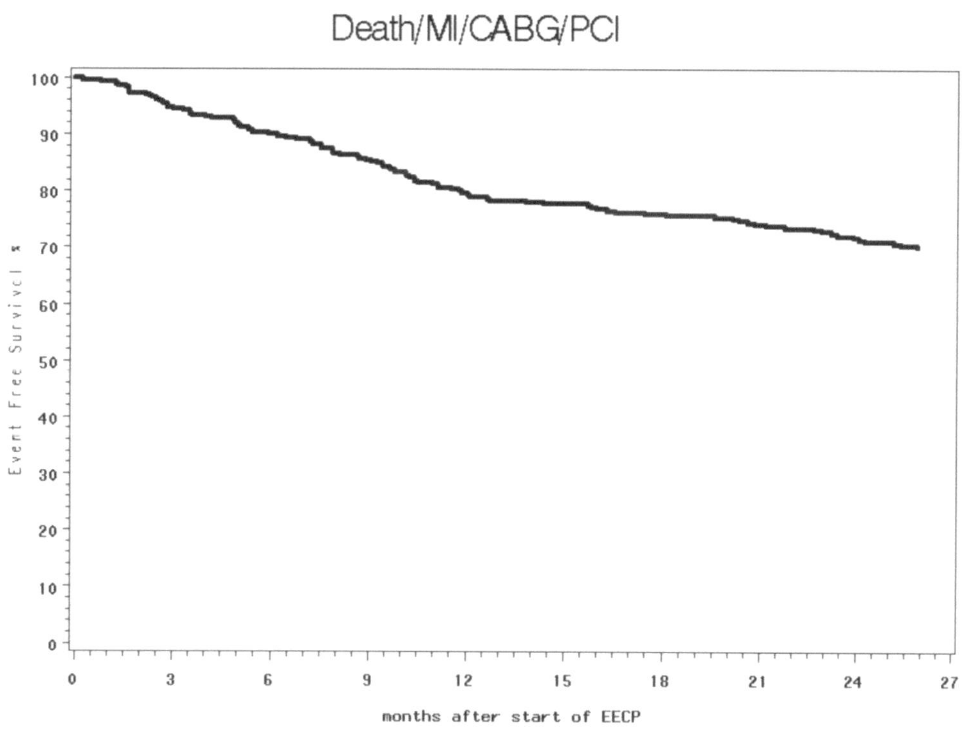

Event (CABG; PCI; MI) free survival rate at 2 years post EECP therapy in patients with coronary artery disease and SLVD (With permission from Dr. Soran; Soran et al 2006)
CABG: Coronary Artery Bypass Grafting Surgery, MI: Myocardial Infarction,
PCI: Percutaneaus Coronary Intervention, SLVD: Severe left ventricular dysfunction

Fig. 5. Event Free Survival Rate at 2 years -Post EECP

survival was 70%. Forty-three percent had no cardiac hospitalization; 81% had no congestive heart failure event (Fig.5). They concluded that EECP therapy for angina is safe and effective in patients with SLVD who are not considered good candidates for revascularization by CABG or PCI.

Estahbanaty et al., evaluated the effects of EECP on systolic and diastolic cardiac function using echocardiography to measure left ventricular EF, end-systolic volume, end-diastolic volume, systolic wave (Sm), early diastolic wave (Ea), Vp, E/Ea, E/Vp, and diastolic function grade in 25 patients before and after 35 hours of EECP. EECP reduced end-systolic volume and end-diastolic volume and increased EF significantly in patients with baseline left ventricular EF ≤ 50%, baseline E/Ea ≥ 14 , baseline grade II or III diastolic dysfunction (decreased compliance) , baseline Ea <7 cm/s and baseline Sm <7 cm/s. These results demonstrated improved systolic and diastolic function in selected patients. (Estahbanaty et al., 2007)

Lawson et al. evaluated CAD patients with preserved left ventricular function (PLV; EF > 35%) and with SLVD (EF≤ 35%) who were treated with a 35-hour course of EECP. Bioimpedance measurements of cardiovascular function were obtained before the first and after the 35th hour of EECP therapy. Twenty-five patients were enrolled, 20 with PLV and 5 with SLVD. Angina class improved similarly in both groups. The SLVD group, in contrast to the PLV group, had increased cardiac power (ie, mean arterial pressure × cardiac output/451), stroke volume, and cardiac index and decreased systemic vascular resistance with treatment. This study suggests that EECP may benefit patients experiencing CAD with SLVD directly by improving cardiac power and indirectly by decreasing systemic vascular resistance (Lawson et al. 2002).

Patients with CAD and left ventricular dysfunction exert an enormous burden on health care resources, primarily because of the number of recurrent emergency department visits and hospitalizations. Improvements in symptoms and laboratory assessments in these patients may not correlate with a reduction in emergency room visits and hospitalizations. Soran et al. assessed the impact of EECP therapy on emergency department visits and hospitalization rates at 6-month follow up. In this prospective cohort study, clinical outcomes, number of all-cause emergency department visits, and hospitalizations within the 6 months before EECP therapy were compared with those at 6-month follow-up. The mean number of emergency department visits per patient decreased from 0.9 ± 2.0 before EECP to 0.2 ± 0.7 at 6 months ($P < 0.001$), and hospitalizations were reduced from 1.1 ± 1.7 to 0.3 ± 0.7 ($P < 0.001$) (Soran et al. 2007).

Scientific data indicates that EECP provides a safe and effective treatment option for patients with CAD and left ventricular dysfunction.

4. Mechanism of action

Upon diastole, cuffs inflate sequentially from the calves, raising diastolic aortic pressure proximally and increasing coronary perfusion pressure. Compression of the vascular beds of the legs also increases venous return. Instantaneous decompression of all cuffs at the onset of systole significantly unloads the left ventricle, thereby lowering vascular impedance and decreasing ventricular workload. This latter effect, when coupled with augmented venous return, raises cardiac output. In summary, EECP therapy increases venous return, raises cardiac preload, increases cardiac output, and decreases systemic vascular resistance (Michaels et al. 2002).

Mechanism of action of EECP therapy is not through one pathway, but several pathways affecting each other. (Fig.6)

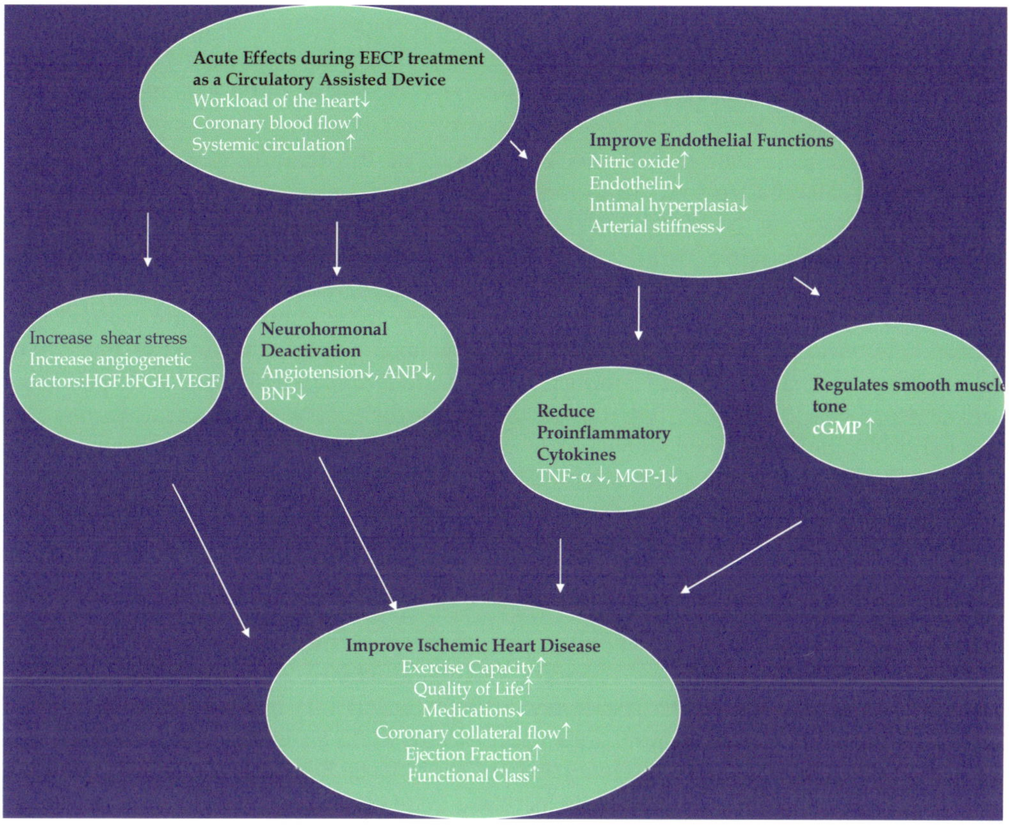

Possible mechanisms responsible for the clinical benefit associated with EECP therapy. Acute hemodynamic and neurohormonal changes, prolonged stimulus to increase sheer stress which promotes endothelial function improvement is thought to promote myocardial collateralization via opening of latent conduits, arteriogenesis, and angiogenesis.
HGF: hepatocyte growth ***factor, bFGF:*** basic Fibroblast Growth ***Factor, VEGF:*** Vascular endothelial growth ***factor, TNF:*** Tumor necrosis factor-***alpha,*** MCP-1: Monocyte chemotactic protein-1, cGMP: Cyclic guanosine monophosphate

Fig. 6. Mechanism of EECP Therapy

4.1 Collateral development

One of the mechanisms of action is through collateral development. Mode-of-action studies have shown that EECP therapy increases angiogenesis factors such as human growth, basic fibroblast growth, and vascular endothelial growth factors. Enhanced diastolic flow increases shear stress, increased shear stress activates the release of growth factors, and augmentation of growth factor release activates angiogenesis.(Soran et al., 1999)
To clarify the mechanism of action of EECP therapy, Masuda et al used (13) N-ammonia positron emission tomography to evaluate myocardial perfusion. Eleven patients (mean age: 61 years) with angina pectoris underwent EECP therapy for 35 1 h sessions. Treadmill

exercise test and (13) N-ammonia positron emission tomography, both at rest and with dipyridamole, before and after EECP therapy were performed. Neurohumoral factors and nitric oxide were also evaluated. Myocardial perfusion increased significantly at rest after therapy. In ischemic regions, particularly the anterior region, myocardial perfusion at rest and with dipyridamole and coronary flow reserve improved significantly after therapy. Exercise time was prolonged and the time to 1-mm ST depression improved markedly. After therapy, nitric oxide levels increased significantly and neurohumoral factors decreased. These results suggest that one of the mechanisms of the therapy is development and recruitment of collateral vessels. (Masuda et al., 2001).

To test the hypothesis that EECP augments collateral function Gloekler et al randomized patients with chronic stable angina to EECP therapy or sham treatment. Before and after 30 h of randomly allocated EECP or sham EECP, the invasive collateral flow index (CFI) was obtained in 34 vessels. CFI was determined by the ratio of mean distal coronary occlusive pressure to mean aortic pressure with central venous pressure subtracted from both. Additionally, coronary collateral conductance (occlusive myocardial blood flow per aorto-coronary pressure drop) was determined by myocardial contrast echocardiography and brachial artery flow-mediated dilatation was obtained. CFI significantly improved in the EECP group but not in the sham treatment. EECP appeared to be effective in promoting coronary collateral growth. The extent of collateral function improvement was related to the amount of improvement in the systemic endothelial function (Gloekler et al. 2010).

4.2 Endothelial function improvement

Another mechanism of action of EECP therapy is through endothelial changes. EECP therapy improves endothelial function and enhances vascular reactivity. Akhtar et al examined the effects of EECP on plasma nitric oxide and endothelin-1 (ET-1) levels. Plasma nitrate and nitrite (NOx) and ET-1 levels were measured serially in 13 patients with coronary artery disease who received 1-hour daily treatments of EECP over 6 weeks. During the course of EECP therapy, plasma NOx progressively increased and plasma ET-1 progressively decreased. After 36 hours of EECP, there was a 62 % increase in plasma NOx compared with baseline ($p < 0.0001$) and a 36% decrease in plasma ET-1 ($p < 0.0001$). At 3 months after completion of EECP, NOx remained 12% above baseline ($p = 0.002$), and ET-1 remained 11% below baseline ($p = 0.0068$). This data provides neurohormonal evidence to support the hypothesis that EECP improves endothelial function.(Akhtar Am J Cardiol 2006)

Braith et al investigated the effects of EECP on peripheral artery flow-mediated dilation in a randomized placebo-controlled study. Symptomatic patients with CAD were randomized (2:1 ratio) to thirty-five 1-hour sessions of either EECP or sham EECP . Flow-mediated dilation of the brachial and femoral arteries was performed with the use of ultrasound. Plasma levels of nitrate and nitrite, 6-ketoprostaglandin, F1α, endothelin-1, asymmetrical dimethylarginine, tumor necrosis factor-α, monocyte chemoattractant protein-1, soluble vascular cell adhesion molecule, high-sensitivity C-reactive protein, and 8-isoprostane were measured. EECP significantly increased brachial and femoral artery flow-mediated dilation, the nitric oxide turnover/production markers nitrate and nitrite and 6-keto-prostaglandin F1α, whereas it decreased endothelin-1 and the nitric oxide synthase inhibitor asymmetrical dimethylarginine in treatment versus sham groups, respectively. EECP significantly decreased the proinflammatory cytokines tumor necrosis factor-α, monocyte chemoattractant protein-1 , soluble vascular cell adhesion molecule-1, high-sensitivity C-reactive protein, and the lipid peroxidation marker 8-isoprostane in treatment versus sham groups, respectively. EECP also significantly reduced angina classification in treatment versus sham groups, respectively. Findings from this study provide novel mechanistic evidence that EECP has a beneficial effect on peripheral artery flow-mediated dilation and endothelial-derived vasoactive agents in patients with symptomatic CAD (Braith et al. 2010). It is known that cGMP regulates vascular smooth muscle tone that may improve arterial function. French investigators assessed the effect of a single session of EECP on plasma and platelet Cyclic GMP (cGMP) in asymptomatic subjects with cardiovascular risk factors and in patients with CAD. Fifty-five subjects were randomized into two groups to receive either sham (control) or active EECP during 1 h. Plasma and platelet cGMP were measured immediately before and after EECP by radioimmunoassay. One hour of EECP increased cGMP plasma concentration by 52% ± 66% (SD) ($P < .001$) and platelet content by 19%± 28% ($P < .01$). The increase in plasma cGMP was particularly marked in CAD patients receiving active EECP ($P<.01$), mainly in those with low LDL cholesterol. Platelets, inhibition of nitric oxide synthesis by NG-monomethyl-L-arginine (L-NMMA) reduced cGMP by 23% ± 31% (*P* _ .001), whereas presence of superoxide dismutase and inhibition of phosphodiesterase-5 increased cGMP by 46% ± 49% and 70% ± 77%, respectively ($P <.001$). In all of the cases EECP increased additional platelet cGMP content, which suggests nitric oxide synthase activation. These acute results showed that very early treatment increases the cGMP production that may participate in the mechanism by which EECP exerts its clinical benefit. Analysis of the modulation of platelet cGMP content suggests that EECP activated the nitric oxide-dependent pathways. (Levenson et al., 2006)

4.3 Neurohormanal changes

As with athletic training, the vascular effects of EECP therapy may be mediated through changes in the neurohormonal milieu. Wu et al. showed that EECP therapy has a sustained, dose-related effect in stimulating endothelial cell production of the vasodilator nitric oxide (NO) and in decreasing production of the vasoconstrictor endothelin. (Wu et al. 1999). In another study, Qian et al. showed that the NO level increased linearly in proportion to the hours of EECP treatment.(Qian X et al. 1999). Urano et al. further showed that plasma brain natriuretic peptide levels decreased after EECP therapy and were positively correlated with left ventricular end diastolic pressure and negatively correlated with peak filling rate. They concluded that EECP therapy reduces exercise-induced myocardial ischemia in association with improved left ventricular diastolic filling in patients with CAD. (Urano et al. 2001)
Another possible mechanism explaining EECP's mode of action is that it may affect changes in ventricular function independent of changes in cardiac load. Gorcsan et al. evaluated the effects of EECP therapy on left ventricular function in New York Heart Association class II or III heart failure patients with an EF less than 40%. Their results showed that EECP treatment was associated with improvements in preload adjusted maximal power, a relatively load-independent measure of left ventricular performance and EF, along with a decrease in heart rate in these heart failure patients. (Gorcsan et al. 2000)

4.4 Anti-inflammatory effect

A recently published randomized controlled study examining the effect of EECP therapy on inflammatory and adhesion molecules in patients with CAD indicated that EECP therapy has an anti-inflammatory effect in patients with angina pectoris. Patients were randomly assigned to receive active EECP or sham treatment. Plasma tumor necrosis factor- α, monocyte chemoattractant protein-1, and soluble vascular cell adhesion molecule-1 were measured before and after a full course of 35 1-hour sessions of EECP or sham treatment. Patients in the EECP group demonstrated reductions in tumor necrosis factor-α and monocyte chemoattractant protein-1 after treatment, whereas those in the sham therapy group showed no changes. EECP therapy decreased circulating levels of proinflamatory biomarkers in patients with symptomatic CAD (Casey et al. 2008).

5. Patient selection

5.1 Indications

FDA Labeled indications for the use of EECP include treatment of patients with:

- Stable or unstable angina pectoris
- Congestive heart failure
- Acute MI
- Cardiogenic shock

5.2 Which group of patients may benefit from EECP therapy?

Patients with angina or angina equivalent symptoms such as shortness of breath and/or fatigue who:

- have coronary anatomy unsuitable for surgical or catheter-based revascularization
- inadequately respond to optimum medical therapy
- underwent incomplete invasive revascularization
- are considered inoperable or at high risk of operative/interventional complications
- have comorbid conditions that increase the risk of revascularization procedures, such as diabetes, heart failure, pulmonary disease, and renal dysfunction
- are unwilling to undergo additional invasive revascularization procedures
- have stable (NYHA class II or III) heart failure; patients with any evidence of decompensation should not be treated until they are stable with the use of medical therapy
- have ischemic or idiopathic cardiomyopathy
- have cardiac syndrome X or microvascular ingina
- have LVD (EF < 35%)

5.3 Contraindications and side effects

It is important to point out that EECP therapy is not for everyone. This noninvasive outpatient procedure can be somewhat uncomfortable for patients because of the highpressure sequential compression of the cuffs. It is not recommended for certain types of valvular heart disease (especially aortic insufficiency), or for those with recent cardiac catheterization, an irregular heart rhythm, severe hypertension, significant blockages in the leg arteries, or a history of deep venous thrombosis. For anyone else, however, the procedure seems to be quite safe.

5.4 Contraindications

- Moderate to severe aortic insufficiency (regurgitation would prevent diastolic augmentation)
- Arrhythmias that may interfere with EECP system triggering (uncontrolled atrial fibrillation or fl utter or very frequent premature ventricular contractions)

- Coagulopathy with an INR of prothrombin time greater than 2.5
- Severe hypertension: greater than 180/110 mm Hg (the augmented diastolic pressure may exceed safe limits)
- Cardiac catheterization or arterial puncture (risk of bleeding at femoral puncture site) within the past 2 weeks
- Decompensated heart failure
- Severe peripheral arterial disease (reduced vascular volume and muscle mass may prevent active counterpulsation)
- Aortic aneurysm (≥ 5 mm) or dissection (diastolic pressure augmentation may be deleterious)
- Pregnancy or being of childbearing age (effects of EECP therapy on the fetus have not been studied)
- Venous disease (phlebitis, varicose veins, stasis ulcers, prior or current deep vein thrombosis or pulmonary embolism)
- Severe chronic obstructive pulmonary disease (no safety data in pulmonary hypertension)

5.5 Side effects

- Skin abrasion or ecchymoses
- Bruises (especially in patients using warfarin in whom the international normalized ratio [INR] is not adjusted)
- Paresthesias
- Leg or waist pain
- Worsening of heart failure in patients with severe arrhythmias

6. Future research

Throughout the world, EECP therapy has been studied for various potential uses other than heart disease ((Offergeld et al 2000; Rajaram et al 2006; Hilz et al 2004; Myhre et al 2004).

*__Cardiac Syndrome X__: its role in improving endothelial function might be beneficial in the treatment of patients with Cardiac Syndrome X, which is marked by severe chest pain caused by myocardial dysfunction, often without detectable atherosclerosis. Investigators have reported successful treatment of Cardiac Syndrome X with severely symptomatic coronary endothelial dysfunction in the absence of obstructive CAD with standard 35-h course of EECP therapy (Bonetti et al 2004).

*__Acute M/Cardiogenic Shock:__ Based on its acute haemodynamic effects, comparable to those of IABP, EECP can be proposed as a potential treatment for coronary syndromes in acute setting, as an inpatient therapy for patients with IABP contraindications. Recently developed mobile EECP Therapy system, enables its use in the catheter laboratory and operation room settings.

*__Erectile dysfunction__: Studies looking at EECP therapy and erectile dysfunction have shown a 200% increase in penile artery flow and reported improvement in erectile function [Froschermaier et al 1998; Lawson et al 2007; El-Sakka AI et al 2007

*__Hepatorenal syndrome:__ Werner et al. assessed the potential role of EECP therapy in diuresis and increased urinary fl ow in patients with endstage liver disease awaiting a transplant. They found that EECP therapyincreased mean arterial pressure as well as urinary production (urinary flow rate) in patients with end-stage cirrhosis and hepatorenal syndrome. (Werner et al 2005.)Studies involving larger sample sizes are necessary to confirm the effectiveness of EECP therapy in erectile dysfunction and hepatorenal syndrome.

* **Ischemic stroke: Investigators** sought to determine effect of EECP on middle cerebral artery blood flow augmentation in normal controls as a first step to support future clinical trials in acute stroke. (Alexandrow et al.,2008)

* **Primary /Secondary Prevention:** New studies are under way to explore the role of EECP therapy in primary and secondary prevention of coronary artery disease and its potential use in failing fontan operation.

7. Conclusion

Scientific data indicates that EECP provides a safe and effective treatment option for patients with CAD. Its different mode of action complements the invasive revascularization treatment. Currently, The American College of Cardiology/ The American Heart Association recommends EECP Therapy as a Class IIb (Level of Evidence: B) intervention for treatment of CAD. Due to the volume and quality of scientific data now available and per the descriptions of the rating and evidence levels as defined by American College of Cardiology and American Heart Association guidelines it is believed that EECP therapy has earned a Class IIa treatment recommendation with level of evidence A.

8. References

American Heart Association. Heart Disease and Stroke Statistics 2010- Update. Amsterdam EA, Banas J, Criley JM, Loeb HS, Mueller H, Willerson JT, Mason DT. 1980. Clinical assessment of external presuure circulatory assistance in acute myocardial infarction. Report of a cooperative clinical trial. *Am J Cardiol*, 45:349-356.

Alexandrov AW, Ribo M,Wong KS, Sugg RM, Garami Z, Jesurum JT,Montgomery B,Alexandrov A.2008. Perfusion Augmentation in Acute Stroke Using Mechanical Counter-Pulsation–Phase IIa Effect of External Counterpulsation on Middle Cerebral Artery Mean Flow Velocity in Five Healthy Subjects. *Stroke,39*:2760.) Arora RR, Chou TM, Jain D Fleishman B, Crawford L, McKiernan T, Nesto RW. 1999. The Multicenter Study of Enhanced External Counterpulsation (MUST-EECP):effect of EECP on exercise-induced myocardial ischemia and anginal episodes. *J Am Coll Cardiol*, 33:1833–1840.

Arora RR, Chou TM, Jain D, Fleishman B, Crawford L, McKiernan T, Nesto R, Ferrans CE, Keller S. 2002. Effects of enhanced external counterpulsation on health-related quality of life continue 12 months after treatment: a substudy of the multicenter study of enhanced external counterpulsation.*J Investig Med*, 50:25–32.

Bagger JP, Hall RJ, Koutroulis G, Nihoyannopoulos P. 2004. Effect of enhanced external counterpulsation on dobutamine-induced left ventricular wall motion abnormalities in severe chronic angina pectoris. *Am J Cardiol*, 15;93(4):465-7.

Birtwell WC, Ruiz U, Soroff HS, DesMarais D, Deterling RA Jr .1986. Technical consideration in the design of a clinical system for external left ventricular assist. *Trans Am Soc Artif Intern Organs*,14:304–310.

Bonetti PO, Gadasalli SN, Lerman A, Barsness GW. 2004. Successful treatment of symptomatic coronary endothelial dysfunction with enhanced external counterpulsation. *Mayo Clin Proc*, 79:690 -2

Braverman, DL. 2009. Enhanced external counterpulsation: An innovative physical therapy for refractory angina. *PM&R, 1:268-76.*

Braith RW, Conti CR, Nichols WW, Choi CY, Khuddus MA, Beck DT, Casey DP. 2010.Enhanced External Counterpulsation Improves Peripheral Artery Flow-Mediated Dilation in Patients with Chronic Angina. A Randomized Sham-Controlled Study. *Circulation*,122:1612-1620.

Cohen LS, Mullins CB, Mithell JH. 1973. Sequenced external counterpulsation and intra aortic balloon pumping in cardiogenic schock. *Am J Cardiol*,32: 656-661.

Casey DP, Conti CR, Nichols WW, Choi CY, Khuddus MA, Braith RW. 2008. Effect of enhanced external counterpulsation on infl amatory cytokines and adhesion molecules in patients with angina pectoris and angiographic coronary artery disease. *Am J Cardiol*, 101:300–302.

El-Sakka AI, Morsy AM, Fagih BI, et al.: Enhanced external counterpulsation in patients with coronary artery disease-associated erectile dysfunction. Part II: impact of disease duration and treatment courses. *J Sex Med* 2007, 4:1448–1453.

Froschermaier SE, Werner D, Leike S, et al.: Enhanced external counterpulsation as a new treatment modality for patients with erectile dysfunction. *Urol Int* 1998, 61:168–171.

Gorcsan J, Crawford L, Soran OZ. 2000. Improvement in left ventricular performance by enhanced external counterpulsation in patients with heart failure. *J Am Coll Cardiol*, 35:230A.

Gloekler S, Meier P, Marchi SF, Rutz T, Traupe T, Rimoldi SF, Wustmann K, Steck H, Cook S, Vogel R, Togni M & Seiler C.2010. Coronary Collateral Growth by External Counterpulsation: A Randomized Controlled Trial. *Heart*, 96: 202-207

Hilz MJ, Werner D, Marthol H, Flachskampf FA, Daniel WG.Enhanced external counterpulsation improves skin oxygenation and perfusion. Eur J Clin Invest 2004,34:385–91.

Holubkov R, Kennard ED, Foris JM, Kelsey SF, Soran O, Williams DO, Holmes DR.2002. Comparison of Patients Undergoing Enhanced External Counterpulsation and Percutaneous Coronary Intervention for Stable Angina Pectoris. *Am J Cardiol*,89: 1182-1186.

Katz WE, Gulati V, Feldman AM, Crawford L, Peron M, Soran O, Gorcsan III J. 1998. Effects of enhanced external counter pulsation on internal mammary artery flow; Comparison with intraaortic balloon counterpulsation. *J Am Coll Cardiol* (Supp A); 31: 85A.

Lakshmi MV, Kennard ED, Kelsey SF, Holubkov R, Michaels AD.2002. Relation of the pattern of diastolic augmentation during a course of enhanced external counterpulsation (EECP) to clinical benefit (from the International EECP Patient Registry [IEPR]). *Am J Cardiol*. 89(11):1303-5.

Lawson WE, Hui JCK, Soroff HS, Zeng SZ, Kayden DS, Sasvary D, Atkins H, Cohn PF.1992. Efficacy of enhanced external counterpulsation in the treatment of angina pectoris. *Am J Cardiol,* 70:859–862.

Lawson WE, Hui JCK, Cohn PF.2000. Long-term prognosis of patients with angina treated with enhanced external counterpulsation: five-year follow-up study. *Clin Cardiol,* 23:254–258.

Lawson WE, Pandey K, Hui JCK. 2002. Benefit of enhanced external counterpulsation in coronary patients with left ventricular dysfunction: cardiac or peripheral effect? *J CardFail,* 8(Suppl 41):146

Lawson WE, Hui JC, Kennard ED.2007. Effect of enhanced external counterpulsation on medically refractory angina patients with erectile dysfunction. *Int J Clin Pract,* 61:757–762.

Loh PH, Cleland JG, Louis AA, Kennard ED, Cook JF, Caplin JL, Barsness GW, Lawson WE, Soran OZ, Michaels AD.2008. Enhanced external counterpulsation in the treatment of chronic refractory angina: a long-term follow-up outcome from the International Enhanced External Counterpulsation Patient Registry. *Clin Cardiol,* 31:159–164.

Masuda D, Nohara R, Hirai T, Kataoka K, Chen LG, Hosokawa R, Inubushi M, Tadamura E, Fujita M, Sasayama S. 2001. Enhanced external counterpulsation improved myocardial perfusion and coronary flow reserve in patients with chronic stable angina. *Eur Heart J,* 22:1451–1458.

Manchanda A, Soran O. 2007.Enhanced external counterpulsation and future directions: step beyond medical management for patients with angina and heart failure. *J Am Coll Cardiol.* 50:1523–1531.

Masuda D, Nohara R, Kataoka K. 2001. Enhanced external counterpulsation promotes angiogenesis factors in patients with chronic stable angina. *Circulation,* 104:II445.

Michaels AD, Kennard ED, Kelsey SE, Holubkov R, Soran O, Spence S, Chou TM.2001. *Clin Cardiol,* Does higher diastolic augmentation predict clinical benefit from enhanced external counterpulsation?: Data from the International EECP Patient Registry (IEPR). 24(6):453-8.

Michaels AD, Accad M, Ports TA, Grossman W. 2002. Left ventricular systolic unloading and augmentation of intracoronary pressure and Doppler fl ow during enhanced external counterpulsation. *Circulation,*106:1237–1242.

Michaels AD, Tacy T, Teitel D, Shapiro M, Grossman W.2009. Invasive left ventricular energetics during enhanced external counterpulsation. *Am J Ther,*16(3):239-46.

Myhre LG, Muir I, Schutz RW, Rantala B, Thigpen T. 2004. Enhanced external counterpulsation for improving athletic performance. Paper presented at: *Experimental Biology April 17–21, 2004; Washington,DC*

Nichols WW, Estrada JC, Braith RW, Owens K, Conti CR.2006. Enhanced external counterpulsation treatment improves arterial wall properties and wave reflection characteristics in patients with refractory angina. *J Am Coll Cardiol,*19;48(6):1208-14.

Offergeld C, Werner D, Schneider M, Daniel WG, Hüttenbrink KB.Pneumatic external counterpulsation (PECP): a new treatment option in therapy refractory inner ear disorders?2000. *Laryngorhinootologie;* 79:503–9.

Pettersson T, Bondesson S, Cojocaru D, Ohlsson O, Wackenfors A, Edvinsson L. 2006. One year follow-up of patients with refractory angina pectoris treated with enhanced external counterpulsation. *BMC Cardiovasc Disord* , 6:28.

Rajaram SS, Shanahan J, Ash C, Walters AS, Weisfogel G. 2006. Enhanced external counter pulsation (EECP) for restless legs syndrome (RLS): preliminary negative results in a parallel double-blind study. *Sleep Med*, 7:390 -1.

Soran O, Crawford LE, Schneider VM, Feldman AM. 1999.Enhanced external counterpulsation in the management of patients with cardiovascular disease.*Clinical Cardiol*,22: 173-178.

Soran O, Michaels AD, Kennard ED, Kelsey SF, Holubkov R, Feldman AM.2001. Is Diastolic Augmentation an Important Predictor of treatment Completion for Patients with Left Ventricular Dysfunction Undergoing enhanced External Counterpulsation for Angina. J. *Cardiac Failure*,(Suppl 2);7: 99.

Soran O, Kennard ED, Kfoury AG, Kelsey SF; IEPR Investigators. 2006. Two-year clinical outcomes after enhanced external counterpulsation(EECP) therapy in patients with refractory angina pectoris and left ventricular dysfunction (report from The International EECP Patient Registry). *Am J Cardiol*, 97:17–20.

Soran O, Kennard ED, Kelsey SF, Holubkov R, Strobeck J, Feldman AM. 2002. Enhanced external counterpulsation as treatment for chronic angina in patients with left ventricular dysfunction: a report from the International EECP Patient Registry (IEPR). *Congest Heart Fail*, 8:297–302.

Soran O, Kennard ED, Bart BA, Kelsey SF; IEPR Investigators.2007. Impact of external counterpulsation treatment on emergency department visits and hospitalizations in refractory angina patients with left ventricular dysfunction. *Congest Heart Fail*,13:36–40

Soran O, Kennard L, Kelsey SF, On behalf of IEPR Investigators.2010. Comparison of six-month clinical outcomes, event free survival rates of patients undergoing enhanced external counterpulsation (EECP) for coronary artery disease in the United States and Europe. *European Heart J;* (Suppl 31);24:353.

Stys TP, Lawson WE, Hui JCK, Fleishman B, Manzo K, Strobeck JE, Tartaglia J, Ramasamy S, Suwita R, Zeng ZS, Liang H, Wener D. 2002. Effects of enhanced external counterpulsation on stress radionuclide coronary perfusion and exercise capacity in chronic stable angina pectoris. *Am J Cardiol*. 89:822–882.

Taguchi I, Ogawa K, Kanaya T, Matsuda R, Kuga H, Nakatsugawa M. 2004. Effects of enhanced external counterpulsation on hemodynamics and its mechanism. *Circ J*,68(11):1030-4.

Urano H, Ikedah H, Ueno T, Matsumoto T, Murohara T, Imaizumi T. 2001. Enhanced external counter pulsation improves exercise tolerance, reduces exercise-induced myocardial ischemia and improves left ventricular diastolic filling in patients with coronary artery disease. *J Am Coll Cardiol*, 37:93–99.

Qian X, Wu W, Zheng ZS. 1999. Effect of enhanced external counterpulsation on nitric oxide production in coronary disease. *J Heart Disease*,1:193

Werner D, Tragner P, Wawer A, et al.: Enhanced external counterpulsation: a new technique to augment renal function in liver cirrhosis. *Nephrol Dial Transplant* 2005, 20:920–926.

Wu GF, Qiang SZ, Zheng ZS. 1999. A neurohormonal mechanism for the effectiveness of the enhanced external counterpulsation. *Circulation*,100:I832.

Zeng ZS, Li TM, Kambic H, Chen GH, Yu LQ, cai Sr, Zhan CY, Chen YC, Wo SX, Chen GW, Ma H, Chen PJ, Huang BJ, Nose Y. 1983. Sequential external counterpulsation in China. *Trans Am Soc Artif Intern Organs,29:593-603.*

7

Alternative Non-Medical, Non-Surgical Therapies for the Treatment of Angina Pectoris

Maryam Esmaeilzadeh, Bahieh Moradi and Nasim Naderi
Tehran University of Medical Sciences,
Shaheed Rajaei Cardiovascular Medical and Research Center
Iran

1. Introduction

The treatment of angina pectoris as an important symptom of coronary artery disease is usually focused on restoring the balance between myocardial oxygen demand and supply by administration of drugs interfering in heart rate, preload, afterload, and coronary vascular tone. For non responders to drug therapy or for those with jeopardized myocardium, revascularization procedures such as coronary artery bypass graft surgery (CABG) and percutaneous transluminal coronary angioplasty (PTCA) are at hand. However, these therapies cannot stop the disease process and, at longer terms, angina may recur. It is not always possible to revascularize all the patients who do not sufficiently react to medical treatment. In these group patients alternative therapies are more effective. A major difference between alternative therapies versus traditional therapies is that alternative therapy tends to look at the entire patient rather than simply treating a disorder as traditional treatments do. Some kinds of these therapies are applicable in all patients with coronary artery disease irrespective of their symptoms and the other ones would be considered in patients with refractory angina who are not suitable for revascularization.

2. General alternative therapy

These therapies are applicable in all patients with coronary artery disease whether they are symptomatic or not.

2.1 Heart healthy lifestyle

2.1.1 Goals

Preventing heart disease, living heart healthy, and overcoming stress-related heart illness requires more than just a physical approach to heart problems. Whether or not patients had an interventional angioplasty or bypass surgery, it's obvious that some changes in lifestyle will need to be made. To continue living a normal active life, one needs to begin making heart healthy lifestyle changes that include eating a heart healthy diet. Maintaining a healthy diet and lifestyle offers the greatest potential of all known approaches for reducing the risk for CVD in the general public. Specific goals are to consume an overall healthy diet;

aim for a healthy body weight; recommended levels of low-density lipoprotein cholesterol, high-density lipoprotein cholesterol, and triglycerides; normal blood pressure; normal blood glucose level; be physically active and avoid use of and exposure to tobacco products.

Consume a Healthy Diet:

An emphasis on whole diet should be done to ensure nutrient adequacy and energy balance. Hence, rather than focusing on a single nutrient or food, individuals should aim to improve their whole or overall diet. (1) The American Heart Association has provided dietary recommendations and recommendations for an overall healthy lifestyle to the American public with the goal of reducing risk for cardiovascular diseases. (1)

Achievement or maintaining an ideal body weight:

A healthy body weight is currently defined as a body mass index (BMI) of 18.5 to 24.9 kg/m^2. Overweight is a BMI between 25 and 29.9 kg/m^2, and obesity is a BMI 30 kg/m^2. Achieving and maintaining a healthy weight throughout life is particularly difficult and are critical factors in reducing CVD risk in the general public. Great emphasis should be put on prevention of weight gain (2), because achievement and maintenance of weight loss, although certainly possible, require more difficult behavioral changes ie, greater calorie reduction and more physical activity, than prevention of weight gain in the first place.

Prevention of excess weight gain:

Prevention of excess weight gain relies on the maintenance of energy balance, whereby energy intake equals energy consumption over the long term.(1, 2) This means maintaining a relatively stable weight across life stages. A positive imbalance will increase energy storage, deposited as body fat and observed as weight gain. Although the concept is seemingly simple, the physiological systems that regulate body weight through energy intake and consumption mechanisms are complex, interactive, homeostatic, and still poorly understood. Furthermore, the components of energy balance are not weighed easily or with adequate precision to be practical as a guide to help individuals maintain energy balance. In theory, a small persistent energy imbalance of 50 kcal per day could result in a 5-lb weight gain in 1 year, provided that all other things being equal. (2)

Treatment of obesity:

Although prevention and treatment of obesity both depends on the same principles of energy balance, the application of the principles is completely different. For treatment of obesity, a large reduction in calorie intake of about 500 to 1000 kcal per day, along with increased physical activity, can result in a loss of approximately 8- 10% of body weight over the relatively short period of about 6 months. Although the types of low-calorie diets that best promote weight loss are the subject of current investigations, behaviors for weight loss focused on caloric reduction such as decreasing overall food intake, reducing portion sizes, substituting lower-calorie for higher calorie foods, and increasing physical activity. Weight loss is best achieved by participation in a behavioral program using self-monitoring, goal-setting, and problem-solving techniques. Motivation levels may be high for appearance reasons or if adverse health consequences and quality of life impairments associated with obesity are readily perceived.(2) However, because weight regain after weight loss is common, motivations and strategies to maintain weight may differ largely from those initiating weight loss.(2)

A diet rich in vegetables and fruits:

Most vegetables and fruits are rich in nutrients, low in calories, and high in fiber. Diets high in fiber, especially from cereal sources, substantially reduce the risk of coronary heart disease. Short-term randomized trials have shown that diets rich in vegetables and fruits not only provide micronutrient, macronutrient, and fiber requirements, but also lower BP and improve other CVD risk factors. Vegetables and fruits that are deeply colored, for example, spinach, carrots, peaches and berries, ought to be emphasized because they tend to be higher in micronutrient contents compared to other vegetables and fruits such as potatoes and corn. Equally important is the method of preparation which includes techniques preserving nutrient and fiber content without adding unnecessary calories, saturated or trans fat, sugar, and salt.(1)

2.2 Supplements

It is ideal to get the body nutritional needs in foods .When that is not enough, a registered dietitian may also start a series of supplements to make up for nutrients not getting through the diet. Some of the more popular supplements for both healthy and those at risk for coronary artery disease include antioxidants such as vitamins C and E, B-complex, omega-3 fish oil and coenzyme Q10. The American Heart Association recommends 2-4 grams of Omega-3 per day for anyone with high triglycerides and at least 1 gram per day for anyone with documented coronary heart disease. (1) According to the results of many clinical trials performed to clear the role of dietary supplements in the prevention and /or slowing the progression of cardiovascular diseases , the long-term effects of most dietary supplements other than for vitamins and minerals are not known, so these agents should be prescribed under professional supervision of physician or a registered dietitian.

Essential Fatty Acids
Omega-3 and Flaxseed oil

Flaxseed oil comes from the seeds of the flax plant ***(Linum usitatissimum, L.)*** which contains both omega-3 and omega-6 fatty acids, which are vital for health. They are composed of essential fatty acid alpha-linolenic acid (ALA), which the body turns into eicosapentaenoic acid (EPA) and docosahexaenoic acid (DHA), the omega-3 fatty acids found in fish oil. Some researchers argue that flaxseed oil might have some of the same usefulness as fish oil, but the body is not very efficient at converting ALA into EPA and DHA, however, the benefits of ALA, EPA, and DHA are not necessarily the same. The human body is not able to make its own omega-3 fatty acids, so it is important that they are part of everyone's dietary intake. (3) The consumption of 2 servings (8 ounces) per week of fish high in EPA and DHA can result in a reduction of risk of mortality and morbidity from coronary artery disease. In addition to providing EPA and DHA, regular fish consumption may facilitate the displacement of other foods higher in saturated and trans fatty acids from the diet, such as fatty meats and full-fat dairy products.(1) Omega-3 fatty acids seem to have a small, dose-dependent, hypotensive effect, the extent of which seems to be dependent on the degree of hypertension.(4) In a meta-analysis, Morris et al found a significant reduction in blood pressure of ≤ 3.4/ 2.0 mmHg in studies with hypertensive subjects who consumed 5.6 g/d of omega-3 fatty acids.(4) Likewise, Appel et al found that blood pressure was decreased ≤ 5.5/ 3.5 mmHg in trials of untreated hypertensives given 3 g/d of omega-3 fatty acids. DHA seems to be more effective than EPA in lowering blood pressure. (4) Getting a good balance of omega 3 and 6 fatty acids in the diet is important which are examples of polyunsaturated fatty acids (PUFAs). Omega 3 fatty acids help reduce inflammation, while most omega 6 fatty acids tend to contribute to inflammation. A healthy diet should consist of roughly 2 to 4 times fewer omega 6 fatty acids than omega 3 fatty acids. Some species of fish may contain significant levels of methylmercury, polychlorinated biphenyls (PCBs), dioxins, and other environmental contaminants which is a potential concern for using them.(1,4) Subgroups of the population, primarily children and pregnant women are advised by the FDA to avoid eating those fish with the potential for the highest level of mercury contamination. Eating up to 12 ounces (2 average meals) per week of a variety of fish and shellfish that are lower in mercury is also recommended. (1) The American Heart Association recommends inclusion of omega 3 fatty acids in patients with stable CAD because of evidence from randomized controlled trials. The recommended daily dose in patients with stable coronary artery disease is 1 gram of eicosapentaenoic acid/docosahexaenoic acid (EPA/DHA) by capsule supplement, the equivalent amount in alpha-linolenic acid (LNA) from vegetable source, or by eating daily fatty fish(1). Since maintaining daily fish meals can be difficult, capsule supplements may be preferred although there is no uniformity of EPA/DHA content or purity.

Niacin

Niacin (nicotinic acid) is a B vitamin that has been used in high doses (1.0–4.5 grams per day) as a treatment for hyperlipidemia which is associated with increased risk of CAD. Niacin reduces cholesterol and TG levels, and increases the concentration of high-density lipoprotein (HDL). (5) It is also effective at modulating blood lipids, but side effects sometimes dampen enthusiasm for therapy. Although side effects are dose-related, few studies have determined an optimal dose of nicotinic acid that alters lipid levels with the fewest side effects. Martin-Jadraque et al. (6) found improvement in blood lipid levels in 75% of subjects who tolerated low-dose nicotinic acid therapy. Nicotinic acid may also be useful in combination drug therapy for prevention of CAD if higher doses cannot be tolerated. Use of a lower dose should still be beneficial for producing a moderate rise in HDL levels. Women seem to have a greater LDL response to niacin, but experience more side effects at higher dosages. (7)

Long-term treatment with nicotinic acid (4 g/day for 6 weeks) not only corrects serum lipoprotein abnormalities, but also reduces the fibrinogen concentration in plasma and stimulates fibrinolysis. (8) Although most medications used to treat dyslipidemias will raise HDL levels modestly; however, niacin appears to have the greatest potential to do so, increasing HDL up to 30%. (9)

Vitamin C

A widely publicized study showed that men who took 800 mg daily of vitamin C lived about 6 years longer than those consuming of 60 mg per day. (10) A study of elderly subjects; being supplemented by vitamin C and vitamin E to subjects using no vitamin supplements showed that use of vitamin E alone reduced death from myocardial infarction (MI) by 63% and overall mortality by 34%. When the vitamin C and E were used together, overall mortality was reduced by 42%. (11)

A proper supply of nutrients will allow the cellular damage to vascular walls to be repaired properly and prevent further cracks and lesions. The results of a clinical studies, published in the Journal of Applied Nutrition (12), determine the effect of a nutritional supplement program, consisting of vitamin C therapy, on the natural progression of coronary artery disease. The study used Ultrafast Computed Tomography to document the level of coronary artery disease and the sample of patients composed of people with early and advanced stages of the disease. During the course of the 12-month study, the rate of coronary artery calcification decreased in all patients by an average of 15%. In the subset of early stage patients, the progression of calcification was stopped completely. In some cases, calcification was actually reversed, including a case of the disappearance of all calcification deposits.

Vitamin E

Evidence demonstrates that vitamin E protects against development of atherosclerosis by reducing oxidation of LDL, inhibiting proliferation of 4smooth muscle cells, decreasing platelet adhesion and aggregation, and changing the expression and function of adhesion molecules. The biological functions of vitamin E (attenuating the synthesis of leukotrienes and potentiating release of prostacyclin) which reduces platelet aggregation and acts as a vasodilator may protect against the development of atherosclerosis. (13)

A large study that examined the relationship between the intake of dietary carotene, vitamin C, and vitamin E and subsequent coronary mortality found an inverse association between dietary vitamin E and coronary mortality, supporting the hypothesis that antioxidant vitamins provide protection against CAD. (14) Large epidemiological studies revealed that higher vitamin E levels in plasma result in a reduced incidence of CAD. Dose-response studies in humans have demonstrated that 400 IU per day of vitamin E increased vitamin E plasma levels twofold and delayed oxidation of LDL, while the length of time was more important than the amount of the nutrient used. (15) The type and blend of vitamin E selected for supplementation can affect the end results. Studies show that α-tocopherol may offer better protection against CAD when it is combined with gamma tocopherol, which has a greater activity. Unfortunately, gamma tocopherol is poorly retained in body because it is excreted in urine following liver metabolism, whilst α-tocopherol is more abundant in body tissues which does not provide for maximum protection against free radical attack. So complexing α-tocopherol (80%) with gamma tocopherol (20%) is an ideal blend for individuals seeking protective cardiovascular effects from vitamin E tocopherol.

Coenzyme Q10

Coenzyme Q10 (CoQ10; ubiquinone) is a fat-soluble cofactor substance. It is a naturally occurring substance that prevents cell damage due to myocardial ischemia (hypoxia) or subsequent to reestablishment of blood flow to the heart after temporary ischemia. CoQ10 is involved in several key enzymes in energy production within a cell, and has membrane-stabilizing activity. Numerous studies provide details of the efficacy of CoQ10 in the prevention and treatment of heart disease, as detailed below. Oral CoQ10 (150 mg daily in 3 doses) was given for 4 weeks to exercising angina patients. Average levels of CoQ10 in plasma increased after CoQ10 treatment and were significantly related to an increase in exercise duration. The study suggested that: "CoQ10 is a safe and promising treatment for angina pectoris". (16) Pretreatment with intravenous CoQ10 minimized myocardial injury caused by cardiac bypass graft (CABG) surgery and improved heart function. In patients undergoing CABG pretreatment with intravenous CoQ10 (5 mg/kg, intravenously 2 hours before cardiopulmonary bypass) prevents left ventricular depression in early reperfusion and minimizes myocardial cellular injury during CABG following reperfusion. (17)

In comparison with younger individuals, the outcome of surgery in the elderly, is compromised by age-related reduction of cellular energy production in the myocardium during surgery. Fibers from subjects over age 70 showed poor recovery of force after simulated ischemia compared to younger patients. This age-associated effect was prevented by pretreatment with CoQ10 (18), in addition CoQ10 pretreatment prior to stress improved recovery of the myocardium after stress (19). Because of the popular use of "statin" drugs (Zocor, Lipitor, Pravachol, Lescol, and Mevacor) it is important to emphasize that statins act by inhibiting HMG-CoA reductase, the rate-limiting enzyme in cholesterol biosynthesis. Drugs inhibiting HMG-CoA reductase activity decrease CoQ10 levels (20) because HMG-CoA reductase is required for CoQ10 synthesis. Individuals using statins ought to increase their intake of CoQ10 to negate the decrease in CoQ10 biosynthesis caused by the statin drugs. So it is recommended to administer it with statin therapy. CoQ10 is free of toxicity and typically produces no side effects and may change the insulin requirements of people with diabetes.

2.3 Mind-body relaxation techniques

While living a type A lifestyle isn't typically categorized as a main risk factor for heart disease, learning how to deal with life and lower stress levels can help down road to recovery.

Mind-body approach aimed at diminishing excess activation in the nervous system and thereby improving one's own ability to modulate emotional and behavioral responses.

Relaxation therapy is a broad term used to describe a number of techniques that promote stress reduction, the elimination of tension throughout the body, and a calm and peaceful state of mind.

Relaxation techniques include behavioral therapeutic approaches that differ widely in philosophy, methodology, and practice. There are two basic methods, deep methods include autogenic training, progressive muscle relaxation, and meditation (although meditation is sometimes distinguished from relaxation based on the state of "thoughtless awareness" that occurs during meditation). Brief methods include self-control relaxation, paced respiration, and deep breathing. Brief methods generally are less time consuming and often represent a summarized form of a deep method. In order to be able to evoke the relaxation, several months of practice (at least three times per week) is required.

Some of the more popular relaxation techniques include massage therapy, yoga, listening to music, pray and meditation.

Massage therapy

Massage therapy is the scientific manipulation of the soft tissues of the body, consisting primarily of manual (hands-on) techniques such as applying fixed or movable pressure, holding, and moving muscles and body tissues.

Various forms of therapeutic superficial tissue manipulation have been practiced for thousands of years across cultures. Chinese use of massage dates to 1600 BC, and Hippocrates made reference to the importance of physicians being experienced with "rubbing" as early as 400 BC. There are references to massage in ancient records of the Chinese, Japanese, Arabic, Egyptian, Indian, Greek, and Roman nations. Many different therapeutic techniques can be classified as massage therapy. Most involve the application of fixed or moving pressure or manipulation of the muscles/connective tissues of clients. Practitioners may use their hands or other areas such as forearms, elbows, or feet. Used techniques during massage therapy include (1) superficial stroking away from the heart or deep stroking towards the heart; (2) kneading in a circular pattern using fingers and thumbs; (3) deep muscle stimulation; (4) rhythmic movements such as slapping or tapping; and (5) vibration. Scientific research of massage is limited, and existing studies use a variety of techniques and trial designs. Firm evidence-based conclusions about the effectiveness of massage cannot be drawn at this time for any health condition.

Shiatsu

Shiatsu literally means 'finger pressure'. Shiatsu is based on the same principles as acupuncture concentrating on meridians or energy lines but without the needles. Everything is related to the five elements that correspond to different parts of the body: *Heart: Fire, Kidney: Water, Spleen: Earth, Lungs: Metal, Liver: Wood.*

The idea, as in acupuncture, is to balance the life energy in the body which is disturbed when we become ill. Through a series of finger pressures all over the body along the specific pathways, Shiatsu can rebalance the body's energies, regulate the organs' function and improve circulation. Shiatsu last up to 1 hour during which practitioners often use their elbows, knees and feet as well as their fingers for palpation of the abdomen and other areas which may be lacking energy , but they seldom use the hands' palms unlike other traditional Western contact therapies.

Yoga

The term "Yoga" comes from a Sanskrit word meaning "union." Yoga combines physical exercises, mental meditation, and breathing techniques to strengthen the muscles and relieve stress.The first known work is "The Yoga Sutras," written more than 2,000 years ago, although yoga may have been practiced up to 5,000 years ago. Yoga has been described as "the union of mind, body, and spirit," which addresses physical, mental, intellectual, emotional, and spiritual dimensions towards an overall harmonious state of being. It works towards self-realization and control of mental, physiological, and psychological parameters. Yoga is often practiced by healthy individuals with the aim to achieve relaxation, fitness, and a healthy lifestyle. Yoga has also been recommended and used for a variety of medical conditions and consists 30 to 90 minutes sessions.

Meditation

Meditation is usually suggested as a stress management technique used to cause a tranquil and relaxed state of mind. However, researchers have lately found that meditation offers other significant health benefits by changing deeper and more dynamic processes in the body, even so far as being able to strengthen the heart. Researchers at the Margaret and H.A. Rey Laboratory, Boston, USA discovered that meditation impacts prominent heart rate variability traditionally associated with practicing slow breathing during specific traditional forms of Chinese Yoga meditation techniques. (21) The magnitude of this variability during meditation was much far greater than when compared to those not practicing any meditation in healthy young adults and even elite athletes during sleep. These results uncovered that meditation can have a profound effect on the heart and its activity. The researchers observed that the variability of beat-to-beat heart rate was directly affected by meditation. The report concluded that meditation should not be seen as just a method of relaxation and stress management, but also as an aid to strengthen the heart and create a more active state in the body.(21)

2.4 Cardiac rehabilitation and exercise training

I. Cardiac rehabilitation definition

Cardiac rehabilitation (CR) is welcomed not only as integral in the management of patients with coronary artery disease, but also as the primary means in delivering secondary prevention which consists of a number of activities or measures that may be adapted by patients so as to reduce the symptoms or the risk of a further event.

More recently CR has been redefined as follows: "Cardiac rehabilitation is the process by which patients with cardiac disease, in partnership with a multidisciplinary team of health professionals, are encouraged and supported to achieve and maintain optimal physical and psychosocial health". (22,23)

According to guidelines, CR including exercise training, patient education, psychological support, risk factor management, and clinical assessment, is indicated for patients with ischemic heart disease (IHD), chronic heart failure, patients with a high risk for developing IHD (24-27), patients with valvular heart diseases, cardiac transplantation, Implanted cardioverter defibrillators, and congenital heart diseases (23).

II. Cardiac rehabilitation phases

Cardiac rehabilitation is divided into four phases, ranging from the acute hospital admission stage to long-term maintenance of lifestyle changes, as follows (23,25,26):

Phase I (in patient period): is started after a 'step change' in cardiac condition including myocardial infarction, onset of angina, any emergency hospital admission for coronary heart disease, cardiac surgery or angioplasty and/or stenting, and first diagnosis of heart failure. This should begin as soon as possible after admission. Phase I consists of assessment, education, exercise/mobilization.

Phase II (Early post-discharge): exercise consultation and behavior change strategies are benefecial at this stage to improve adherence to both lifestyle change and maintenance of exercise in phase II and uptake of phase III in the future. This is the stage for risk factors modification and goal setting in phase I (lasting over a period of between 8 and 12 weeks).

Phase III (supervised out-patient): at this stage, risk factor changes and education are continued. Phase III is usually consists of at least two supervised exercise sessions per week, lasting over a period of between 6 and 12 weeks. Patients may be provided with one session of education per week. Physical training is often the essential part of phase III, while psycho-social counseling and education considering risk factors and lifestyle are of primary importance. In addition to the aerobic conditioning phase, resistance training is part of CR exercise. Home-based exercise is also prescribed with self monitoring skills being used by the patients.

Phase IV (long-term maintenance of exercise and other lifestyle changes): For the benefits of physical activity and lifestyle change to be sustained, the available evidence suggests that both are necessary to be retained. As clinically indicated, referral to specialist clinicians, such as smoking cessation or psychological support, may still be needed. Continuation and progression of appropriate physical activities are persuaded outside the hospital setting. By this time it is looked forward that individuals will be aware of their exercise capabilities and be able to monitor themselves properly.

III. Cardiac rehabilitation and exercise training in Ischemia

There are several mechanisms by which regular exercise training exercise training may improve myocardial oxygen supply and thereby result in an anti ischemic effect. Exercise training reduces cardiac workload at a given (sub maximal) exercise level by improved adaptation of the peripheral circulation. A alternative external work can be gained with a lower heart rate and blood pressure, thereby reducing myocardial oxygen demands and coronary blood flow requirements in areas with a potentially critical perfusion deficit. Since myocardial perfusion is related to the length of the diastole, the time for perfusion of the myocardium decreases with increasing heart rate. Thus, exercise training improves the economy of the heart work and facilitates myocardial perfusion in patients with coronary artery stenoses. A lower heart rate and a lower systolic blood pressure during exercise is a usual though somewhat transient phenomenon after exercise training in normal persons as well as in patients with CAD. To maintain this training effect exercise needs to be incorporated into the daily routine - such as medication. (22, 25) Many studies have revealed that the symptomatic improvement as a result of exercise training is mainly owing to a decrease in the rate–pressure product at sub maximal workloads with no change in the rate–pressure product at the onset of angina (22, 28) Later reports also showed a rise in the rate–pressure product at the onset of angina along with a reduction in the ischemic response measured as angina or ST-segment depression, at a given rate–pressure product, suggesting that exercise training improves myocardial oxygen delivery. There are controversial aspects about improvement in angiographic collateralization or regression of coronary atherosclerosis- that might be a reason for less ischemia- despite the endurance exercise training program. However, some surveys showed a significant tendency toward decreasing progression after prolonged rather intense, particularly in those patients who took part more sessions of the structured training program (22,29,30).

The question whether ischemia should be avoided during endurance training in stable patients is open to question. The studies of Ehsani et al. suggest that in selected patients significant ST-segment depression can be borne without adverse effects (31). However, for safety reasons it is usually recommended to avoid ischemia during endurance training in order to minimize risks and maximize benefits. In patients with symptoms suggesting instability, exercise is not recommended until the phase of instability has resolved. (32)

Randomized clinical trials (RCTs) and meta-analyses have demonstrated significant (14% to 24%) relative reductions in all-cause mortality over 1 to 2 years in patients with coronary artery disease randomized to cardiac rehabilitation programs. Women, elderly patients, low-income groups, and ethnic minorities tend to be under-represented in RCTs. (33 - 35) CR also resulted in a comparable effects in terms of cardiac overall survival, event-free survival and other secondary outcome measures like cardiac morbidity. (36,37) Stukel et al argued whether the true size of the effect is 10% or 30%, but both are large when translated into absolute population numbers .(38)

The effects of Cardiac rehabilitation on Endothelial function

One of the positive effects of exercise is the improvement of endothelial dysfunction. Endothelial dysfunction is a precursor of clinically significant atherosclerotic disease and is a signal for an increased cardiovascular event rate.(39-41)

Different efforts have been made to correct the impaired endothelium-dependent vasodilatation. In recent years it has become apparent that exercise affects the functional activity of the vascular endothelium.Whereas normal coronary arteries dilate, atherosclerotic coronary arteries often exhibit a paradoxical vasoconstriction in response to exercise, thereby causing critical ischemia even in moderate epicardial stenosis. Endothelium-derived NO is the main mediator of improved endothelial function and enforces a multitude of anti atherosclerotic functions. Acting on the endothelial cell itself, NO inhibits endothelial cell apoptosis, suppresses inflammatory activation, and increases the activity of oxygen radical-scavenging enzymes. Furthermore NO inhibits platelet aggregation via luminal release from the endothelium and also inhibits vascular smooth muscle cell proliferation and promotion of positive arterial remodeling. Studies using cultured endothelial cells and animal experiments suggest that increases in endothelial NO synthesis expression and protein phosphorylation are possible mechanisms. Exercise training in stable CAD leads to an improved agonist-mediated endothelium-dependent vasodilatory capacity. (42-45) Exercise training induces adaptations in cellular mechanisms of nitric oxide regulation in collateral-dependent coronary arteries of chronically occluded vessels that contribute to enhanced nitric oxide production (46). Also arterial production of reactive oxygen species could significantly reduced by exercise training.

Improvement in Exercise Capacity

Physical activity is seen as a behavior that generally has advantages on exercise capacity and many of the physiologic processes involved in the development of primary prevention of coronary artery disease. (26) Lavie et al reported a 34% improvement in exercise capacity after cardiac rehabilitation participation. (47) Some newer studies showed every one MET increase in exercise capacity can induce more than 17% improvement in survival rate, it is especially important in heart failure patients .(25,26)

Improvement in Left Ventricular Function (systolic and diastolic)

Ehsani et al studied 25 patients, 52 (±2) years old with coronary artery disease and mildly impaired LV function (ejection fraction 53%)[31], They compared these to 14 patients with comparable maximal exercise capacities and ejection fractions who did not undergo an exercise training program. The exercise group completed a 12- month program of very intense endurance exercise training of progressively increasing intensity, frequency, and duration. Ejection fraction did not change during maximal supine exercise before training (52 ± 3%),but after training it increased during exercise to 58 ±3% (P<0.01), despite a higher rate-pressure product during maximal exercise, providing some evidence for an improvement in contractile state after training - or also for improved perfusion with less ischemic impairment of myocardial function during exercise. (22,31)

In one of the first small prospective studies of endurance training in HF patients, Sullivan et al confirmed that 4 to 6 months of training did not deteriorate LV ejection fraction and tended to improve maximal cardiac output. (48) Another larger randomized clinical trial provided evidence for a training- induced reverse remodeling with modest improvements of LVEF and reductions of LV end-diastolic diameter in a mixed population of ischemic and dilated cardiomyopathy.(49)

Heart failure with preserved left ventricular ejection fraction (HFPEF) is the most popular form of HF in the older population. Exercise intolerance is the primary chronic symptom in patients with HFPEF and is a strong determinant of their reduced quality of life (QOL). Exercise training improves exercise intolerance and diastolic function and QOL in patients with HF with preserved and reduced ejection fraction. (50)

Improvement of quality of life

Cardiac rehabilitation is increasingly known as an integral part of comprehensive cardiac care. The evidence supporting its effectiveness in reducing morbidity and mortality and improving quality of life (51) Frank suggested that those who have greater physical functionality, the confidence to perform physical activities, and are not restricted clinically, may more readily adjust to cardiac rehabilitation and progress more rapidly. Those patients with the poorest exercise capacities at entrance to the program tended to make the greatest gains in health related quality of life. (52)

Improvement in risk factors profile

Regular physical activity is associated with favorable modification of cardiovascular risk factors such as hypercholesterolemia, hypertension, diabetes, and obesity. (22,53-57)

Cost- benefit

Cardiac rehabilitation is one of the most effective treatments of secondary prevention for patients with heart disease. These standard training programs are safe and cost-effective. (37)

IV. Cardiac rehabilitation components

IV.a Exercise program

Not only a universal understanding of patient's medical history, current status, and medication regimen need to be taken into account, while prescribing an exercise, but also a solid understanding of exercise physiology as relates to recreational and vocational activities. Experience and individualization of exercise prescription are essential for optimal success in activity programming. A staged exercise test (preferably Ramp protocols) is recommended for exercise prescription. Every activity program should be consist of a warm-up, conditioning, and cool-down periods. (25,58)

Warm up: is a 5 to 15 minutes period, during which the musculature and joint structures are stimulated gently with a series of static stretches and dynamic range of motion (ROM) activities. A large group of muscle is involved in the warm-up stretches. The stretch should be maintained 15-30 seconds and should not result in discomfort or pain. Patients should be encouraged to continue to breathe to avoid Valsalva maneuver that can cause exaggerated BP responses.

Conditioning period: The conditioning period may be designed to focus on the following activities:

1. To increase caloric expenditure to aid with weight management
2. To improve overall functional capacity
3. To delay the onset of symptom
4. To improve muscle tone and strength
5. To optimize job or vocational abilities
6. To optimize recreational activity performance
7. To optimize ability to perform activities of daily living (ADL)

It must address 5 keys factors: Frequency, Intensity, Mode, Duration, Rate of progression

Frequency: Typically, the exercise stimulus must be done at least three times per week. It is recommended that the sessions be allocated equally throughout the week. From an FC improvement standpoint, there is trivial achievement by extending the program beyond 5 days per week. It is recommended that the average rehabilitation program being with an exercise frequency of 3 times per week for at least the first 3-6 months, if after this time the patient has remained free of musculoskeletal complications and expresses an interest in increasing the frequency, the program can reach to four to five times per week.

Intensity: According to ACSM guideline the intensity threshold for healthy adults is between 60-90% of HR max in a staged exercise test or 50-85% of Vo2max or heart rate reserve (HRR).The typical range of exercise intensity for patients involved in cardiac rehabilitation is between 40% and 85%. Exercise intensity is not static. The cost of the activities varies slightly from day to day, depending on the time of day, environmental

factors, and time since medications were last taken. Medications, especially β-blockers, can alter the patient's FC significantly. If significant stable ischemic changes or symptoms occur with activity, the exercise intensity must be established at a level adequately below the threshold for these findings (usually 10-15 beat/min below the onset of ischemic changes).
If possible, to minimize any flaw in prescribing exercise intensity, it is advised to carry out the exercise test for exercise prescription on all usual medications and the same approximate time of day as patients exercise.
Mode: Any activity that ingages a mass of muscle group in a rhythmic and repetitive fashion (dynamic exercises) at the approximate intensity and duration leads to improved FC. The most common sorts of the activity used in CR are walking and appropriate jogging. Cycling, swimming, rowing, stair climbing, and aerobic dancing are other popular activities used in CR programs. Recent studies, however, have demonstrated the safety and benefit of isotonic and weight training programs. Strengthening is recommended 2-3 times per week.
Duration: The duration of conditioning period is typically 15 and 60 minutes. A minimum of 15 minutes is necessary to achieve an improvement in FC. The optimal duration is 20-40 minutes. It can be extended if the intensity is reduced and a goal of the program is increased caloric consumptions. Patients with significant claudication, low FC, or marked weakness may require an interval program (limited by symptoms), until the total time of all intervals equals the prescribed duration.
Rate of progression: The first scale developed by Borg ranges from 6 to 20 and is linear, with word anchors that describe the exercise intensity equally spaced along the length of the scale. On average, a perceived exertion of 12 to 14(somewhat hard), on the 6 to 20 scale, corresponds with a HR response of between 60% and 85%, respectively. The second scale has an exponential design to the spacing of the word anchors and runs from 0 to 10. For ratings on the 10 point scale; values between 3 and 6 correspond to a similar HR response.
Cool- down: this period should promptly follow the conditioning period in an activity session. It lasts 3-10 minutes. The patients should perform low- level, rhythmic, aerobic activities during period. After the active aerobic cool- down, static stretching and fine ROM activity included again. Stretching exercises are essential segment in each training session.

IV.b Education

Patient education can play an integral role in acomplishment of any CR program, provided that it is done properly. The inclusion of the patient education program changes, depending on the background of the patient and on the phase of CR. Some topics which should be taken into consideration are the following: management of risk factors through lifestyle modifications of smoking, diet, stress management and exercise behavior; return to work; medications; sexual activity; exercise prescription and psychological issue.

IV.c Psychological consideration and stress management

Depression: The relationship between depression and CAD is well atated. Depression is highly prevalent in cardiac patients, and is a considerable risk factor for cardiac outcomes. Patients should be screened for depression at entry to CR programs, using either a few verbal screening questions or a standardized depression questionnaire. Depressed patients enrolled in CR programs will need more attention to insure continued adherence and close monitoring to rapidly intervene provided that depressive symptoms worsen. (22,23,25,59) Several treatments have shown some success in treating depression in cardiac patients, including antidepressant medication (sertraline), psychological interventions (such as cognitive behavioral therapy), and exercise training. Other psychological disorders such as type A personality behavior, anger and hostility should be managed in CR setting. (23, 25, 26) Treatment with cardiac rehabilitation can improve mental health related quality of life in a significant way. (60)

Stress management: The previous researches has indicated that mental and emotional stress can result in myocardial ischemia and is associated with a several fold increase in occurrence of subsequent fatal, and nonfatal, cardiac events. Although the efficacy research on stress management in cardiac rehabilitation is fraught with methodological issues, it appears that psychological interventions that are successful in reducing distress are also successful in reducing morbidity and mortality. Key components for providing sufficient stress management interventions include envolving patients through joining the process of heart disease to their own experiences, assissting them to understand the ability they have in slowing or reversing the process through the choices they make in dealing with responses, providing adequate training and opportunities for guided practice in producing the relaxation response, and teaching patients to shift perceptions and beliefs that tend to increase stress and effect healthy coping.

Relaxation Training: Relaxation training has also been found to reduce heart rate, respiratory rate and muscle tension. The patients can take advantage of relaxation training that instructs them to use abdominal breathing and visual imagery to focus attention on healing stimuli, memories, or fantasies.

V. Home- based cardiac rehabilitation

Home-based secondary prevention programs for CAD are an effective and fairly low-cost alternative measure to hospital-based CR and should be noticed for stable patients unlikely to access or adhere to hospital-based services.(61,62)

VI. Safety of exercise training

In the meanwhile, the benefits of comprehensive cardiac rehabilitation have been obviously demonstrated, but the exercise training-induced complications and benefit-risk ratio of cardiac rehabilitation remains poorly understood. Screening procedures can be used to identify subjects at increased risk for an exercise-related cardiac event. These are patients who are generally at increased risk of sudden cardiac death; particularly patients with severe LV dysfunction or ischemia at low levels of exercise. The results of studies reporting the risks of sudden cardiac arrest during exercise training depict that this risk is low even during vigorous exercise. These studies strongly suggest that the incidence of sudden cardiac arrest across a variety of activities, with the exception of jogging, is similar to that expected by chance alone. In summary, the risk of cardiac events during exercise testing and training appears to be very low, but such events seem difficult to for see. Finally, although risk stratification remains necessary at the beginning of a CR program, the occurrence of a severe cardiac event seems to be difficult to predict in most cases. This difficulty emphasizes the role of the cardiologist in the prescription and supervision of CR sessions. (63-66)

VII. Problems exist in cardiac rehabilitation

Underutilization of cardiac rehabilitation

Unfortunately despite the obvious benefits and effectiveness of CR on quality of life and mortality, and regardless of the class I indication from AHA/ACC (67-69), the majority of people who would benefit from this program fails to participate in it and right now the main present problem with exercise-based cardiac rehabilitation is its underutilization. (37,70,71)

Barrier to cardiac rehabilitation

There are multiple interrelated factors that influence a patient's decision to use cardiac rehabilitation services. These factors divided into environmental and individual categories. (72) The healthcare delivery systems and policies within hospitals and cardiac rehabilitation programs represent factors within the internal environment. These factors are amenable to improvement. The external environment which includes factors that affect the patient's ability to use healthcare services are not as amenable to change, such as where they reside or their access to these services. Individual factors (at the patient and provider level) are composed of 4 categories. 1) Predisposing factors are socio-demographic characteristics and prior experiences with cardiac rehabilitation. 2) Enabling factors are any skill or resource required to enroll and participate regularly (income, social support, work/personal schedules, transportation, knowledge, attitude, and beliefs). 3) Reinforcing factors strengthen or lessen the motivation for program attendance and adherence (strength of physician endorsement, encouragement and support of healthcare providers, family, and friends). 4) Need factors in term of physician's and patient's perceptions are influenced by the clinical condition, psychological factors, and anticipated benefits of the service. Many of the barriers that arise from these categories provide opportunities for healthcare professionals to attempt to improve rates of CR referral, registration, and completion. (72-79)

3. Specific alternative therapy

Treatment of patients with refractory angina pectoris has still remained challenging in patients with end-stage coronary artery disease not suitable for revascularization (even bypass surgery or angioplasty with stent).

3.1 ESMR (Extracorporeal Shockwave Myocardial Revascularization)

Extracor Extracorporeal Shock Wave Therapy (ESWT) was introduced in the early 1990s as a spin-off of urological lithotripsy.(80) Since then, ESWT has been applied to treat various musculoskeletal conditions. Right now Shockwave Myocardial Revascularization (ESMR) is a breakthrough in management of refractory angina pectoris with end-stage coronary artery disease not suitable for revascularization (81). The treatment is performed using a special generator that produces low intensity shockwaves, a kind of sound waves similar to, but of lower strength than Extracorporeal Shock Wave Lithotripsy (ESWL) that is used in the treatment of kidney stones . These acoustic shock waves are not dissolving plaque in the same way that lithotripsy breaks up a stone, instead, these waves result in release substances which stimulate the formation of new blood vessels in the heart.(82) The shock wave schedule consists of three 20-minute sessions per week over nine weeks.

The patient must first undergo cardiac SPECT (single photon emission computed tomography) testing to identify the location of the ischemic areas. Afterwards a handheld device called a transducer is placed over the skin and shockwaves will then be delivered directly to the ischemic region under echocardiographic guidance. (83)The therapy sessions that have already been conducted have yielded positive results among treated patients who claim they have had their pain alleviated since the beginning of the treatment. ESMR is an alternative therapy for patients who have angina, even though they take medicine, and are not suitable candidates for coronary angioplasty or bypass surgery.

3.2 EECP (Extracorporeal Electrical Counter pulsation)

EECP is sometimes known as a "natural bypass" since it optimizes the body's ability to develop new vessels around stenotic arteries. EECP seems to be a noninvasive, well-tolerated therapeutic option for patients with coronary artery disease (CAD) and refractory angina who are not amenable to standard revascularization procedures. (84-86)The EECP device consists of three paired pneumatic cuffs applied to the lower extremities. Patients are typically treated for 1 hour daily program for a total of 35 sessions over 7 weeks. The cuffs are inflated in sequence, placing pressure on the legs which pushes blood flow from the lower limbs up towards the heart. The inflation of the cuffs occurs during diastole so it increases blood flow delivery to the heart at the precise moment it is relaxing. Then, just before the heart pumps, the cuffs deflate, reducing resistance and decreasing the heart's workload.

Prospective clinical trials and large treatment registries have shown major reductions in anginal symptoms and improvements in objective measures of myocardial ischemia in response to EECP in patients with symptomatic CAD. Its potential role in heart failure management, which improves quality of life and reduces symptoms, has been also shown.(84)

EECP treatment is associated with an immediate increase in blood flow in multiple vascular beds including the coronary artery circulation and causes acute changes in hemodynamics including an increase in preload and a decrease in afterload.(87-90) Several published studies were designed to assess objective evidence of improvement in myocardial perfusion and beneficial hemodynamic effects. They have also shown improvements in various organ system perfusions and LV diastolic filling after EECP treatment and it is even recommended as initial revascularization treatment for refractory angina. The abrupt drop in intra-aortic pressure unloads the left ventricle during systole, thus reducing the cardiac workload in ejection period and reducing myocardial oxygen demands.

EECP greatly accelerates the formation of collateral vessels, helping restore adequate circulation to organs and tissues that have been deprived of blood and oxygen. EECP was developed at Harvard University almost 50 years ago as a therapy for angina. Several studies have shown that patients who undergo a course of EECP experience fewer episodes of angina, experience less intense episodes of angina, need less anti-angina medication, can walk farther without experiencing angina, and resume work and enjoy more social activities.(86, 91)

In a recent study by Esmaeilzadeh et.al, the effects of EECP on regional myocardial function were evaluated. Given their findings, EECP can improve global and regional LV systolic and diastolic functions by means of strain and strain rate imaging.(91)

Unlike drugs that are prescribed for angina, EECP is completely safe and without side effects. And unlike angioplasty and bypass surgery, EECP can be done on an outpatient basis and requires no post-treatment recovery period. Patients suffering a heart attack or enduring one or even several surgeries for coronary artery disease are best candidates for this kind of treatment. In some cases, EECP is their only option. Yet this noninvasive therapy is so safe and effective that it should be considered as a first-line treatment for angina, not just a last resort after surgery has been ruled out.

For a growing number of patients, who are imposed a potentially dangerous surgical procedure, recommending EECP is a wise decision; because in less time than it takes to recover from bypass surgery, these patients can complete a full course of EECP and begin enjoying an active, pain-free life.

3.3 Neurostimulation

For the first time healing power of electric current was described by Scribonius Largus, the physician of the Roman emperor Claudius, in the treatment of headache and gout.(92)

Because of the very promising results of neurostimulation in different ischemic syndromes, it seemed obvious to try electrical neurostimulation therapy as an adjuvant therapy in patients suffering from medically refractory angina pectoris. The beneficial effects of transcutaneous electrical nerve stimulation (TENS) were described by Mannheimer and colleagues. (93,94)

For patients not responding to adequate medication and not being suitable anymore for revascularization and suffering from refractory angina pectoris, neurostimulation has been described repeatedly as an effective and safe therapy.(95,96) The mechanism of action of neurostimulation is not completely known, however, recent studies suggest that anti-ischemic effect expressed by decrease in the serum catecholamine level, exerted by reducing sympathetic tone. (97-99)

The effect of TENS on coronary flow was not accomplished in patients with a heart transplant which suggests that neurostimulation employs its effect through neural mechanisms employed at the microcirculatory level. (100) Considering the lack of resting heart rate and blood pressure variability under neurostimulation, it's unlikely that beta-adrenergic mechanisms are involved. (101) Moreover, beta-mediated coronary dilatation is of less importance in the ischemic myocardium. (102) On the other hand, alpha- adrenergic receptors may play a role in the anti-ischemic mechanism of action of neurostimulation. Inhibition of the alpha receptors may cause relative vasodilation at the subendocardial coronary level,(103) which in turn may cause a redistribution effect.

At present it is unknown which neural pathways are involved in neurostimulation for angina pectoris. It is discovered that angina begins with stimulation of cardiac nerve endings.(104,105) by visceral afferent nerve fibers, converging in common pathways into the dorsal spinal cord at C7-T5 level, where they have synaptic connections with other neurons.(106) Afferent fibers from the heart and cutaneous input are assumed to cover specific interneurons in the same segment of the spinal cord, explaining the ensuing referred projection of pain to the related dermatome.(107, 108) Consequently, angina is felt in areas of the chest that refer to the dermatome from which afferent nerves project to the same segment of the spinal cord (C7-T5) as the heart. For an optimal clinical result of neurostimulation it is of great importance to achieve paresthesia in the same dermal regions.

Although there is increasing evidence that neurostimulation is effective in angina pectoris, its safety needs to be established. In a 5-year follow-up study of 23 patients on spinal cord stimulation (SCS), Sanderson reported that it is a safe therapy based on the fact that; (109) only three patients died during this follow-up. In another follow up study, out of 46 patients with severe coronary artery disease who were treated at the Groningen University Hospital Department of Cardiology with SCS; only six patients died during a7- year period. (110)

However, despite declining mortality rates in patients with coronary artery disease, little is known about mortality rates in patients with refractory angina due to severe coronary artery disease. It is estimated that 3% (about 7 million) of Americans have active coronary artery disease implying an annual death rate of 7 %. (111)

Another important issue which needs further attention before the general acceptance of neurostimulation as an alternative therapy in angina pectoris is its complication rate. Because of the high skin impedance, TENS is frequently complicated by persistent skin irritation, which makes adequate continuation of therapy difficult. Meanwhile, SCS has a rather high incidence of dislocation of the epidural lead,(112) and this often impairs its effect.

Once the safety of neurostimulation in angina pectoris is convincingly established and the aforementioned side effects can be further reduced, both TENS and SCS may be commonly used as alternatives in the therapeutic spectrum of intractable angina pectoris.

3.4 Acupuncture

Acupuncture involves the insertion of extremely thin needles in skin at strategic points of body. Acupuncture originated in China six thousands of years ago, but during the past three decades it was grown significantly as a popular therapy within the world.

It works by stimulating the body to naturally correct the imbalances of energy. This is done by inserting ultra-fine, disposable needles, underneath the skin at specific points of the body. (113) These acupuncture points are related to energy pathways that run throughout the entire length of the body. Acupuncture points are also related to specific internal organs. The earliest known text on acupuncture was published more than 4,500 years ago.

Acupuncture has been traditionally used to treat a wide variety of cardiovascular diseases, and recent controlled studies have demonstrated that it is particularly beneficial for angina pectoris by offering a proven option to drug therapy.

Traditional Chinese theory explains acupuncture as a technique for balancing the flow of energy through specific pathways (meridians) in the body. In contrast, many Western practitioners believe the acupuncture points as places to stimulate nerves, muscles and connective tissue. This stimulation seems to boost the activity of natural painkillers and increase blood flow. (114)

Basically, acupuncture is a method of encouraging the body to enhance its own natural healing. The idea is to balance overall energy in order to establish or re-establish well-being. Research has shown that the body response to acupuncture is releasing endorphins (neurotransmitters that stop pain), increasing blood cell counts, and heightening the immune system. Acupuncture is used worldwide both as a primary and complementary form of medical treatment. The frequency of treatment depends greatly on the condition. Most people will begin to see results from acupuncture in approximately 4-10 treatments. Treatments are generally administered once per week until improvement is made and then follow-up appointments may range from a few times per year to monthly to bi-weekly.

In one study (115) at the Human College of Traditional Chinese Medicine, forty patients with stable type of angina pectoris were assessed during and after acupuncture treatments and compared to a control group. After only one acupuncture treatment, 15 (37.5%) of the patients were already noticing a marked improvement in degree and area of pain, but after 7 treatments 25 (63%) of the patients recorded significant reductions both in extent and area of pain, and they also experienced a reduction in the number and the duration of attacks. Furthermore the patients in the acupuncture group who did get angina attacks recovered much faster than the patients in the control group.

Similar findings were reported in another study, this time in Sweden (116), where 21 patients with stable effort angina pectoris were treated with acupuncture. All of the patients had a history of at least five anginal attacks per week despite intensive conventional medical treatment. They were given three acupuncture treatments per week which led to a 40% reduction in the number of anginal attacks and the researchers also observed that the patients were able to exercise for longer before the onset of pain. All the patients completed a life quality questionnaire which confirmed that they all felt better as a result of the acupuncture treatment. The report concluded that acupuncture should be considered a beneficial treatment even for patients with severe, intensively treated angina pectoris.

Other studies have come to the same conclusion (117,118) in the treatment of angina. In one research project at the Nanjing Medical College involving 267 patients, all suffering from angina pectoris, acupuncture treatment was shown to have a 93.3% success rate with no harmful side effects (119).

There are some possible side effects and risks that could be involved in patients and depend completely upon the experience and expertise of the acupuncturist, but these are relatively less when compared to other forms of treatment. Some of the common acupuncture side effects or inconveniences experienced during or after acupuncture are: a regular sensation of warmth, tenderness, and tingling when the acupuncture needles reach the acupoint or trigger point, mild bruising and bleeding, temporary drop in blood pressure which may result in fatigue and rarely fainting, allergic reactions to stainless steel acupuncture needles, infections, and perforation of some of the vital organs by needles.

Acupuncture is safe and complications are extremely rare and side effects, if any, are limited. There are a number of guidelines, however, which govern the use of particular acupuncture points. A precaution may be related to use in certain conditions, with particular techniques, or because of a points location, however, in some cases, practitioner may still use a point or technique even if it is listed as a precaution.

4. References

[1] Lichtenstein AH, Appel LJ, Brands M, Carnethon M, Daniels S, Franch HA, Franklin B,et al. Diet and Lifestyle Recommendations Revision 2006: A Scientific Statement From the American Heart Association Nutrition Committee. Circulation 2006;114;82-96

[2] Kumanyika SK, Obarzanek E, Stettler N, Bell R, Field AE, Fortmann SP. Population-Based Prevention of Obesity. The Need for Comprehensive Promotion of Healthful Eating, Physical Activity, and Energy Balance. A Scientific Statement From American Heart Association Council on Epidemiology and Prevention, Interdisciplinary Committee for Prevention (Formerly the Expert Panel on Population and Prevention Science) Circulation 2008;118;428-464.

[3] Gebauer SK, Psota TL, Harris WS, and Kris-Etherton PM. N-3 Fatty acid dietary recommendations and food sources to achieve essentiality and cardiovascular benefits. Am J Clin Nutr 2006;83(suppl):1526S–35S

[4] Kris-Etherton PM, Harris WS, Appel LJ. Fish Consumption, Fish Oil, Omega-3 Fatty Acids, and Cardiovascular Disease. Circulation 2002;106;2747-2757

[5] Crouse JR. New developments in the use of Niacin for treatment of hyperlipedemia. Coron Artery Dis 1996; 7:321-326.

[6] Martin-Jadraque R, Tato F, Mostaza JM, Vega GL, Grundy SM. Effectiveness of Low-Dose Crystalline Nicotinic Acid in Men With Low High-Density Lipoprotein Cholesterol Levels. Arch Intern Med. 1996;156(10):1081-1088.

[7] Goldberg AC. Clinical trial experience with extended-release niacin (Niaspan): Dose-escalation study. Am J Cardiol. 1998; 82:35U-38U.

[8] Johansson JO, Egberg N,Carlson AA, Carlson LA. Nicotinic Acid Treatment Shifts the Fibrinolytic Balance Favourably and Decreases Plasma Fibrinogen in Hypertriglyceridaemic Men. European Jour of Cardiovascular Prevention & Rehabilitation 1997;4:165-171.

[9] Kwiterovich PO. The antiatherogenic role of high-density lipoprotein cholesterol. Am J Cardiol. 1998;82:13Q-21Q

[10] Enstrom JE, Kanim LE, Klein MA. Vitamin C Intake and Mortality among a Sample of the United States Population. Epidemiology 1992;3(3): 194-202.

[11] Losonczy KG, Harris BT, Havlik JR. Vitamin E and vitamin C supplement use and risk of all cause mortality and coronary heart disease in older persons: the Established Populations for Epidemiologic Studies of the elderly. Am J Clin Nutr 1996;64:190-6.

[12] Rath M, Niedzwiecki A. Nutritional Supplements program halts progresion of early coronary atherosclerosis documented by ultrafast computed tomography. Journal of Applied Nutrition 1996; 48 (3):1-11.

[13] Chan AC, Wagner M, Kennedy C, Mroske C, Proulx, P, Laneuville O, Tran K, Choy PC. Vitamin E up-regulates phospholipase A2, arachidonic acid release and cyclooxygenase in endothelial cells. Akt. Ernahr. Med 1998;23: 1-8.

[14] Knekt P, Reunanen A, Järvinen R, Seppänen R, Heliövaara M, Aromaa A. Antioxidant vitamin intake and coronary mortality in a longitudinal population study. Am. J. Epidemiol. 1994; 139:1180–1189.

[15] Suzukawa M et al, Effect of supplementation with vitamin E on LDL oxidizability and prevention of atherosclerosis. Biofactors. 1998;7:51-4.

[16] Kamikawa T, Kobayashi A, Yamashita T, et al. Effects of coenzyme Q10 on exercise tolerance in chronic stable angina pectoris. Am J Cardiol 1985;56:247-251.

[17] Sunamori M, Tanaka H, Maruyama T, Sultan I, Sakamoto T, Suzuki A, Clinical experience of coenzyme Q10 to enhance intraoperative myocardial protection in coronary artery revascularization, *Cardiovasc. Drugs Ther.* 1991;2(Suppl.): 297-300

[18] Rosenfeldt FL, Pepe S, Ou R, Mariani JA, Rowland MA, Nagley P, Linnane AW. Coenzyme Q10 improves the tolerance of the senescent myocardium to aerobic and ischemic stress: studies in rats and in human atrial tissue. Biofactors. 1999;9:291-299.

[19] Rosenfeildt FL,Pepe S, Linnane A,Nagley P,Rowland M,Ou R,Marasco S,Lyon W,Esmore D.Coenzyme Q10 Protects the Aging Heart against Stress,Studies in Rats, Human Tissues, and Patients. Ann. N.Y. Acad. Sci. 2002;959: 355–359

[20] Folkers k, Langsjoen P, Willis R, Richardson P, Xia LJ, YE CQ, Tamagawa H. Lovastatin decreases coenzyme Q levels in humans, Proc. Nat. Acad. Sci.1990; 87:8931-8934.

[21] Peng CK, Mietus JE, et al. Exaggerated heart rate oscillations during two meditation techniques.Int J Cardiol 1999;70 (2):101-107.

[22] Perk J, Mathes P, Gohlke H, Monpère C, Hellemans I, McGee H, Sellier P, Saner H. Cardiovascular Prevention and Rehabilitation

[23] Morag K. Thow Dip. Exercise Leadership in Cardiac Rehabilitation. An evidence-based approach

[24] Ann-Dorthe Olsen Zwisler, Anne Merete Boas Soja, Søren Rasmussen, Marianne Frederiksen, Sadollah Abadini Jon Appel, et al. Hospital-based comprehensive cardiac rehabilitation versus usual care among patients with congestive heart failure, ischemic heart disease, or high risk of ischemic heart disease: 12-Month results of a randomized clinical trial Am Heart J 2008; 155:1106-1113.
[25] Pashkow FJ, Dafoe W A. clinical cardiac rehabilitation, a cardiologist's guide. Second edition, 1999
[26] Kraus WE, Keteyian SJ. Cardiac rehabilitation.2008
[27] Goble AJ., Worcester MUC. Best Practice Guidelines for cardiac rehabilitation and secondary prevention, Published by Department of Human Services Victoria April 1999.ISBN: 0 7311 5258 1
[28] Thompson A. Exercise and physical activity in the prevention and treatment of atherosclerotic cardiovascular disease. Circulation 2003;107:3109-3116.
[29] Schuler G, Hambrecht R, Schlierf G, Niebauer J, Hauer K, Neumann J, et al. Physical exercise and low fat diet: effects on progression of coronary artery disease. Circulation 1992;86(1):1-11.
[30] Niebauer J,Hambrecht R,Velich T, et al.Attenuated progression of coronary artery disease after 6 years of multifactorial risk intervention - role of physical exercise. Circulation 1997; 96:2534-2541.
[31] Ehsani AA,Heath GW,Hagberg JM, Sobel BE,Holloszy JO. Effects of 12 months of intense exercise training on ischemic ST-segment depression in patients with coronary artery disease. Circulation 1981;64:1116-1124.
[32] Fletcher GF, Balady GJ,Amsterdam EA, et al. Exercise standards for testing and training: a statement healthcare professionals from the AmericanHeart Association. Circulation 2001;104:1694-1740.
[33] Therese A. Stukel, and David A. Analysis Methods for Observational Studies: Effects of Cardiac Rehabilitation on Mortality of Coronary Patients, J. Am. Coll. Cardiol. 2009;54;34-35.
[34] Clark AM, Hartling L, Vandermeer B, McAlister FA. Meta-analysis: secondary prevention programs for patients with coronary artery disease. Ann Intern Med 2005;143:659 -72
[35] Suaya JA, Stason WB, Ades PA, Normand S-LT, Shepard DS. Cardiac rehabilitation and survival in older coronary patients. J Am Coll Cardiol 2009; 54:25-33
[36] Steinacker JM, Liu Y, Muche R, Koenig W, Hahmann H, Imhof A, et al. Long term effects of comprehensive cardiac rehabilitation in an inpatient and outpatient setting. Swiss Med Wkly. 2011;140:w13141
[37] Dorosz J. Updates in cardiac rehabilitation. Phys Med Rehabil Clin N Am. 2009;20(4):719-736.
[38] Stukel TA, Fisher ES, Wennberg DE, et al. Analysis of observational studies in presence of treatment selection bias: effects of invasive cardiac management on AMI survival using propensity score and instrumental variable methods. JAMA 2007; 297:278-285.

[39] Schächinger V, Britten MB, Zeiher AM. Prognostic impact of coronary vasodilator dysfunction on adverse long-term outcome of coronary heart disease. Circulation 2000;101:1899–1906

[40] Suwaidi JA, Hamasaki S, Higano ST, Nishimura RA, Holmes DR, Lerman A. Long-term follow-up of patients with mild CAD and endothelial dysfunction. Circulation 2000; 101:1002-1006.

[41] Laughlin MH. Endothelium-mediated control of coronary vascular tone after chronic exercise training. Med Sci Sports Exerc. 1995 ; 27(8):1135-44

[42] Hambrecht R, Adams V, Erbs S, et al. Regular physical activity improves endothelial function in patients with coronary artery disease by increasing phosphorylation of endothelial nitric oxide synthase. Circulation 2003; 107:3152-3158.

[43] Laughlin MH Effects of exercise training on coronary circulation. Med Sci Sports Exerc. 1994; 26(10):1226-1229.

[44] Kuru O, Sentürk UK, Koçer G, Ozdem S, Başkurt OK, Cetin A, et al. Effect of exercise training on resistance arteries in rats with chronic NOS inhibition. J Appl Physiol. 2009; 107(3):896-902

[45] Griffin KL, Laughlin MH, Parker JL. Exercise training improves endothelium-mediated vasorelaxation after chronic coronary occlusion. J Appl Physiol. 1999; 87(5):1948-56

[46] Zhou M, Widmer RJ, Xie W, Jimmy Widmer A, Miller MW, Schroeder F, et al. Effects of exercise training on cellular mechanisms of endothelial nitric oxide synthase regulation in coronary arteries after chronic occlusion. Am J Physiol Heart Circ Physiol. 2010; 298(6):H1857-69

[47] Lavie CJ, Milani RV, Littman AB. Benefits of Cardiac Rehabilitation and Exercise Training in Secondary Coronary Prevention in the Elderly. J Am Coll Cardiol. 1993; 22:678–683

[48] Sullivan MJ, Higginbotham MB, Cobb FR. Exercise training in patients with severe left ventricular dysfunction: hemodynamic and metabolic effects. Circulation.1998; 15:801-9

[49] Hamberchet R, Gielen S,Linke A, Fiehn E, Yu J, et al. Effects of exercise training on left ventricular function and peripheral resistance in patients with chronic heart failure: a randomized trial: JAMA 2003; 283:3095-3101

[50] Kitzman DW, Brubaker PH, Morgan TM, Stewart KP, Little WC. Exercise training in older patients with heart failure and preserved ejection fraction: a randomized, controlled, single-blind trial. Circ Heart Fail. 2010;3(6):659-67

[51] Thompson DR, Clark A M. Cardiac rehabilitation: into the future. Heart. 2009; 95(23):1897-900

[52] Frank AM, McConnell TR, Rawson ES, Fradkin A. Clinical and Functional Predictors of Health-Related Quality of Life During Cardiac Rehabilitation. J Cardiopulm Rehabil Prev. 2011 Jan 13. [Epub ahead of print]

[53] Balducci S, Zanuso S, Nicolucci A, De Feo P, Cavallo S, Cardelli P, et al. Effect of an intensive exercise intervention strategy on modifiable cardiovascular risk factors in subjects with type 2 diabetes mellitus: a randomized controlled trial: the Italian Diabetes and Exercise Study (IDES). Arch Intern Med. 2010; 170(20):1794-1803.

[54] Grima-Serrano A, García-Porrero E, Luengo-Fernández E, León Latre M. Preventive Cardiology and Cardiac Rehabilitation. Rev Esp Cardiol. 2011;64S1:66-72
[55] Deskur-Smielecka E, Borowicz-Bienkowska S, Maleszka M, Wilk M, Nowak A, Przywarska I. Early Phase 2 Inpatient Rehabilitation after Acute Coronary Syndrome Treated with Primary Percutaneous Coronary Intervention: Short- and Long-Term Effects on Blood Pressure and Metabolic Parameters.Am J Phys Med Rehabil. 2011 Jan 7. [Epub ahead of print]
[56] Kamakura T, Kawakami R, Nakanishi M, Ibuki M, Ohara T, Yanase M, Aihara N. et al. Efficacy of out-patient cardiac rehabilitation in low prognostic risk patients after acute myocardial infarction in primary intervention era. Circ J. 2011; 75(2):315-21
[57] Toufan M, Afrasiabi A. Benefits of cardiac rehabilitation on lipid profile in patients with coronary artery disease. Pak J Biol Sci. 2009 Oct 1;12(19):1307-13
[58] D'hooge R, Hellinckx T, Van Laethem C, Stegen S, De Schepper J, Van Aken S, et al.Clin Influence of combined aerobic and resistance training on metabolic control, cardiovascular fitness and quality of life in adolescents with type 1 diabetes: a randomized controlled trial.Rehabil. 2010 Nov 26. [Epub ahead of print]
[59] Milani RV, Lavie CJ, Mehra MR, Ventura HO.Impact of exercise training and depression on survival in heart failure due to coronary heart disease. Am J Cardiol. 2011; 107(1): 64-8
[60] Oneil A, Sanderson K, Oldenburg B, Taylor CB. Impact of Depression Treatment on Mental and Physical Health-Related Quality of Life of Cardiac Patients: A META-ANALYSIS. J Cardiopulm Rehabil Prev. 2010 Dec 9. [Epub ahead of print]
[61] Clark AM, Haykowsky M, Kryworuchko J, MacClure T, Scott J, DesMeules M, e al. A meta-analysis of randomized control trials of home-based secondary prevention programs for coronary artery disease. Eur J Cardiovasc Prev Rehabil. 2010 ;17(3):261-70
[62] Schweikert B, Hahmann H, Steinacker JM, Imhof A, Muche R, Koenig W. Intervention study shows outpatient cardiac rehabilitation to be economically at least as attractive as inpatient rehabilitation. Clin Res Cardiol. 2009;98(12):787-95
[63] Keteyian SJ et al. Safety of symptom-limited cardiopulmonary exercise testing in patients with chronic heart failure due to severe left ventricular systolic dysfunction. Am Heart J 2009; 158:S72-S77
[64] O'Connor C M, Whellan D J,Lee K L,et al.Efficacy and Safety of Exercise Training in Patients with Chronic Heart Failure: HF-ACTION Randomized Controlled Trial. JAMA 2009;301(14):1439-1450
[65] Pavy B, Christine Iliou M, Meurin P, Tabet J, Corone S. Safety of Exercise Training for Cardiac Patients Results of the French Registry of Complications during Cardiac Rehabilitation . Arch Intern Med. 2006;166:2329-2334
[66] Goto Y, Sumida H, Ueshima K, Adachi H , Nohara R, Itoh H.Safety and Implementation of Exercise Testing and Training After Coronary Stenting in Patients With Acute Myocardial Infarction. Circulation J 2002; 66: 930–936
[67] Thomas R J., King M., Lui K.,Oldridge N., Ileana L. P., Spertus J., Masoudi F A., DeLong E., Erwin III P.J., Goff Jr D C., Grady K., Green L A., Heidenreich, PA.,

Jenkins K J, Loth A R., Peterson E D, Shahian D M. Reprint-AACVPR/ACCF/AHA 2010 Update: Performance Measures on Cardiac Rehabilitation for Referral to Cardiac Rehabilitation/Secondary Prevention Services A Report of the American Association of Cardiovascular and Pulmonary Rehabilitation and the American College of Cardiology Foundation/American Heart Association Task Force on Performance Measures (Writing Committee to Develop Clinical Performance Measures for Cardiac Rehabilitation). J Am Coll Cardiol. 2010;56;1159-1167

[68] Piepoli M F, Corra` U, Benzer W, Bjarnason-Wehrens B, Dendale P, Gaita D, McGee H, Mendes M, Niebauer J, Olsen Zwisler A Schmid J. Secondary prevention through cardiac rehabilitation: physical activity counselling and exercise training. European Heart Journal 2010; 31:1967-76

[69] Ghannem M. [Cardiac rehabilitation after acute myocardial infarction]. [Article in French]. Ann Cardiol Angeiol (Paris). 2010;59(6):367-79

[70] Piepoli M F, Corra` U., Benzer W., Bjarnason-Wehrens B., Dendale P., Gaita D., McGee H., Mendes M., Niebauer J., Olsen Zwisler A Schmid J. Secondary prevention through cardiac rehabilitation: physical activity counselling and exercise training. European Heart Journal 2010; 31:1967-76

[71] Scott IA,Lindsay KA,Harden HE.Utilisation of outpatient cardiac rehabilitation Queensland.Med J Aust 2003;179:341-345

[72] Parkosewich J A. Cardiac rehabilitation barriers and opportunities among women with cardiovascular disease, Cardiology in Review; 2008; 16 :36-52

[73] Brown T M., Hernandez A F., Bittner V., Cannon C P., Ellrod G., Liang L., Peterson E D. Predictors of cardiac rehabilitation referral in coronary artery disease patients. J Am Coll Cardiol Vol. 54, No. 6, 2009:515-21

[74] Andersen RM. Revisiting the behavioral model and access to medical care: does it matter? J Health Soc Behav. 1995; 36:1-10

[75] Sanderson BK. The ongoing dilemma of utilization of cardiac rehabilitation services. J Cardiopulm Rehabil. 2005; 25:350 -353

[76] Grace SL, Krepostman S, Brooks D, et al. Referral to and discharge from cardiac rehabilitation: key informant views on continuity of care.J Eval Clin Pract. 2006;12:155-163

[77] Scott LB, Allen JK. Providers' perceptions of factors affecting women's referral to outpatient cardiac rehabilitation programs: an exploratory study. J Cardiopulm Rehabil. 2004; 24:387-391

[78] Grace S L., Grewal K., Stewart D E. Factors affecting cardiac rehabilitation referral by physician specialty, J Cardiopulm Rehabil 2008;28:248-252

[79] Sharp J., DClinPsy, Freeman C., Patterns and predictors of uptake and adherence to cardiac rehabilitation, J Cardiopulm Rehabil 2009;29:241-247.

[80] Wild C, Khene M, Wanke S. Extracorporeal Shock Wave Therapy in Orthopedics. Assessment of an emerging health technology. International Journal of Technology Assessment in Health Care. 2000;16(1):199-209.

[81] Caspari GH, Erbel R. Revascularization with extracorporeal shock wave therapy: first clinical results. Circulation 1999;100(Suppl 18):84-89.

[82] Nishida T,Shimokawa H et al. Extracorporeal cardiac shock wave therapy markedly ameliorates ischemia-induced myocardial dysfunction in pigs in vivo. Circulation 2004;110: 3055-3061.
[83] Faber L, Lindner O, Prinz C, Fricke E, Hering D, Burchert W, Horstkotte D. Echo guided extracorporeal shockwave therapy for refractory angina improves regional myocardial blood flow as assessed by PET imaging. J. Am. Coll. Cardiol. 2010;55:A120.E1125
[84] Soran O, Kennard ED, Kfoury AG and Kelsey SF. Two-year clinical outcomes after enhanced external counterpulsation (EECP) therapy in patients with refractory angina pectoris and left ventricular dysfunction (report from the international EECP patient registry). Am J Cardiol 2006;97:17-20.
[85] Soran O. A New treatment modality in heart failure enhanced external counterpulsation (EECP). Cardiology in Review 2004;12:15-20.
[86] Lawson WE, Hui JCK, Lang G. Treatment benefit in the enhanced external counterpulsation consortium. Cardiology 2000; 94: 31-35.
[87] Taguchi I, Ogawa K, Kanaya T, Matsuda R, Kuga H, Nakatsugawa M. Effects of enhanced external counterpulsation on hemodynamics and its mechanism. Circ J 2004; 68(11):1030-1034.
[88] Michaels AD, Accad M, Ports TA, Grossman W. Left ventricular systolic unloading and augmentation of intracoronary pressure and Doppler flow during enhanced external counterpulsation. Circulation 2002;106(10):1237-1242.
[89] Bonetti PO, Gadasalli SN, Lerman A, Barsness GW. Successful treatment of symptomatic coronary endothelial dysfunction with enhanced external counterpulsation. Mayo Clin Proc 2004;79:690-692.
[90] Lawson WE, Hui JCK, Kennard ED, Barsness G, Kelsey SF. Predictors of benefit in angina patients one year after completing enhanced external counterpulsation: Initial responders to treatment versus nonresponders. Cardiology 2005;103:201-206.
[91] Maseri A, Crea F, Kaski JC, Davies C. Mechanisms and significance of cardiac ischemic pain. Prog Cardiovasc Dis 1992; 35(1): 1-18
[92] Esmaeilzadeh M, Khaledifar A, Maleki M, Sadeghpour A,Samiei N, Moladoust H, Noohi F, Ojaghi Haghighi Z , Mohebbi A. Evaluation of left ventricular systolic and diastolic regional function after enhanced external counter pulsation therapy using strain rate imaging. Eur J Echocardiogr 2009;10 (1): 120-126.
[93] Mannheiiner C, Carlsson C-A, Eriksson K, Vedin A, Wilhelinsaon C. Transcutaneous electrical nerve stimulation in severe angina pectoris. Eur Heart J 1982;3: 297 -302.
[94] Mannheimer C. Carlsson CA, Emanuelsson H. Vedin A. Waagstein F. Wilhemsson C. The effects of transcutaneous electrical nerve stimulation in patients with severe angina pectoris. Circulation 1985; 71:308-316.
[95] Sanderson JE. Electrical neurostimulators for pain relief in angina. Br Heart J 1990; 63: 14 1- I43.

[96] Mulcahy D, Knight C, Stables R, Fox K. Lasers. burns, cuts, tingles and pumps: A consideration of alternative treatments for intractable angina. Br Heart J 1994; 71: 406-407.
[97] Augustinsson LE, Carlsson CA. Fall M. Autonomic effects of electrostimulation. Appl Neurophysiol 1982; 45: 185- 189.
[98] Mannheirner C, Emanuelsson H, Waagstein F. The effect of transcutaneous nerve stimulation (TENS) on catecholamine metabolism during pacing induced angina pectoris and the influence of naloxone. Pain 1990; 41: 27-34.
[99] Emmanuelsson H, Mannheimer C,Waiigstein F, Wilhelmsson C. Catecholamine metabolism during pacing-induced angina pectoris and the effect of transcutaneous electrical nerve stimulation. Am Heart J 1987;114: 1360-1366.
[100] Chauhan A, Mullins PA, Thuraisingham SI, Taylor G,Petch MC, Schotield PM. Effect of transcutaneous electrical neive stimulation on coronary hlood flow. Circulation 1994;89:694-702
[101] DeJongste MJL, Haaksma J, Hautvast RWM, Hillege JL, Meyler WJ, Staal MJ. Sanderson JE, Lie KI. Effects of spinal cord stimulation on myocardial ischemia during daily life in patients with severe coronary artery disease-a prospective ambulatory electrocardiographic study. Br Heart J 1994;71: 413-418.
[102] Heusch G. Control of coronary vasomotor tone in ischemic myocardium by local metabolism and neurohumoral mechanisms. Eur Heart J 1991;12, (suppl F): 99-106.
[103] Heusch G. α-adrenergic mechanisms in myocardial ischemia. Circulation 1990; 81: 1 - 13
[104] Malliani A. The link between transient myocardial ischemia and pain. In Silent Myocardial Ischemia and Angina (Ed. Singh BS). Pergamon Press, New York, 1988:34-47.
[105] Vancew WH, Bowkcr RC: Spinal origins of cardiac afferents from the region of the left anterior descending artery. Brain Res 1983; 258: 96-103.
[106] Foreman RD, Ohata CA: Effects of coronary artery occlusion on thoracic spinal neurons receiving viscerosomatic inputs. Am J Physiol 1980;218: H667-673.
[107] Kennard MA, Haugen FP: The relation of subcutaneous focal sensitivity referred pain of cardiac origin. Anesthesiology 1955;16:297
[108] Selzer M, Spencer WA: Interactions between visceral and cutaneous afferents in the spinal cord: Reciprocal primary afferent fiber depolarization. Brain Res 1969;14:349
[109] Sanderson JE, Ibrahim B, Waterhouse D, Palmer RBG: Spinal electrical stimulation for intractable angina-long term clinical outcome and safety. Eur Heart J1994; 15: 810-814 .
[110] Hautvast RWM, DeJongste MJL,Ter Horst GJ, Blanksma PK,Lie KI. Angina pectoris refractory for conventional therapy-Is neurostimulation a possible alternative treatment? Clin Cardiol 1996(19);531-535
[111] National Heart, Lung and Blood Institute: Morbidity from coronary heart disease in the United States. NHLBI Data Fact Sheet, June 1990
[112] DeJongste MJL. Nagelkerke D. Hooijschuur CAM, Jourmee LH. Meyler WJ. Staal MJ. de Jonge P, Lie KI. Stimulation characteristics, complications, and efficacy of spinal

cord stimulation systems in patients with refractory angina: A prospective feasibility study. PACE1994;17:1751-1760.
[113] Smith FW Jr. Acupuncture for cardiovascular disorders. Cardiopet, Inc., Floral Park, New York. Probl Vet Med 1992; 4 (1) :125-131.
[114] Vickers A, et al. ABC of complementary medicine: Acupuncture. British Medical Journal. 1999;319:973
[115] Zhou XQ, Liu JX. Metrological analysis for efficacy of acupuncture on angina pectoris. Changsha. Chung Kuo Chung Hsi I Chieh Ho Tsa Chih (CHINA) 1993; 13 (4):212-214.
[116] Richter A, Herlitz J, Hjalmarson A. Effect of acupuncture in patients with angina pectoris. Fur Heart J Feb 1991; 12 (2):175-178.
[117] Wang WT, Wei WL, Liu DG. Acupressure on the zhiyang point in patients with acute anginal attack. Chung Hsi I Chieh Ho Tsa Chih Apr 1987; 7(4) :206-7, 195
[118] Ballegaard C, Jensen C, Pedersen F, Nissen VH. Acupuncture in severe, stable angina pectoris: a randomized trial. Acta Med Scand 1986; 220 (4) :307-313
[119] Ballegaard C, Meyer CN, Trojaborg W. Acupuncture in angina pectoris: does acupuncture have a specific effect? Intern Med 1991; 229 (4) :357-362.